ix Acet. adducts mentioned? ✓105, x?
fellow paper alcohol?
FAS?

Clinical Biochemistry of Alcoholism

CONTEMPORARY ISSUES IN CLINICAL BIOCHEMISTRY

In preparation

Therapeutic drug monitoring
B. Widdop

Clinical biochemistry nearer the patient
V. Marks K.G.M.M. Alberti

Clinical biochemistry of hospital nutrition
A. M. J. Woolfson

Developmental clinical biochemistry
J. B. Holton

Acid-base equilibrium and blood gases
H. F. Weisberg

Clinical Biochemistry of Alcoholism

EDITED BY

Sidney B. Rosalki MD, FRCP, FRCPath
Consultant Chemical Pathologist
Royal Free Hospital and School of Medicine, London, UK

CHURCHILL LIVINGSTONE
EDINBURGH LONDON MELBOURNE AND NEW YORK 1984

CHURCHILL LIVINGSTONE
Medical Division of Longman Group Limited

Distributed in the United States of America by
Churchill Livingstone Inc., 1560 Broadway, New York,
N.Y. 10036, and by associated companies, branches and
representatives throughout the world.

First published 1984

ISBN 0 443 02582 7
ISSN 0265 6701

British Library Cataloguing in Publication Data
Clinical biochemistry of alcoholism. —
(Contemporary issues in clinical biochemistry)
1. Alcoholism
I. Rosalki, Sidney B. II. Series
616.86'1 RC 565

Library of Congress Cataloging in Publication Data
Clinical biochemistry of alcoholism.
Includes index.
1. Alcohol—Physiological effect. 2. Alcoholism.
3. Biological chemistry. I. Rosalki, Sidney B.
[DNLM: 1. Alcoholism—Metabolism. 2. Alcohol, Ethyl—
Pharmacodynamics. 3. Alcoholism—Complications.
WM 274 C6417]
QP801.A3C55 1984 616.86'1 83-26285

Printed in Hong Kong by
Sing Cheong Printing Co Ltd

Preface

With more than two per cent of the population consuming harmful quantities of alcohol, and alcoholism on the increase, the clinical and biochemical consequences of alcohol abuse are assuming expanding importance in medical practice.

Alcohol excess can damage any organ and can give rise to a vast array of biochemical abnormalities. With this in mind, it seemed timely to bring clinicians and biochemists together, to examine some of the origins and effects of ethanol over-indulgence. This volume commences with a broad view of alcoholism in the community, concentrating on predisposing factors and the recognition of alcohol intake and alcoholism. The effects of alcohol on metabolism and on individual body systems are then considered in detail, paying particular attention to the biochemical consequences.

Each chapter is comprehensive in scope, and combines to give a very full account of the clinical and biochemical features of alcoholism and its major complications.

1984 S.B.R.

Contributors

Abdulla A-B. Badawy PhD, MIBiol, MRCPath
Principal Research Biochemist, Addiction Unit Research, Whitchurch Hospital, Cardiff, UK

D.G. Cramp PhD
Senior Lecturer, Department of Chemical Pathology, Royal Free Hospital and School of Medicine, London, UK

Ronald C. Denney BSc, PhD, CChem, FRSC
Senior Lecturer in Analytical Chemistry, Thames Polytechnic, London, UK

Richard Fink MD, MRCP
Consultant Chemical Pathologist, West Middlesex Hospital, Isleworth, Middlesex, UK

Sir Abraham Goldberg MD, DSc, FRCP, FRSE
Regius Professor of the Practice of Medicine, University of Glasgow, Glasgow, UK

Odette Guy PhD
Maitre de Recherche au CNRS, Institût National de la Santé et de la Recherche Médicale, Marseille, France

William Jenkins MD, MSc, MRCP
Lecturer, Department of Medicine, Royal Free Hospital and School of Medicine, London, UK

G. Lake-Bakaar BSc, MD, MRCP
Medical Advisor/Research Physician, Janssen Pharmaceutical Ltd, Wantage, Oxfordshire, UK

Kenneth E.L. McColl MD, MRCP
Lecturer in Medicine, Gardiner Institute, Western Infirmary, Glasgow, UK

Neil McIntyre BSc, MD, FRCP
Professor, Department of Medicine, Royal Free Hospital and School of Medicine, London, UK

Vincent Marks DM, FRCP, FRCPath
Professor of Clinical Biochemistry, University of Surrey, Guildford, UK

Michael R. Moore BSc, PhD
Senior Lecturer in Medicine, Gardiner Institute, Western Infirmary, Glasgow, UK

Sidney B. Rosalki MD, FRCP, FRCPath
Consultant Chemical Pathologist, Royal Free Hospital and School of Medicine, London, UK

Peter Ryle BSc, MIBiol
Research Biochemist, Department of Chemical Pathology, Greenwich District Hospital, London, UK

Henri Sarles DSc, MD
Professor of Gastroenterology, Faculty of Medicine, University of Aix-Marseille, Marseille, France

Marc A. Schuckitt MD
Professor of Psychiatry, University of California, San Diego, California, USA

Allan D. Thomson BSc, MD, ChB, PhD, MRCP
Consultant Physician, Department of Gastroenterology/Liver Unit, Greenwich District Hospital, London, UK

John Wright MSc, MRCP, MRCPath
Reader in Metabolic Medicine, Department of Biochemistry, University of Surrey, Guildford, UK

Contents

SECTION ONE

The alcoholic in the community

1 *Sidney B. Rosalki*

Alcoholism — an overview

INTRODUCTION

Clinical biochemistry requires an understanding of both the clinical features and the biochemical abnormalities associated with disease. In order to set the scene of this volume, this introductory chapter will provide an overview of alcoholism in the community. Alcoholism will be defined, the size of the alcoholism problem indicated, and comment made on its origins, social concomitants and outcome. Additionally, the clinical characteristics of alcoholism and its complications will be described.

DEFINING ALCOHOLISM

There is no universally agreed criterion of what constitutes alcoholism or problem drinking, and the definition of alcoholism has been and continues to be a subject of controversy (Lancet, 1977a). The term alcoholism has been variously related to the quantity of alcohol consumed (De Lint & Schmidt, 1971), the frequency and the drinking pattern (Jellinek, 1960; Keller, 1960), the presence of social, psychological or physical damage from alcohol (Jellinek, 1952), or a serious life problem related to drinking (Schuckit, 1978), or to psychological and physical dependence on alcohol (synonym: alcohol addiction) evidenced by the alcohol dependency syndrome (Jellinek, 1952; Edwards & Gross, 1976; Edwards et al, 1977). This latter is characterised by high alcohol consumption, drink-orientated behaviour, alcohol craving, tolerance to alcohol, continued drinking despite harm and withdrawal symptoms on abstinence.

Excessive use of alcohol is also difficult to define, for it varies with geographic, ethnic, and cultural factors (Lelbach, 1974). Daily intakes of greater than 150 ml of ethanol (120 g) have been considered as excessive (De Lint & Schmidt, 1971; Glatt, 1977) because of the high risk of dependency at this level (Kendell, 1979), others have set lower levels of around 80 g per day (Hetzel, 1975; Spratley & Pollak, 1977) because of the risk of organ damage. Women, however, are more susceptible than men to liver damage from alcohol (Pequignot, 1974), and although daily intakes above 80 g may be considered excessive for males, for women 60 g ethanol per day would seem a more appropriate figure. Most upper reference limits in biological studies are set to include some 98 per cent of the healthy population, and until recently an intake of 80 g ethanol per day was exceeded by only 2 per cent of the total adult UK population (Kendall, 1979; Spratley & Pollak, 1977). However, if men and women are considered separately, a daily intake of 80 g is now exceeded by 6 per cent of men, but an intake of 60 g by only 1 per cent of women (Wilson, 1980).

Excess alcohol consumption may be considered as synonymous with 'heavy drinking' but should not be equated with 'problem' drinking or alcoholism, though it is important to recognise that heavy drinkers are potential alcoholics and that heavy drinking is a prerequisite of alcoholism. 'Problem drinking' and alcohol dependence ('addiction') are both included in the original (1952) World Health Organisation Definition of Alcoholism (Jellinek, 1952) where alcoholics are defined as 'those excessive drinkers whose dependence on alcohol has attained such a degree that it shows a noticeable mental disturbance or an interference with their bodily and mental health, their interpersonal relations, and their smooth social and economic functioning; or who show the prodromal signs of such development'. Problem drinking and dependence are, however, separated in the World Health Organisation (1977) report's use of the terms 'alcohol-related diability' and 'alcohol dependence syndrome' (Edwards et al, 1977). The definition of alcoholism as 'the repeated (intermittent or continual) ingestion of alcohol leading to dependency, physical disease or other harm' (Davies, 1973; Paton & Saunders, 1981), would include problem drinkers, alcohol 'addicts' and different drinking patterns, and would seem a useful brief definition of the disorder.

HOW MANY ALCOHOLICS?

In the UK, with a population of 55 million, there are now thought to be in excess of three quarters of a million alcoholics (Paton, Potter & Saunders, 1981). There are more than half a million alcoholics in England and Wales alone (Lancet, 1977c; Donnan & Haskey, 1977; Glatt 1977), representing some 2 per cent of the adult population. In some parts of England e.g. the North East, alcoholism is especially prevalent (Lancet, 1977), and in Scotland (British Medical Association News Review, 1979), and Ireland (O'Connor, 1978), the incidence of alcoholism is four times as frequent as in England. For every alcoholic there are at least a similar number of subjects whose drinking is at such a level ('excessive drinkers', 'excessive users', 'problem drinkers') that they are at high risk of alcoholism (Wilkins, 1975; Glatt, 1977) even if not yet completely fulfilling some accepted criterion for its definition.

It is also interesting to examine the contribution of alcoholism to general hospital admissions and attendance. Thus in recent studies in Manchester, alcoholism was present in 15 per cent of male general medical admissions (Owens, 1977), and was a direct or contributory factor in 27 per cent of all acute general medical hospital admissions (Jariwalla, Adams & Horne, 1979). In Glasgow, 19 per cent of acute admissions to a male general medical unit had illnesses related to alcohol (Quinn & Johnston, 1976). A recent study from a London Teaching Hospital reported 19.5 per cent of hospital patients (medical and orthopaedic in-patients and casualty out-patients) to have an unsuspected drinking problem (Jarman & Kellett, 1979). One third of patients attending hospital accident and emergency departments in the evening hours have blood ethanol levels above 80 mg/dl (Holt et al, 1980).

In the United States of America, there are an estimated 9 million alcoholics, with 10 per cent of the urban population above the age of 20 having an 'alcohol problem', and 4–10 per cent of hospital admissions associated with alcohol (Nolan, 1965; Dolan 1976).

ALCOHOLISM IS ON THE INCREASE

Alcoholism is increasing, as evidenced by the increasing incidence of liver cirrhosis and hospital admissions for treatment of alcoholism, and as reflected by the increasing levels of alcohol consumption, of convictions for drunkenness, convictions for driving under the influence of alcohol, and of road accidents where alcohol is involved. This increase in alcoholism is worldwide (see for example Lancet, 1978a for an account of alcoholism in Australia, and the reviews of Smith, 1982a for Poland; 1982b for the Third World, and 1982c for New Zealand), it may be exemplified by considering the situation in the UK.

Two-thirds of cirrhosis of the liver is now believed to be alcoholic in origin (Hodgson & Thompson, 1976). Deaths from cirrhosis in Britain now approximate to some 2500 per annum or 0.3 per cent of all deaths (Central Statistical Office, 1979). A cirrhosis mortality of 3.7 per 100 000 population was recorded in England and Wales for 1975, having increased by almost 30 per cent in the preceding 10 years (Royal College of Psychiatrists, 1979). For comparison, in France, the leading alcohol consumer in Europe, with a per head annual alcohol consumption of approximately 25 litres of ethanol, cirrhosis mortality is more than ten times that in Britain (Popham, Schmidt & de Lint, 1975).

Alcohol-related psychiatric admissions in England and Wales increased some 120 per cent in the 10 year period up to 1975 (Royal College of Psychiatrists, 1979), to reach 35.5 per 100 000 population over 15 (Lancet, 1978b). There are now some 20 000 such admissions annually in the United Kingdom constituting more than 10 per cent of total psychiatric admissions (Paton, Potter & Saunders, 1981).

Consumption of wine and spirits has doubled during the last decade and beer consumption has increased by one third (Central Statistical Office, 1979). Some 70 million gallons of wine, 35 million gallons of proof spirit, and 40 million bulk barrels of beer are now consumed annually in Britain. Expenditure on alcoholic beverages occupies some 5 per cent of average total weekly household expenditure and a quarter of the amount spent on food. The average consumption of alcohol per head of the adult population approximates to 20 g ethanol per day or between 7 and 8 kg (9 to 10 litres) of ethanol per year (Levi & Chalmers, 1978) with a 50 per cent increase in the last 10 years (Royal College of Psychiatrists, 1979).

Convictions for drunkenness in Britain doubled in the 25 year period preceding 1975 (Glatt, 1977), increasing in the last six years of this period by 28 per cent in England and Wales but by 91 per cent in Scotland (Kendall, 1979). Such convictions approximate to 300 per 100 000 population over 15, and exceed 100 000 per annum. Similarly, convictions for driving with an excess of alcohol in the blood or urine increased more than sevenfold in the decade preceding 1975 (Glatt, 1977) and now exceed 70 000 per annum. A 1979 review (British Medical Journal, 1979), reported that 38 per cent of drivers and 28 per cent of pedestrians killed in road traffic accidents had blood alcohol levels above the legal limit (80 mg/dl). Similar figures have been reported for road traffic accidents in the USA (Kaye, 1976).

PRONOUNCED INCREASE IN ALCOHOLISM IN WOMEN AND YOUTHS

Patterns of drinking behaviour and of alcoholism have also shown evidence of change, with drinking and cirrhosis and alcoholism showing a more pronounced rate of increase in females and in youths. This pattern has been observed in the USA (Westwood, Cohen & McNamara, 1978) and Canada (Smart, 1980) as well as the UK, but will again be illustrated by numerical data from British studies. Thus convictions for drunkenness under the age of 21 trebled in the 15 years preceding 1974 compared with an overall doubling in the preceding 25 years (Glatt, 1977). In males aged 18–20, convictions increased by 90 per cent in the decade preceding 1975 compared with 400 per cent for females (Donnan & Haskey, 1977). Overall, in the period 1970–1978 convictions for drunkenness in England and Wales rose by 27 per cent in males but by 64 per cent in females, the cirrhosis death rate increased by 36 per cent in males and by 243 per cent in females, and psychiatric hospital admissions for alcoholism increased by 77 per cent in males but by 130 per cent in females (British Medical Journal, 1980a), the increase being fastest in women under 25 (Donnan & Haskey, 1977). The proportion of women joining Alcoholics Annonymous, the drinker's self-help organisation is also steadily rising, with one third of its 1979 membership women, compared with one-fifth in 1972. The average age of members dropped from 47 to 44 during this period (Daily Telegraph, 1979). It has been claimed that currently 13 per cent of men and 4 per cent of women between the ages of 18 and 24 are regular heavy drinkers (Wilson, 1980).

THE COST OF ALCOHOLISM

This year we may anticipate that the 55 million population of the United Kingdom will spend some £9000 million on alcoholic beverages (Office of Health Economics, 1981). The Government will earn £3500 million of revenue from their sale but at least £1000 million of this will be lost to the nation because of the cost of alcoholism, this latter made up of some £500 million lost to industry in early death, absenteeism and accidents at work, and £500 million in the provision of medical and social services for alcoholics and their families (Tucker, 1977; Lancet 1978b; Holterman & Burchell, 1981). By extrapolation, comparable figures relative to population size and drinking habits (Popham, Schmidt & de Lint, 1975) might be expected in other countries. For example, the annual economic loss from alcoholism in the USA has been estimated as 15–25 billion dollars (Lundberg, 1976). These figures reflect the cost to the nation of alcoholism, but not the disruption and damage to the individual or his family that can result from alcohol excess.

WHO ARE THE ALCOHOLICS?

Currently, alcoholism shows the highest incidence in middle-aged males. It is more frequent in urban than in rural communities, and in the highest (professional and managerial) and the lowest (unskilled) social classes. It is particularly associated with those occupations where alcohol is cheap and and readily available, where heavy alcohol consumption is traditional and uncensured, where there is separation from normal social and sexual relationships, or where the occupation is particularly stressful or hazardous (Mellor, 1967; Smith, 1981c). Thus, it is most frequent in those involved with the manufacture, distribution or retailing of drinks, in merchant seamen, naval and other service personnel, in journalists, commercial travellers, actors, managing directors and those on expense accounts (Plant, 1981). Doctors also have an increased incidence (Murray, 1977). There is the possibility that there may be (unconscious) preselection of such high-risk occupations in potential alcoholics.

In the UK there is a higher incidence of alcoholism in the Scots and Irish than in the English and Welsh. Its prevalence is higher in Catholics than in Protestants, possibly because of a large Irish contribution to the former religion (Mellor, 1967). It is lowest in Jews and Moslems (Clare, 1979). These variations reflect differences in ethnic, religious, social and cultural attitudes to alcohol.

Alcoholism is especially common in the unmarried, in the divorced and separated. As previously indicated, the pattern of alcoholism is changing, with an increasing proportion of women and young people.

WHY DO PEOPLE DRINK?

No single cause accounts for excessive drinking. People drink alcohol to counter anxiety, loneliness or boredom, to ease relationships, in response to peer pressure, from curiosity or because they like the taste or the effect. The excess drinking resulting in alcoholism is believed to develop from the combined effects of biological or psychological vulnerability and of opportunity (Ritson, 1975; Lindberg, 1976).

Biological vulnerability postulates that pre-existing metabolic factors may enhance the risk of alcoholism. There is considerable evidence of genetic differences in alcoholic compared with normal populations and these support a partial role for a metabolic cause (McCord & McCord, 1960; Mellor, 1967; Schuckit, 1978; Clare, 1979; see also Ch. 2). Most observed metabolic abnormalities in alcoholics, however, appear to be secondary to alcohol abuse, though they may act to perpetuate drinking.

Psychological vulnerability suggests that poor personality development in the alcoholic, or enhanced need of alcohol for anxiety relief may result in excessive drinking, alcohol providing behavioural reward in the form of stress relief, personality support, and alleviation of withdrawal symptoms (Clare, 1979).

Vulnerability and opportunity are both strongly influenced by socio-cultural factors, (ethnic, occupational, familial) which govern the availability and acceptability of alcohol and the stress upon the individual. In women, alcoholism shows an increased frequency in association with alteration in domestic role, particularly the departure of the children from the home. In young people, excessive paternal punishment may be contributory (O'Connor, 1978; Clare, 1979).

Whatever the factor or factors which initiate the drinking process there is no doubt that high alcohol intake in excess of 120 g per day for a prolonged period, itself produces dependence (Kendall, 1979), and serves to perpetuate the susceptibility produced by genetic, psychological and socio-cultural influences.

BORN TO DRINK?

Alcoholism is at least twice as frequent in the sons of alcoholic fathers as in the sons of non-alcoholic fathers. Though environmental example may contribute to this higher incidence (McCord & McCord, 1960; Winokur et al, 1970), adoption, half-sibling and twin studies indicate an important role for genetic factors in alcoholism.

Adoption studies have shown that the adopted sons of alcoholics when separated from their biological parents in early childhood and raised by foster parents, are more likely to be alcoholics than adoptees from non-alcoholic biological parents (Goodwin et al, 1973), and show an incidence of alcoholism comparable to their non-adopted brothers (Goodwin et al, 1974). Similarly the half-sibs of alcoholics with alcoholic biological parents have been found to have three times the rate of alcoholism of those with non-alcoholic biological parents, but raised by alcoholic non-biological parents (Schuckit, Goodwin & Winokur, 1972). In male twins, if one twin is an alcoholic, the other is twice as likely to be an alcoholic if the twins are mono-zygotic (identical) than if they are di-zygotic (fraternal) (Kaij, 1960). In addition, similar drinking habits have been observed in reared-apart mono-zygotic twins (Shields, 1977).

Though the daughters of alcoholics also show an increased incidence of alcoholism (Goodwin et al, 1978), evidence of genetic influence in female alcoholism has been less convincing than in the male, possibly because of the small numbers of females hitherto included in such studies. Some studies have suggested that genetic associations in the male correlate more closely with alcohol dependence or the medical complications of alcohol than with heavy drinking or social disability (Kaij & McNeil, 1979), but most workers believe that the principal influence of genetic factors is to affect the frequency and amount of drink consumed (Partanen, Bruin & Markannen, 1966; Clifford et al, 1981).

Largely from twin studies it has been suggested that an autosomal dominant gene with partial penetrance may contribute to the development of dependence or damage in those with high alcohol intakes (Kaij & McNeil, 1979) though intake levels appear to be primarily influenced by non-genetic factors (British Medical Journal, 1977). Simple Mendelian inheritance has, however, been considered unlikely (British Medical Journal, 1980b), because of studies showing similar alcoholism rates in first-degree and second-degree relatives of alcoholics. Two recent adoption studies (Cloninger, Bohman & Sigvardson 1981; Bohman, Sigvardson & Cloninger, 1981) have postulated two distinct patterns of alcohol abuse with different inheritance patterns. A common mild type affecting males and females, with minimal evidence of parent-offspring transmission, and a more severe type in male, with a strong inheritance pattern.

Biochemical and other evidence of possible genetic abnormalities predisposing to alcoholism is considered fully in Chapter 2.

BIOCHEMICAL ORIGINS OF ADDICTION

Attempts have been made to relate the development or persistence of the alcohol dependency syndrome ('addiction') to alterations in brain biochemistry (Lancet, 1972). They mostly postulate that alcohol excess produces altered cerebral concentrations or imbalance of stimulatory or inhibitory neuro-amines, with desirable psychic effects. Abstinence will then result in psychically undesirable effects.

These cerebral effects may be mediated by acetaldehyde produced from ethanol oxidation. This compound inhibits the oxidation of the aldehyde products of stimulatory neuro-amines (dopamine and nor-adrenaline) and serotonin so that these or their psycho-active metabolites accumulate (Lahti & Machrowitz, 1967; Davis et al, 1967; Walsh, Truitt & Davis, 1970). Acetaldehyde may also combine with neuro-amines such as dopamine to give tetrahydroisoquinolines (e.g. salsolinol) or with tryptophan derivatives to yield tetrahydro-β-carbolines, (componds which are themselves stimulatory; Cohen, Mytilineou & Barrett, 1972). In addition, acetaldehyde may inhibit the further metabolism of the aldehyde product of dopamine so that this combines with dopamine itself to yield an addictive opiate-like compound (tetrahydropapaveroline) (Davis & Walsh, 1970).

Impaired cerebral synthesis of noradrenaline, serotonin, and the inhibitory neurotransmitter γ-aminobutyrate (GABA) may also be a consequence of Vitamin B_6 defiency, which is common in alcoholics (Davis & Smith 1974), this vitamin being required as a co-enzyme for the proper functioning of the enzyme systems controlling neuroamine synthesis (Rosalki, 1979). Experiments carried out by the author in rabbits (Nicholson, Rosalki & Gilliland, 1979) also suggest that alcohol ingestion may cause a reduction in the activity of a brain enzyme (γ-glutamyltransferase) responsible for the catabolism of stimulatory neuroamines or the formation of GABA. A recent suggestion postulates that increased antidepressive activity from increased prostaglandin E_1 production by alcohol may be relevant to addiction (Horrobin & Manku, 1980). Possible biochemical origins of addiction are further considered in Chapter 2.

CLINICAL CLUES TO ALCOHOLISM

The alert physician may suspect alcoholism in the patient presenting with, or referred because of, marital, family or work problems (especially work deterioration and Monday morning absenteeism), psychiatric disturbance or the features of any disease associated with alcohol. This suspicion may be reinforced if there is a family history of the disease, if the patient's occupation or environment is such as to encourage drinking, or there is a history of road traffic or other accidents or of minor brushes with the law e.g. for assault or drunkenness (Wilkins, 1975; Spratley & Pollak, 1977; Hore, 1977). The alcoholic may be a frequent visitor to the doctor's surgery with minor complaints, his attendance being some 3 times the national average (Hospital Doctor, 1978).

A hoarse voice, a bloated face, tremulousness, the smell of drink, an unkempt appearance or an overfamiliar manner, may all suggest the disorder. Changes in the hands: clubbing, transverse white bands, furrows or opacity of the nails, reddening of the palms (palmar erythema), and contraction of the palmar fascia (Dupuytren's contracture) and changes in the skin (bruising, telangectasia) are also suggestive (Silverfarb, 1976). The presence of any one of the complications of alcoholism may indicate its presence. Of these, gastro-intestinal symptoms (dyspepsia, morning anorexia or nausea, diarrhoea), liver disease with liver tenderness or enlargement, neuropathy (sensory disturbance) and neuro-psychiatric disturbance (poor concentration, amnesia, fits) and pancreatitis (pain, diarrhoea) are the most frequent (Craig, 1976). Hypertension, mild diabetes mellitus, gout and lipid disorders may also be secondary to alcoholism. Finally, the alcoholic may admit to a level of alcohol intake that is clearly excessive.

The principal clinical features, early physical signs and complications of alcoholism are summarised in Tables 1.1, 1.2 and 1.3.

COURSE AND CONSEQUENCES OF ALCOHOLISM

During their drinking life, alcoholics show a marked fluctuation in their drinking with periods of abstinence or modest drinking alternating with heavier consumption, following which the patient presents with some drink-related disorder. The first major medical problems may be anticipated after some 10 years or more drinking, with the average age of presentation in the late 20s or early 30s. Infections, gastritis, trauma, neurological and psychiatric complications may be early modes of presentation. Liver disease and

Table 1.1 Some early physical signs of alcoholism (Annals of Internal Medicine, 1972; Silverfarb, 1976)

1. *General*:	Unkempt, overfamiliar, smell of alcohol
2. *Voice*:	Hoarse
3. *Face*:	Bloated, flushed, bloodshot eyes
4. *Skin*:	Bruising, dilated blood vessels
5. *Hands*:	Red palms, tremor, rapid pulse
6. *Trunk*:	Obese, pot-belly, male breast enlargement

Table 1.2 Clinical features of alcoholism (Annals of Internal Medicine, 1972; Silverfarb, 1976; Hore, 1977; Hospital Doctor, 1978)

1. *At-risk factors present*
   Occupation, family history etc.
2. *Social difficulties*
   Marital, family, work
   Law contravention (assault, drunkenness etc.)
   Accidents (work, traffic)
3. *Psychiatric disturbance*
   Anxiety, depression, etc.
4. *Symptoms of addiction*
   Craving, withdrawal symptoms
   (fits, hallucinations, amnesia)
5. *Features of diseases associated with alcohol*
   See Table 1.3

Table 1.3 Features of complications of alcoholism (Annals of Internal Medicine, 1972)

Hepatic/gastro-intestinal/pancreatic
(Leevy, Tamburro & Zetterman, 1975; Sarles, 1975; Krasner, 1977; Lake-Bakaar, 1982)
Pain, nausea, vomiting, diarrhoea, bleeding, hepatomegaly, jaundice

Neuropsychiatric
(Lees, 1967; Pearce, 1977; Hore, 1977; Glatt, 1977; Rail & Swash, 1982; Cutting, 1982)
Poor concentration and memory, insomnia, blackouts, sweating, numbness, tingling

Cardiovascular
(Brigden, 1977; Goodwin, 1977)
Palpitations, dyspnoea, raised blood pressure

Musculoskeletal
(Perkoff et al, 1967)
Pain, weakness, fractures, gout

Endocrine/metabolic/reproductive
(Marks & Chakraborty, 1975; Isselbacher, 1977; Hanson, 1977)
Obesity, breast swelling, glycosuria, impotence, infertility, fetal abnormality

Immunological/neoplastic
(Hurley, 1977; Green & Trawbridge, 1977)
Chest infections, upper gastro-intestinal cancer

Note: References in brackets refer to useful reviews

pancreatitis are also frequent and important modes of presentation, though generally first appearing in the mid 40s (Mellor, 1967; Schuckit, 1978).

Liver disease is a presenting feature in one third, and is present in two-thirds of hospitalised alcoholics (Leevy, Tamburro & Zetterman, 1975; Potek et al, 1975; Bruguera, Bordas & Rodes, 1977). Pancreatitis and peripheral neuropathy are found in some 10 per cent of alcoholics with a history of 10 years daily ingestion of 120 g ethanol (Popper et al, 1974), with an increased incidence with more pronounced or prolonged consumption (Eghoje and Juhl, 1973) so that a 50 per cent incidence may result from 25 years daily consumption of 180 g (British Medical Journal, 1976). It may be noted that, worldwide, the average daily ethanol intake of the established alcoholic is approximately 180 g (Lelbach, 1974). 5 year survival with cirrhosis averages some 80 per cent in those who abstain compared with 50 per cent in those who continue to drink, with lower survival rates in females (Brunt et al, 1974; Williams & Davis, 1977).

There is a strong correlation between alcoholism and male mortality (Mellor, 1967). Overall mortality in alcoholics is more than twice the national average, with a markedly increased risk of death from cirrhosis of the liver and self-poisoning (Health Trends, 1977). Leading causes of death include heart disease and cancer in the elderly, accidents in the young (Schuckit, 1978). These latter make such a strong contribution to the excess deaths in young alcoholics that in the 15 to 39 age group, mortality is more than 17 times the national average in females and more than 11 times the national average in males (Health Trends, 1977).

It may be noted in passing that in middle-age, mortality is 50 per cent lower in modest alcohol consumers (less than 30 g daily, average 20 g) than in complete abstainers, largely due to a decrease in cardiovascular deaths, and possibly a consequence of the effect of alcohol on elevating 'protective' high-density lipoprotein cholesterol (Klatsky, Friedman & Siegelaub, 1981; Marmot et al, 1981; see also Ch. 8). With intakes of 30–60 g ethanol daily, mortality increases to the level found in abstainers.

HOW MUCH ALCOHOL IS HARMFUL?

A statistical increase in cirrhosis of the liver is seen with 5 years' intake of 60–80 g of ethanol per day in the male, representing some 3–4 pints of beer or 6–8 glasses of wine or sherry or 3–4 double measures of spirit daily. In women, the corresponding figure is 20–40 g daily (Pequignot, 1974). This may be regarded as a risk threshold for the disorder, though most patients with alcoholic cirrhosis have consumed at least double this amount for double this duration. Convincing evidence of damage to other organs at low levels of intake is scanty, though the incidence of hypertension may be enhanced by prolonged intake exceeding 30 g daily (Klatsky et al, 1977) and increased fetal morbidity has been observed with maternal intakes between 30 and 50 g (Kaminski, Rumeau-Rauquette & Schwartz, 1976). The full fetal alcohol syndrome (growth retardation, neurological disorder and abnormal facial appearance) is in general associated with regular daily maternal intakes exceeding 60 g. However, it has also been suggested that minor congenital abnormalities may be produced by the occasional maternal intake of 60 g ethanol, superimposed on a daily intake as low as 15 g (Smith, 1981b), and current advice favours complete abstinence during pregnancy (Edwards, 1983).

Most patients with organ or psychiatric damage have a history of daily intakes in excess of 150g (Turner, Mezey & Kimball, 1977). Prolonged daily consumption in excess of 120 g may result in the alcohol dependency syndrome independent of predisposition (Kendall, 1979). Brain atrophy visible by computed tomography (CT) scanning and accompanied by intellectual impairment has been noted in some 50 per cent of young males with intakes greater than 100 g daily for three years (average 200 g for 10 years) being twice as frequent as cirrhosis in the group studied (Lee et al, 1979). In a recent extensive review of damage resulting from alcohol, it was concluded that 'to show physical or mental disease primarily from long-continued use of alcohol, the critical level of daily intake which must be exceeded by the majority of persons seems to be in the order of 80–100 g of ethanol adjusted up or down from the 70 kg weight' (Turner, Mezey & Kimball, 1977). 80 g ethanol per day for males and 40 g for females is now widely avocated as the upper limit of safe drinking, with 60 g and 30 g daily respectively as the preferred limit (Royal College of Psychiatrists, 1979).

PREVENTING ALCOHOLISM

Whatever the factors which predispose to alcoholism in the individual (see previously), the strong correlation between mortality and morbidity from alcohol and per head alcohol consumption (Schmidt, 1977) and the claimed fixed relation between average and excess consumption (Lederman, 1956), imply that national drinking habits govern the incidence of alcoholism. Waves of alcoholism coincident with the availability of cheap potent alcoholic drink and social deprivation in the mid 18th and 19th centuries support this view and hint at the directions in which effective primary control might lie (Glatt, 1977).

Control of the sale of alcohol by prohibition, limitation of supply, or stringent licensing laws have been ineffective in restricting alcohol consumption (Mellor, 1967), though the restriction of licensing hours has probably been of some value (Glatt, 1977). Most effective has been regulation by price by high taxation (Mellor, 1967; Glatt, 1977; Clare, 1979). Present-day high alcohol intake in the United Kingdom has been correlated with the comparative fall in the price of alcohol and reduced effective taxation in recent years. The price of a bottle of whisky as a percentage of disposable income has fallen from 40 per cent in 1950 to 20 per cent in 1970, with the work time required for a male manual worker to pay for a pint of beer having fallen from 23 minutes in 1950 to 12 in 1976, and for a bottle of whisky from 6 and a half hours to 2 hours. For comparison, the time needed to pay for a large loaf of bread rose from 9 minutes to 11 minutes in this period (Kendall, 1979).

Other measures that have been suggested as a means of reducing national levels of alcohol consumption have aimed at more effective education of the public to the dangers of alcoholism (Glatt, 1974) but the level of educational expenditure (less than £200 000 per annum, Lancet, 1977c) is derisory compared with the annual amount spent in alcohol promotion (variously estimated as between £30 million and £100 million; Lancet, 1977c, 1980b; Smith, 1981a). Because of this, limitation on the advertising of alcohol beverages has been proposed (Clare, 1979). It has been suggested that a total advertising ban would result in a 13 per cent drop in alcohol consumption overall (McGuiness, 1980) and a 25 per cent drop by heavy drinkers (de Lint, 1973). Other proposals have included reduced taxation on beverages of low alcohol content and greater attention to the relief of social stresses which may predispose to drinking (Glatt, 1974).

National attitudes may also colour the effort made to prevent some of the more antisocial consequences of alcohol excess. Thus more rigid enforcement of drinking-driving legislation, and greater individual responsibility for offences committed under the influence of alcohol have been suggested (Havard, 1978).

All these measures may serve to reduce the level of alcoholism in the community; for the individual, counselling and psychiatric support for those at risk of alcoholism and for the heavy drinker before excessive drinking has resulted in harm or dependence, are the most important prophylactic measures. However, their success in preventing alcoholism must depend on being able to recognise those who are consuming alcohol in excess. The earlier this diagnosis can be made and treatment started, the more likely to be effective will be these preventive measures (British Medical Journal, 1974).

TREATMENT

Identifying the heavy drinker or alcoholic (see Ch. 4) is the first step to treatment (Edwards, 1967). Treatment is easier if applied at a stage before dependency is present (Wilkins, 1975), and can prevent its development.

The treatment of established alcoholism includes detoxification ('drying out'), the management of the alcohol withdrawal syndrome which may follow abrupt cessation or lowering of intake (see Ch. 6), the correction of nutritional deficiency (see Ch. 11), the therapy of complications, the use of psychotherapeutic techniques to promote continued abstinence, and the physical, psychological and social rehabilitation of the alcoholic (Edwards, 1967; Glatt, 1974; Ritson, 1975; Wilkins, 1975; Hore, 1977 etc.). Methods for promoting abstinence range from simple individual counselling or group self-help programmes to behaviour and aversion therapy.

Wide disagreement exists as to what constitutes the most effective abstinence-promoting programme for alcoholics, but there is general agreement that sustained sobriety states have a disappointingly low incidence. At two years follow-up only one-third of alcoholics are abstinent, though a further third are improved (Pollak, 1978; Chick, 1982). There are however reports of maintained abstinence rates of up to 70 per cent achieved by intensive programmes applied to subjects of previously high social stability (Von Wiegand, 1972). The earlier the alcoholic is treated, the better are the results of treatment. This particularly applies to the treatment of organ complications.

SUMMARY

This chapter has reviewed the social and medical consequences of chronic alcohol excess, and lists some of the clinical features and complications of alcoholism. The prevention of alcohol dependence and the success of therapy is more likely if the diagnosis of excess drinking and the complications of alcoholism can be made at an early stage. Biochemical procedures which may facilitate this will be described in subsequent chapters.

REFERENCES

Annals of Internal Medicine 1972 Criteria for the Diagnosis of Alcoholism 77: 249–258

Bohman M, Sigvardsson S, Cloninger C R 1981 Maternal inheritance of alcohol abuse. Cross-fostering analyses of adopted women. Archives of General Psychiatry 38: 965–969

Brigden W 1977 Alcoholic cardiomyopathy. British Journal of Hospital Medicine, August: 122–125

British Medical Association News Review 1979 Alcoholism in Scotland, September: 94
British Medical Journal 1974 Alcoholism and its identification. Leading article 2: 132
British Medical Journal 1977 How important are genetic influences in alcohol dependence? Leading article 2: 1371–1372
British Medical Journal 1979 Drinking and drug-taking in road accidents in Great Britain. Medical News 2: 341
British Medical Journal 1980a Alcohol consumption. Questions in the Commons, 2: 464
British Medical Journal 1980b Alcoholism: an inherited disease. Leading article 281: 1301–1302
Bruguera M, Bordas J M, Rodes J 1977 Asymptomatic liver disease in alcoholics. Archives of Pathology and Laboratory Medicine 101: 644–647
Brunt P W, Kew M C, Scheuer P J, Sherlock S 1974 Studies in alcoholic liver disease in Britain: Clinical and pathological patterns related to natural history. Gut 15: 52–58
Central Statistical Office 1979 Annual Abstract of Statistics
Chick J 1982 Do Alcoholics recover? British Medical Journal 285: 3–4
Clare A W 1979 The causes of alcoholism. British Journal of Hospital Medicine April: 403–411
Clifford C A, Fulker D W, Gurling H M D, Murray R M 1981 Genetic and environmental influence on drinking patterns in normal livers. In: Parisi P (ed) Twin research, 3. Alan Liss, New York, p 47
Cohen G, Mytilineou C, Barrett R E 1972 6, 7 dihydroxytetrahydroisoquinoline: uptake and storage by peripheral sympathetic nerve of the rat. Science 175: 1269–1272
Cloninger C R, Bohman M, Sigvardsson S 1981 Inheritance of alcohol abuse. Cross-fostering analysis of adopted men. Archives of General Psychiatry 38: 861–868
Craig J R 1976 Alcohol-associated disease. In: Lundberg G D (ed) The professional and community role of the pathologist in alcohol abuse. US Department of Transportation, Washington pp 15–17
Cutting J 1982 Neuropsychiatric complications of alcoholism. British Journal of Hospital Medicine, April: 335–342
Daily Telegraph 1979 More women drunks, October 18: 11
Davies D L 1973 Implications for medical practice of an acceptable concept of alcoholism. In: Kessel K, Hawker A, Chalke M, Edsall B (eds) Alcoholism — a medical profile. Proceedings 1st International Federal Conference on Alcoholism, London
Davis R E, Smith B K 1974 Pyridoxal and folate deficiency in alcoholics. Medical Journal of Australia 2: 357–360
Davis V E, Walsh M J 1970 Alcohol, amines and alkaloids: a possible biochemical basis for alcohol addiction. Science 167: 1005–1007
Davis V E, Brown H, Huff J A, Cashaw J L 1967 The alteration of serotonin metabolism to 5-hydroxy-tryptophal by ethanol ingestion in man. Journal of Laboratory and Clinical Medicine 69: 132–140
De Lint J 1973 The epidemiology of alcoholism, Substudy 556 (2). Addiction Research Foundation, Ontario
De Lint J, Schmidt W 1971 Consumption averages and alcoholism prevalence: a brief review of epidemiological investigations. British Journal of Addiction 66: 97–107
Dolan W D 1976 In: G D Lundberg (ed) The professional and community role of the pathologist in alcohol abuse. US Department of Transportation, Washington, Preface
Donnan S and Haskey J 1977 Alcoholism and cirrhosis of the liver. Population Trends 7: 18–24
Edwards G 1967 The meaning and treatment of alcohol dependence. Hospital Medicine, December: 272–281
Edwards G 1983 Alcohol and advice to the pregnant woman. British Medical Journal 286: 247–248
Edwards G, Gross M M 1976 Alcohol dependence: provisional description of a clinical syndrome. British Medical Journal 1: 1058–1061
Edwards G, Gross M M, Keller M, Moser J, Room R (eds) 1977 Alcohol related disabilities. Offset publication no 32. World Health Organisation, Geneva
Eghoje K N, Juhl E 1973 Factors determining liver damage in chronic alcoholics. Scandinavian Journal of Gastroenterology 8: 505–512
Glatt M M 1974 Alcoholism. British Journal of Hospital Medicine, January: 111–120

Glatt M M 1977 The English drink problem through the ages. Proceedings Royal Society of Medicine 70: 202–206
Goodwin J F 1977 Alcohol and the heart: alcoholic cardiomyopathy. Journal Royal College of Physicians 12: 5–10
Goodwin D W Schulsinger F, Hermansen L, Guze S B, Winokur G 1973 Alcohol problems in adoptees raised apart from alcoholic biological parents. Archives of General Psychiatry 28: 238–243
Goodwin D W, Schulsinger F, Moller N, Hermansen L, Winokur G, Guze S B 1974 Drinking problems in adopted and non-adopted sons of alcoholics. Archives of General Psychiatry 31: 164–169
Goodwin D W, Schulsinger F, Knop J, Mednick S, Guze S B 1977 Alcoholism and depression in adopted-out daughters of alcoholics. Archives of General Psychiatry 34: 751–755
Green J B, Trawbridge A A 1977 Haematologic and oncologic implications of alcoholism. Postgraduate Medicine 61: 149–154
Hanson J W 1977 Alcohol and the fetus. British Journal of Hospital Medicine, August: 126–130
Havard J D J 1978 Alcohol and the driver. British Medical Journal 1: 1595–1597
Health Trends 1977 Alcoholism and mortality. HMSO, London
Hetzel B S 1975 Tobacco and alcohol. Medicine, series 2, 5: 224–227
Hodgson H J F, Thompson R P H 1976 Cirrhosis in South London. Lancet 2: 118–121
Holt S, Steward I C, Dixon J M J, Elton R E, Taylor T V, Little K 1980 Alcohol and the emergency service patient. British Medical Journal 281: 638–640
Holterman S, Birchell A 1981 The costs of alcohol abuse. Department of Health and Social Security, London
Hore B D 1977 Clinical features and treatment of alcoholism. British Journal of Hospital Medicine, August: 106–116
Horrobin D F, Manku M S 1980 Possible role of prostaglandin E_1 in the affective disorders and in alcoholism. British Medical Journal 1: 1363–1366
Hospital Doctor 1978 Searching for the hidden alcoholic. November 15
Hurley D L 1977 Infectious complications of alcoholism. Postgraduate Medicine 61: 160–162
Isselbacher K J 1977 Metabolic and hepatic effects of alcohol. New England Journal of Medicine 296: 612–161
Jariwalla A G, Adams P H, Hore B D 1979 Alcohol and acute general medical admissions. Health Trends 11: 95–97
Jarman C M B, Kellett J M 1979 Alcoholism in the general hospital. British Medical Journal 2: 469–472
Jellinek E M 1960 The disease concept of alcoholism. Hillhouse Press, New Haven
Jellinek E M 1952 World Health Organisation, Technical Report Series no 48: 26
Kaij L 1960 Alcoholism in twins. Almquist & Wiksell, Stockholm
Kaij L, McNeil T F 1979 Genetic aspects of alcoholism. Advances in Biological Psychiatry 3: 54–65
Kaminski M, Rumeau-Rouquette C, Schwartz D 1976 Consommation d'alcool chez les femmes enceintes et issue de la grossesse. Revue Epidemiologie et Santé Publique 24: 27–40
Kaye S 1976 Alcohol and traffic fatalities. In: Lundberg G D (ed) The professional and community role of the pathologist in alcohol abuse. US Department of Transportation, Washington DC, pp 22–24
Keller M 1960 Definition of alcoholism. Quarterly Journal Studies of Alcohol 21: 125–134
Kendell R E 1979 Alcoholism: a medical or a political problem? British Medical Journal 1: 367–371
Klatsky A L, Friedman G D, Siegelaub A B, Gerard M J 1977 Alcohol consumption and blood pressure: Kaiser-Permanente multiphasic health examination data. New England Journal of Medicine 296: 1194–1200
Klatsky A L, Friedman G B, Seigelaub A B 1981 Alcohol and mortality. Annals of Internal Medicine 95: 139–145
Krasner N 1975 Alcohol and the gastro-intestinal tract. Journal Royal College of Physicians 12: 15–19

Lahti R, Majchrowicz E 1967 The effects of acetaldehyde on serotonin metabolism. Life Sciences 6: 1399–1406
Lake-Bakaar G 1982 Alcohol and the pancreas. British Medical Bulletin 38: 57–62
Lancet 1972 Alcohol addiction a biochemical approach. Leading article 2: 24–25
Lancet 1977a WHO and a new perspective on alcoholism. Leading article 1: 1087–1088
Lancet 1977b The alcoholism treatment package. Leading article 2: 488–490
Lancet 1977c The latest attack on alcoholism. Commentary from Westminster 2: 668–669
Lancet 1978a Alcohol abuse: round the world. Australia. 1: 142
Lancet 1978b Alcoholism: notes and news 2: 747–748
Lancet 1980a The alcoholism endemic. Commentary from Westminster 1: 938–939
Lancet 1980b Alcohol and advertising. Leading article 2: 1175
Lederman S 1956 Alcool, alcoolism, alcoolisation. Presses Universitaires de France, Paris
Lee K, Moller L, Hardt F, Haubek A, Jensen E 1979 Alcohol-induced brain damage and liver damage in young males. Lancet 2: 759–761
Lees F 1967 Alcohol and the nervous system. Hospital Medicine, December: 264–270
Leevy C M, Tamburro C H, Zetterman R 1975 Liver disease of the alcoholic. Medical Clinics North America 59: 909–918
Lelbach W K 1974 Organ pathology related to volume and pattern of alcohol use. In: Gibbons R J (ed) Recent advances in alcohol and drug problems I. Wiley, New York, p 93–198
Levi A J, Chalmers D M 1978 Recognition of alcoholic liver disease in a district general hospital. Gut 19: 521–525
Lundberg G D 1976 Concepts of substance abuse and addiction. In: Lundberg G D (ed) The professional and community role of the pathologist in alcohol abuse. US Department of Transportation, Washington DC, pp 1–2
Marks V, Chakraborty J 1975 The clinical endocrinology of alcoholism. Journal of Alcoholism 8: 94–103
Marmot M G, Rose G, Shipley M J, Thomas B J 1981 Alcohol and mortality; a U-shaped curve. Lancet 1: 580–583
McCord W, McCord J 1960 Origins of alcoholism. Tavistock, London
McGuiness T 1980 An econometric analysis of total demand for alcoholic beverages in the UK 1956–75. Journal of Industrial Economics 29: 85–109
Mellor C S 1967 The epidemiology of alcoholism. Hospital Medicine, December: 284–293
Murray R M 1977 The alcoholic doctor. British Journal of Hospital Medicine, August: 144–149
Nicholson H R, Rosalki S B, Gilliland L 1900 Brain γ-glutamyltransferase in alcohol-fed rabbits. Enzyme 25: 56–59
Nolan J P 1965 Alcohol as a factor in the illness of University service patients. American Journal of the Medical Sciences 294: 135–142
O'Connor J 1978 The young drinkers. Tavistock, London
Office of Health Economics, London 1981 Alcohol: reducing the harm
Owens E P 1977 Cited in Hore B D. Clinical features and treatment of alcoholism. British Journal of Hospital Medicine, August: 106–116
Partanen J, Bruun K, Marknanen T 1966 Inheritance of drinking behaviour. A study on intelligence, personality and use of alcohol in adult twins. In: Finnish Foundation on Alcohol Studies, Helsinki
Paton A, Saunders J B 1981 ABC of alcohol: definitions. British Medical Journal 283: 1248–1250
Paton A, Potter J F, Saunders J B 1981 ABC of alcohol: nature of the problem. British Medical Journal 283: 1318–1319
Pearce J M S 1977 Neurological aspects of alcoholism. British Journal of Hospital Medicine, August: 132–142
Pequignot G 1974 Augmentation du risque de cirrhose en function de la ration d'alcool. Revue d l'alcoolisme 20: 191–202
Perkoff G T, Dioso M M, Bleisch V and Klinkerfuss G 1967 A spectrum of myopathy associaed with alcoholism, 1. Clinical and laboratory features. Annals of Internal Medicine 67: 481–492
Plant M A 1981 Risk factors in employment. In: Hore B D, Plant M A (eds) Alcohol problems in employment. Croom Helm, London
Pollak B 1978 A two year study of alcoholics in general practice. British Journal of Alcoholism 13: 24–33

Popham R E, Schmidt W, de Lint L 1975 The prevention of alcoholism: epidemiological studies of the effects of government control measures. British Journal of Addiction 70: 125–144

Popper H, Sherlock S, Leevy C M, Harris M L 1974 Nomenclature, diagnostic criteria and diagnostic methodology for diseases of the liver and biliary tract. In: Fogarty International Centre Proceedings no 22

Potek A J, Toth I G, Saunders M G, Castro G A M Engel J J 1975 Alcohol and dietary factors in cirrhosis. Archives of Internal Medicine 135: 1053–1057

Quinn M A, Johnston R V 1976 Alcohol problems in acute male medical admissions. Scottish Home and Health Department, Health Bulletin 34: 253–250

Rail D L, Swash M 1982 The neuropsychiatric complications of alcoholism. Hospital Update, April: 463–471

Ritson E B 1975 Treatment of alcoholism. British Medical Journal 2: 124–127

Rosalki S B 1979 Clinical biochemistry of vitamin B_6. In: Taylor D G (ed) The importance of vitamins ot human health. MTP, Lancaster, pp 53–60

Royal College of Psychiatrists 1979 Special committee: alcohol and alcoholism. Tavistock, London

Sarles H 1975 Alcohol and the pancreas. Annals of the New York Academy of Sciences 252: 171–182

Schmidt W 1968 In: Edwards G, Grant M (eds) Alcoholism: new knowledge and new responses. Croom Helm, London, p 15

Schuckit M A 1978 The disease alcoholism. Postgraduate Medicine 64: 78–83

Schuckit A, Goodwin D A, Winokur G 1972 A study of alcoholism in half siblings. American Journal of Psychiatry 128: 1132–1136

Shields J 1977 Genetics and alcoholism. In: Edwards G, Grant M (eds) Alcoholism. New knowledge and new responses. Croom Helm, London, pp 117–135

Silverfarb P M 1976 Recognising alcoholism early by physical signs. Posgraduate Med 59: 79–81

Smart R G 1980 The new drinkers: teenage use and abuse of alcohol. Addiction Research Foundation, Toronto

Smith R 1981a Alcohol and alcoholism. The relation between consumption and damage. British Medical Journal 283: 895–898

Smith R 1981b Alcohol, women and the young: the same old problem. British Medical Journal 283: 1170–1172

Smith R 1981c Alcohol and work: a promising approach. British Medical Journal 283: 1108–1110

Smith R 1982a Polish lessons in alcohol policy. British Medical Journal 284: 98–101

Smith R 1982b Alcohol in the Third World. A chance to avoid a miserable trap. British Medical Journal 284: 183–185

Smith R 1982c Drinking and smoking in the land of the long white cloud. British Medical Journal 284: 1029–1031

Spratley T A, Pollak B 1977 Guide for the recognition of alcohol problems in general practice. Presented at Royal Society of Medicine.

Tucker A 1977 Counting the cost of alcoholism. The Guardian, November 7: 3

Turner T B, Mezey E, Kimball A W 1977 Measurement of alcohol-related effects in man: chronic effects in relation to levels of alcohol consumption. John Hopkins Medical Journal 141: 235–248, 273–286

Von Wiegand R A 1972 Alcoholism in industry. British Journal of Addiction 67: 181

Walsh M J, Truitt E B Jr, Davis V E 1970 Acetaldehyde mediation in the mechanism of ethanol-induced changes. Molecular Pharmacology 6: 416

Westwood M, Cohen M I, McNamara H 1978 Serum γ-glutamyl transpeptidase activity: a chemical determinant of alcohol consumption during adolescence. Pediatrics 62: 560–562

Williams R, Davis M 1977 Alcoholic liver injury. Proceedings of the Royal Society of Medicine 70: 333–336

Watkins R 1975 Alcoholism: the GP's role. Medicine, series 2, 13: 593–594

Wilson P 1980 Drinking in England and Wales. HMSO, London

Winokur G, Reich T, Rimmer J, Pitts F N 1970 Alcoholism 3: Diagnosis and familial psychiatric illness in 259 alcohol probands. Archives of General Psychiatry 23: 104–11

2 *Marc A. Schuckit*

Biochemical markers of a predisposition to alcoholism

INTRODUCTION

This chapter is written looking to the future. Today we have no robust biochemical tests which indicate when an individual is predisposed towards alcoholism. The best predictor of future pervasive alcohol-related problems is the past history of such difficulties and the family history of alcoholism (Schuckit, 1980).

The author of this chapter is not a biochemist but a clinical researcher, whose interest in biochemical markers for a predisposition towards alcoholism grew out of clinical experience in treating alcoholics and, more importantly, the study of possible genetic factors in the development of alcoholism. This in turn led to the need to more closely study biochemical events which might be involved in that predisposition.

In recent years there have been intriguing research results indicating differences between alcoholics and controls in metabolism of alcohol and the related enzymes. Preliminary studies carried out in groups at high risk for alcoholism (usually children of alcoholics) form the basis of speculations about biochemical markers which might correlate with a high future risk.

I will proceed in this chapter through a number of steps to introduce the reader to possible biological markers for a predisposition towards alcoholism. First, I will discuss the concept of alcoholism and the use of diagnosis for prognosis. Second, I will review evidence supporting one way of identifying 'future alcoholics' through a discussion of data supporting a genetic influence in alcoholism. Third, I will introduce our own study approach. Fourth, I will briefly review the important steps in the metabolism of ethanol (ethanol is used here synonymously with beverage alcohol or alcohol) and acetaldehyde (AcH) and go on to discuss the evidence for genetic control of the two most prominent enzymes, alcohol and aldehyde dehydrogenase, tying these into a theoretical framework of how different enzyme patterns might affect the predisposition towards alcoholism. Fifth, I will review a variety of other potentially important markers, trying whenever possible to disentangle those which probably represent the result of heavy drinking (and thus cannot in themselves be looked at as markers for potential heavy drinking or alcoholism in the future) from those which might actually be markers of a predisposition. Finally, I will attempt to summarize the material ard place the findings into perspective.

A brief introduction to the concept of alcoholism

Clinical diagnoses of behavioural disorders are made for a variety of reasons. Some clinicians and researchers use labels to imply aetiology (an approach of theoretical rather than clinical importance), others label to describe an individual's clinical condition at one point in time, while yet others attempt to use labels to indicate prognosis and to help choose between treatments (Goodwin & Guze, 1980; Schuckit, 1979). As a clinical researcher, I use the last named approach which requires that relatively objective terms be applied to populations who are then followed up over time in order to determine their clinical course and response to various treatment approaches.

Applying such a bias to alcoholism helps me to choose between the various diagnostic schemes which have been proposed for this disorder. Due to difficulty in obtaining reliable information on drinking quantity from patients, and major differences for the effects of ethanol in different age groups, I generally do not diagnose the disorder based on quantity and frequency of drinking. The development of an obvious syndrome of physical withdrawal, while diagnostic of alcoholism and indicating future pervasive problems, is too restrictive, as the average middle-class working alcoholic may never drink heavily enough and long enough at one time to demonstrate the more severe and obvious forms of withdrawal (Schuckit, 1979). Finally, while an important component of alcoholism rests with psychological dependence (which might be defined as a state of psychological discomfort when the drug is not available), this concept is too subjective to be of much prognostic value.

Most of the genetic studies cited in this chapter have utilized some form of a social problem approach to diagnosis. Here, the development of serious alcohol-related difficulties is an indication that an individual is drinking a great deal and has continued to drink despite earlier more minor difficulties (i.e. has psychological dependence). In our studies, alcoholism was defined as the occurrence of any single major life problem related to alcohol including a marital separation or divorce, multiple arrests, physical evidence that alcohol harmed health, or a job loss or layoff related to drinking (Schuckit, 1979). To have relevance for genetic studies, it is important that the alcohol related difficulties (or psychological dependence or heavy drinking or alcoholic withdrawal) occur *independently* of any major pre-existing psychiatric disorder such as primary affective disorder (i.e. severe depressive disease) (Schuckit, 1979). In such an instance, alcoholism might be considered secondary to the major pre-existing disorder, making any determination of genetic influences tenuous. Using this approach to diagnosis, we have outlined groups of patients who are very likely to continue to have severe and pervasive alcohol-related difficulties, to run a relatively predictable course of exacerbations and remissions of alcohol-related problems, and to show no evidence of other major psychiatric problems, in the future, independent of their heavy drinking (Schuckit, 1979).

In summary, before discussing biochemical markers for a predisposition towards alcoholism, it is important that the concept of alcoholism be clearly stated. The life problem definition has been shown to correlate with future problems and clinical course, and overlaps greatly with approaches based on quantity of drinking, psychological dependence and physical dependence.

Research attempting to identify biochemical markers of a predisposition towards alcoholism will have to show that the biochemical differences existed before the heavy and persistent alcohol intake and were not a consequence of the heavy drinking. This in turn requires identification of populations at high risk who can then be studied prospectively. Thus, in the next section I will review data supporting one promising approach to identification of high-risk populations, the genetics of alcoholism.

The genetics of alcoholism

It is difficult (some would say impossible) to definitively prove that a human behavioural disorder is genetically influenced. Studies of humans do not allow for adequate control of all possible complicating variables, so that no definitive conclusions can be reached. While animal studies do allow for adequate environmental controls, no universally accepted animal model for human behavioural problems (especially alcoholism) have been developed. Therefore, in viewing the studies presented below, it is more important to look at the pattern of results from different studies using different populations approached through different methodologies than it is to analyze any one investigation in depth (Robins, 1978). In this light, the importance of genetic factors in alcoholism is supported through family studies, animal investigations, genetic marker studies, twin research and adoption type approaches.

Without doubt, alcoholism is a *familial disorder* — i.e. it runs in families. The lifetime risk for alcoholism in children of alcoholics exceeds that of the general population (20–30 per cent vs 5–10 per cent) and alcoholism is more prevalent in the families of alcoholics than it is in the families of individuals with other psychiatric disorders (Cotton, 1979). Alcoholics who have a family history of this disorder may show a more severe clinical deterioration in both social and physical pathology than those lacking such a history (Frances et al, 1980; Penick et al, 1978). These findings point to the possibility that genetic factors may be, at least in part, responsible for the familial nature of alcoholism, but certainly do not prove it.

Animal studies have revealed some of the genetic factors which may influence whether an organism (usually a rat or mouse) chooses to drink (Eriksson, 1975; McClearn, 1979). These may be important clues to biological factors influencing a person's decision to drink, but may have little relevance to why only some drinkers go on to develop alcohol related problems and subsequent alcoholism. In the animal genetic work, different mice and rat strains have been shown to demonstrate divergent propensities in choosing to drink dilute ethanol solutions (rarely over 10 per cent by volume) when pure water is available. In other studies, selective breeding has resulted in new strains with higher drinking propensities and strains which refuse to drink ethanol at any concentration. Investigations of differences in ethanol metabolism, energy utilization, taste threshold and nervous system sensitivity to ethanol have given useful clues to genetic factors influencing an organism's choice to drink (Malila, 1978). However, even the drinking animals do not regularly imbibe enough to become intoxicated, and the information generated may have only limited meaning to human alcoholism. As an aside, these data also underscore the importance of distinguishing between genetic mechanisms determining abstention versus drinking choice, and those which influence the development of alcoholism among drinkers.

A third type of study addressing the possible importance of genetics in alcoholism uses family studies and general population surveys to look for either association or linkage of alcoholism with factors known to be genetically influenced. These *genetic marker studies* have yielded fairly inconsistent results, at least in part because most investigators have looked at association in large populations and rarely gone on to the more sophisticated analyses required to establish actual linkage on a specific chromosome for alcoholism and other genetically controlled biological factors (Hill et al, 1975). Associations have been established between alcoholism and some blood proteins (some of which have been shown to be linked with alcoholism), brain proteins and some enzyme systems (Comings, 1979; Del Villano et al, 1980; Glieberman et al, 1981). Genetic marker studies, therefore, have generally been consistent with the possibility of genetic factors in alcoholism but, at least in part due to methodological shortcomings, have added only limited information.

Twin studies actually attempt to control for environmental factors in humans by comparing the level of similarity for alcoholism within one egg or monozygotic (Mz) twin pairs with the level of similarity or concordance observed within same sex dizygotic (Dz) or fraternal twin pairs. Twin pairs share major childhood environmental events such as death of a parent or financial crisis in the family, whether they are Mz or Dz. Thus, if alcoholism is a genetically influenced disorder and not dependent solely on environmental events, the one egg twin pairs (who share 100 per cent of their genes) should be more similar or concordant for alcoholism than the Dz twin pairs (who share only 50 per cent of their genes). Studies using samples of twins, only a small number of whom are alcoholic, observe drinking patterns (not alcoholism) and have demonstrated a probable heritability for drinking versus abstention and for drinking patterns (Partanen et al, 1966). Studies of alcoholism beginning with large samples of alcoholics and looking at twins have shown a two to three-fold higher level of concordance for alcoholism in Mz than Dz pairs. In a recent study, if one member of an Mz twin pair was alcoholic the other developed alcoholism in 54 per cent of the cases while the same was true for only 28 per cent in Dz pairs (Kaij, 1960). Other studies of twins have shown that genetic factors may help explain a higher concordance for specific alcohol-related problems such as cirrhosis in Mz pairs of alcoholics (Hrubec & Omenn, 1981). The twin studies are not perfect, however, and their shortcomings have been discussed more extensively in another manuscript (Schuckit, 1981b).

The final type of study is based on the premise that if alcoholism is genetically influenced the children of alcoholics separated from their parents near birth and raised without knowledge of their biological parents' problem would have elevated rates of alcoholism, while the adopted-out children of nonalcoholics would not. Studies approaching this problem through a half-sibling methodology and through actual adoption records in the United States and Scandinavia have supported the importance of genetic factors (Bohman, 1978; Cardoret et al, 1980; Goodwin et al, 1974; Schuckit et al, 1972). In most of these investigations the risk for alcoholism in sons of alcoholics adopted out close to birth is four to five times higher than the risk for sons of nonalcoholics adopted out under similar circumstances (e.g. 20 per cent vs five per cent). While most of these studies have been carried out on men, there is at least preliminary evidence indicating that the findings are equally true for daughters of alcoholics (Bohman et al, 1981).

Therefore, all types of genetic studies are consistent with the probability that genetics explain at least some of the variance in whether an individual will develop alcoholism. As demonstrated by the lack of a 100 per cent concordance rate for alcoholism in Mz twins (Kaij, 1960), it is probable that environmental factors also contribute to this development. The most likely model involves an interaction between a genetic predisposition and environmental factors. If this multifactorial model is true, then biochemical markers of a predisposition are traits associated with increased risk for alcoholism but are unlikely to be necessary and sufficient for the development of this problem. In other words, biochemical markers probably identify individuals with a significantly higher risk for alcoholism but, due to the importance of environmental events which can mediate the final expression of the disorder, a 100 per cent correlation between the marker and the final development of alcoholism is unlikely.

The probability that alcoholism is a genetically influenced disorder raises speculations about what might actually be inherited. As demonstrated in Table 2.1, an individual entering a heavy drinking society could carry any one or combination of a series of factors increasing his risk for physical

Table 2.1 Possible biological mediators of an alcoholic predisposition

1. Through metabolism rate or characteristics
2. Through acute reaction to alcohol
3. Via rate or characteristics of tolerance
4. Through personality attributes
5. Via enhanced vulnerability to consequences of chronic drinking

addiction to alcohol, alcoholic social or physical problems, or for being identified as an alcoholic case. These include possible differences in metabolism which might affect either the rate of disappearance of alcohol or accumulation of AcH which in turn might mediate the 'high' or affect the development of tolerance or physical addiction. The enhanced risk might occur through a unique acute reaction to the drug, either resulting in a more pleasant 'high', or less drug so that the drinker takes more to obtain the same effects as those around him. Third, a higher risk individual may show a more rapid development of tolerance to the effects of alcohol with resulting higher levels of intake or, fourth, might demonstrate some unique personality attributes which increases the risk for alcohol-related problems. Finally, higher risk might be associated with a series of independent vulnerabilities to alcohol-related problems which in some persons might increase their risk for cirrhosis, in others increase their chances for developing brain deteriorations such as Wernicke-Korsakoff's syndrome, etc. (Blass & Gibson, 1977). The prospective research approach outlined in the next section attempts to study some of these possibilities in young men at elevated risk for the future development of alcoholism (as determined by their family history of this disorder) and controls.

In summary, family, animal, genetic marker, twin and adoption type studies all point towards the possible importance of genetics in the development of alcoholism. While these investigations are not definitive, they are highly consistent and justify some prospective studies attempting to identify both behavioral and biochemical markers of a predisposition towards alcoholism. Some of these results are of potential importance for enzyme systems under genetic control which might contribute to a predisposition toward alcoholism.

The prospective study design

Our present work is based on the premise that alcoholism is genetically influenced and that young men with first degree (i.e. parent or sibling) alcoholic relatives are at high risk themselves. Each year, all students and nonacademic staff males age 21 to 25 at our university are offered $3.00 to fill out a mailed questionnaire. This age group was chosen because they are old enough to drink but young enough to have a low probability for having yet developed alcoholism (Schuckit, 1979; Haglund & Schuckit, 1977). Through the survey we are able to exclude those men who already fulfil our criteria for alcoholism or other major psychiatric or medical disorders. We then select for testing the remaining drinking but nonalcoholic men with an alcoholic family member who are thus at high risk for the future development of alcoholism themselves. Each family history positive (FHP) or high-risk young man is matched with an individual who lacks a family history of alcoholism (family history negative or FHN), on age, sex, race, socioeconomic stratum, student versus working status, height/weight ratio, and self-reported drinking history using Cahalan's quantity frequency variability index (Schuckit, 1980). FHP and FHN matched pairs are brought individually to the laboratory, where raters blind to their family history status measure baseline cognitive and psychomotor performance, personality attributes, neurological functioning using auditory evoked potentials, and selected blood chemistry tests. After baseline procedures have been completed, the subjects are administered 0.75 ml of pure ethanol/kg body weight as a 20 per cent solution in a sugar-free carbonated beverage and performance measures as well as biochemical markers are followed for five hours to determine if there are any differences between the two family history groups on metabolism of alcohol or acute reaction to ethanol.

In the remainder of this chapter, I will describe our results as they relate to possible biochemical markers for a predisposition towards alcoholism. The next section briefly reviews relevant background information on the metabolism of ethanol, and then goes on to discuss the possible role of the two most relevant alcohol metabolizing enzymes as possible biochemical markers for a predisposition towards alcoholism.

Ethanol metabolizing systems as possible markers of our alcoholic predisposition

General comments

Most organisms have relatively efficient mechanisms for destroying ethanol. This probably results from the body's need to cope with the ingestion of alcohol in fermenting fruit and the production of ethanol from intestinal flora (Veech, 1981). In man, the latter mechanism has been hypothesized to result in between 1 and 10 grams of ethanol per day (10 grams is approximately the amount present in one drink) (Krebs & Perkins, 1970).

After the ingestion of high doses of beverage alcohol in man up to 10 to 15 per cent of the ethanol is excreted directly through the lungs, skin, and kidneys. This changes at different blood alcohol concentrations (BACs), with even less amounts at BACs less than 200 mg/dl, an amount approximately equivalent to 20 mmol/l (Li, 1977).

The vast majority of ethanol metabolism occurs in the liver (Li, 1977). Within this organ, the major pathway of ethanol destruction is via alcohol dehydrogenase (ADH) producing AcH and then through aldehyde dehydrogenase (ALDH) with the subsequent production of acetate and finally

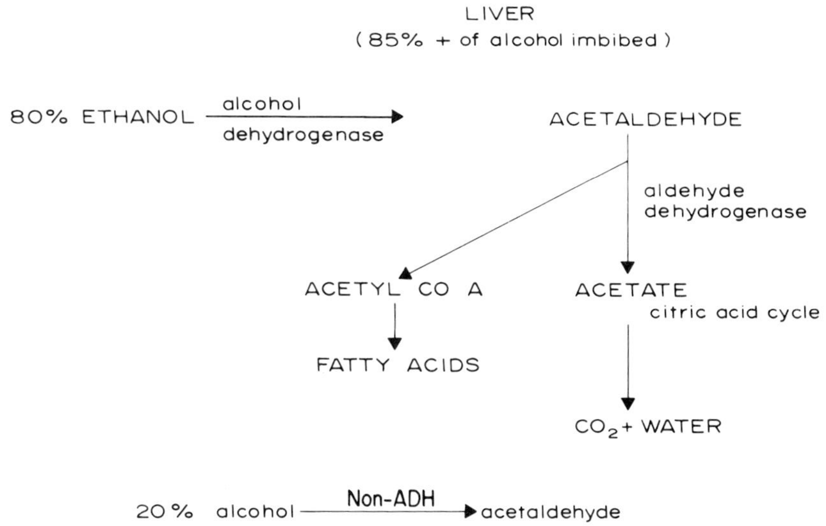

Fig. 2.1 A brief overview of the pathways for ethanol metabolism in humans.

CO_2 and water as shown in Figure 2.1. As a result, at least 75 per cent of the ethanol taken up by the liver is subsequently released as acetate into the circulation, where it is converted to CO_2 and H_2O (Lundquist & Wolthers 1958). Because 70 per cent to 80 per cent of ethanol in the liver is metabolized through ADH and ALDH, their genetic regulation and kinetic properties will be discussed in greater depth below. Before returning to those topics, it is worthwhile to place these enzymes in perspective by briefly reviewing the 'other' or non-ADH pathways which have potential but as yet not fully determined roles in ethanol metabolism.

Non-ADH pathways

The most often discussed non-ADH pathway is the microsomal ethanol oxidizing system (MEOS). This mechanism, first noted by Orm-Johnson 1965, resides in the smooth endoplasmic reticulum and has been hypothesized to metabolize up to 20 per cent or more of ethanol in the liver (Lieber & De Carli, 1970; Li, 1977). The role of this system has been firmly established in vitro, with a Km for ethanol of approximately 10 mmol/l and activity levels which can be induced after exposure to a variety of brain depressants including ethanol and barbituates (Lieber, 1977; Li, 1977). However, the exact importance of this enzyme system in man is still being established (Li, 1977).

The second major non-ADH pathway of potential importance rests with catalase, and appears to be responsible for less than 10 per cent of the liver's oxidation of ethanol (Li, 1977). The Km for ethanol of this relatively ubiquitous system is approximately 10 mmol/l, with it's level of activity dependent upon the rate of production of $H_2 O_2$ (Li, 1977; Lieber & De Carli, 1970). It is likely that the catalase system has no important biological effects at ethanol levels below 20 mmol/l (Li, 1977).

Finally, it is possible that small amounts of ethanol are removed from the circulation through nonenzymatic mechanisms. Conjugation of ethanol to produce ethylsulfate, glucuronides and other products have been noted (Li, 1977). After all is said and done, however, it is likely that the major biochemical events related to a predisposition towards alcoholism probably rest with the ADH and ALDH systems.

The final results of these various alcohol metabolizing pathways is highly complex. Thus, the zero-order kinetic view of ethanol metabolism proposed by Widmark (1934) indicating metabolism of one drink per hour can only be considered an approximation. The different systems mentioned above have divergent kinetics and varying levels of importance at different BACs. As a result, a more accurate overview of ethanol metabolism probably depends upon Michaelis-Menten saturation kinetics (Lundquist & Wolthers, 1958; Wagner, 1976).

In summary, ethanol metabolizing systems are present in almost all higher organisms. In mammals the major focus of metabolism is in the liver, with the vast majority of oxidation occurring through ADH and ALDH. The presence of ancillary ethanol metabolizing systems with differing kinetics mandate a rather complex model of ethanol metabolism. Indeed, as indicated in greater depth in the subsequent subsection, there is great heterogeneity within ADH and ALDH which further adds to the complexity of the system and helps explain the wide interindividual variations in ethanol metabolism which have been observed.

Alcohol metabolism and alcoholism

Whatever the relative importance of ADH and non-ADH pathways, the ethanol elimination rate (reflecting absorption, distribution, excretion, and metabolism) for any one individual remains relatively constant under similar circumstances (Bosron & Li, 1981; Li, 1977). While this does not minimize the shift in metabolic rates which are likely to be observed at different BAC's, it does indicate that for any one individual a relatively stable system is involved (von Wartburg, 1980; Li, 1977). This is of interest because of the two to three fold interindividual differences in ethanol elimination rates and the possibility that ethanol metabolic rates may vary in different ethnic groups, especially American Indians versus Caucasians (Benion & Li, 1976; Reed et al, 1976; Farris & Jones, 1978; Hanna, 1978; 1978; Fenna et al, 1971; Wagner, 1976). All of these factors are consistent with the possibility that ethanol metabolism and some of the major enzyme systems are under genetic control, which, in light of the data on the genetics of alcoholism, raises the question of their importance regarding the development of this serious disorder.

There is more direct evidence that ethanol elimination rates are genetically influenced. There are less intrapair differences in ethanol metabolism for Mz than Dz twin pairs (Vesell et al, 1971; Propping, 1977). As a result, it has been estimated that heredity explains 50 per cent or more of the variance of ethanol metabolic rates (Kopun & Propping, 1977).

However, there is little convincing evidence that the gross ethanol metabolic rate is itself associated with the risk for alcoholism. First, despite the fact that the adopted-out children of alcoholics have a four to five times increased risk for alcoholism (Goodwin et al, 1974) they are no different from controls in their rate of ethanol disappearance (Utne et al, 1977). This conclusion is supported by studies in our laboratory looking at the magnitude and time course of peak BAC and the rate of disappearance of ethanol from the blood after the ingestion of 0.75 ml of alcohol per kg body weight in young men with alcoholic relatives and in controls as related in Figure 2.2 (Schuckit, 1981a). Even though the overall rate of ethanol disappearance does not appear to be important in the genesis of alcoholism, the specific pathways might have such importance as is discussed below.

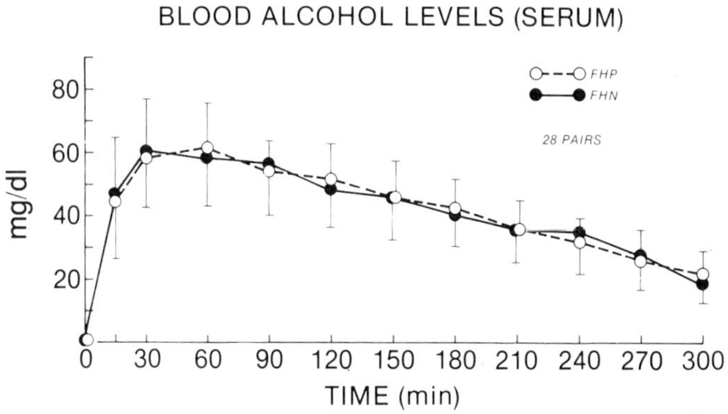

Fig. 2.2 Blood alcohol levels are timed for 28 family history positive (FHP) and negative (FHN) pairs of young men after oral ingestion over five minutes of 0.75 ml ethanol/kg body weight as a 20 per cent by volume solution mixed in room temperature carbonate beverage.

Acetaldehye (AcH) level as a possible marker for a predisposition toward alcoholism

All major pathways of ethanol metabolism result in AcH. The combination of wide distribution in the body and high level of biological activity of this important substance has raised speculation about its possible role as a mediator of the effects of alcohol and as a causative agent in much of the physical pathology associated with alcoholism (Schuckit, in press a). Possible AcH related pathology includes alcoholic myocardiopathy, liver disease, brain deterioration and the fetal alcohol syndrome (Veech, 1981; Eriksson, 1981; Li, 1977).

While the study of AcH might seem relatively simple, there are methodological difficulties which have resulted in a paucity of information on this important substance. First, only about five per cent of the AcH produced by the liver is actually released into the blood stream (Lindros, 1978). Therefore, blood, brain, and breath AcH levels are only poor approximations of what is happening in the liver. The actual blood levels of AcH following ethanol intake even for alcoholics are probably quite low — at most in the 1–2 μg/ml range (about 20–40 μmol/l) when BACs are 50–200 mg/dl (about 11–44 μmol/l) (Lindros, 1978; Veech, 1981). These low levels in more easily studied tissues such as the blood have made it difficult to determine the importance of AcH in the development of alcoholism in man.

AcH brain levels are also a subject of controversy. Early results indicated what appeared to be high concentrations in the brain after an ethanol load (Truitt, 1971; Wescott et al, 1980). These levels probably represent a number of factors including the artifactual production of AcH in tissue samples and differences between studies on animal species used, the presence or absence of pretreatment with an ALDH inhibitor, the ethanol dose, and time allowed for ethanol metabolism (Eriksson, 1980). More recent studies ultilising steps to impair the artifactual production of AcH in brain tissue have demonstrated what appears to be low levels at even high BACs (Wescott, 1980; Eriksson, 1980; Tabakoff et al, 1976).

Difficulties in the accurate measurement of AcH extend to blood as well. These complications have occurred because of marked differences in results between in vitro and in vivo experiments and difficulties in translating between animal and human research (Schuckit, 1980, in press, a). The major problems involve the destruction of AcH within human blood by ALDH in red blood cells (RBCs) and AcH binding to protein. Another problem is the major spurious production of AcH which can occur through ADH present in sample solutions and through release of bound AcH or by 'nonenzymatic' production of AcH which occurs during protein precipitation (Schuckit in press, a; Eriksson, 1980). While this latter problem can be corrected in supernatant solutions over tissue samples (e.g. liver or brain studies in vitro) by the addition of thiourea, with resulting decrease in ascorbic acid which might be involved in oxygen radical related ethanol oxidation, this approach has little effect in blood samples. Many of these difficulties can be minimized by using five to nine-fold dilutions of perchloric acid in saline, keeping blood samples cold, and separating out proteins and red blood cells as rapidly as possible, but no highly dependeble and generally acceptable methodology for measuring AcH in blood has been developed (Mizoi, 1982; Schuckit, in press, a). Newer methods are being proposed but these have not been adequately studied (Knop et al, 1981). As a result, in the genetic studies noted below, absolute AcH levels cannot be accurately compared between different laboratories nor even within the same laboratory using different methods. Therefore, these studies must be viewed with some caution, placing greater emphasis on relative differences between groups than on the specific AcH levels reported.

These problems are of great importance to studies attempting to look at AcH as a possible biochemical marker of a predisposition to alcoholism. Freund & O'Hallarin (1965) demonstrated an almost two-fold increased level of AcH after the administration of ethanol to an alcoholic with neurological damage when compared to physically well alcoholics and nonalcoholics. Subsequently, Truitt (1971) compared alcohol metabolism in alcoholics who had been abstinent approximately a week with staff and students from a medical school and showed a two-fold higher level of AcH in the alcoholics after administration of between 0.5 and 0.75 g of ethanol/kg body weight (the equivalent of three to five drinks). Korsten and colleagues (1975) compared six abstinent chronic alcoholics without evidence of cirrhosis to controls after intravenous (IV) ethanol as a 15 per cent (v/v) solution with resulting BACs of 45 to 53 mmol/l, demonstrating almost two-fold higher AcH levels in the alcoholics. One subsequent report, however, administering ethanol in 10–100 mmol/l ranges, showed no AcH difference between alcoholics and controls (Lindros et al, 1979).

Taken together, these studies show a probable increased AcH in alcoholics, and are generally consistent with a possible role of AcH in either the genesis of alcoholism or in some of the consequences of chronic high ethanol intake. However, it is difficult to draw definite conclusions as most of the investigations did not control for the usual alcohol intake patterns in the groups being compared, most tested alcoholics after only a short period of abstinence and because of the controversy regarding the AcH measurement methodologies.

Our laboratory has compared AcH blood levels in young, nonalcoholic, men, half of whom demonstrated a family history of alcoholism and half of whom did not. Using our usual methodology of administering 0.75 ml of ethanol per kg body weight and observing AcH levels over five hours, we have demonstrated what appears to be two-fold higher AcH levels in the sons of alcoholics than controls (Schuckit & Rayses, 1979; Schuckit, in press, a). While there are no perfect or generally accepted AcH measures and it is likely that much of the AcH measured was produced during PCA precipitation in blood samples, the fact that FHP and FHN subjects were treated in an identical manner and appear to demonstrate different AcH levels implies this substance could have importance in the predisposition towards alcoholism. This in turn implicates both the enzyme systems producing and those destroying AcH as potential biochemical markers for the future development of this disorder.

Even after recognizing the methodological problems, it is interesting to speculate on how increased AcH levels could either decrease or increase the predisposition towards alcoholism. Related to possible lowered alcoholism risks, some ethnic groups demonstrating relatively low alcoholism rates have an increased propensity to develop an AcH related facial flush after drinking even small amounts of ethanol. All comparisons of flushing after drinking in Orientals versus Caucasians have shown significantly higher levels of flushing in the former (Farris, 1978; Reed et al, 1976; Fenna et al, 1971). The mild to moderately unpleasant nature of the facial flush and the associated symptoms have led some authors to speculate that this might be responsible in part for the lowered levels of alcoholism in those groups. As is discussed below, this flush could be mediated by an atypical ADH form producing higher AcH (even though there is no association between the ethanol elimination rate and flushing) (Mizoi et al, 1978) or an isoenzyme of ALDH destroying AcH more slowly (Ewing et al, 1974; Wolff, 1973).

However, the situation is not straight forward. Other ethnic groups with exceptionally high levels of alcoholism (e.g. native Americans and Eskimos) also demonstrate high levels of flushing and associated increases in AcH after drinking (Haglund & Schuckit, 1977). Our own finding of increased AcH levels in young men at elevated risk for alcoholism led us to examine the association between AcH levels and alcoholism risk *within* a Caucasian group. Thus, we used both subjective observer ratings and facial skin optical density change measurement with a plethysmogram to observe facial flushing after 0.75 ml of ethanol/kg body weight in the two family history groups. Recognizing that our investigations were limited to Caucasian subjects, the FHP men demonstrated significantly more flushing than the FHN, a finding consistent with the AcH results (Schuckit & Duby, in press).

In the final analysis, the association between mild increases in AcH, facial flushing, and the development of alcoholism may be highly complex. Thus, elevations in AcH and associated facial flushing may be a deterrent to drinking in some groups with high levels of social controls of drinking (e.g. Orientals), but might have no effect in discouraging drinking in other groups with low levels of social controls and intense social pressures towards heavy drinking and frequent intoxication (e.g. native Americans). In the latter group, the elevated AcH, while having little influence on the decision to drink, may increase the predisposition towards organ damage and/or moderate the type of intoxication and/or increase the formation of beta-carbolines and tetrahydroisoquinolines (TIQs), with subsequent enhanced risk for alcoholism. This discussion underscores the tenuous nature of any overview of biochemical factors of possible importance in the predisposition towards alcoholism.

There are a number of ways that increased AcH levels could theoretically increase the risk for alcoholism (Schuckit & Duby, in press). First, it is possible that higher AcH could increase AcH-related damage of the brain, liver, heart and other vital organs. This in turn could result in the patient being labelled alcoholic because of alcohol-related organ damage. Second, a two-fold increase in AcH, while much lower than those levels seen after drinking while taking the ALDH inhibitor disulfiram (Schuckit, in press, a) has been shown in animal experiments to apparently have reinforcing properties (Amit et al, 1980). Third, AcH has been shown in vitro and possibly in vivo to condense with dopamine or dopaldehyde to produce TIQs or to condense with serotonin to produce beta-carbolines. These substances are opiate precursors with the result that higher AcH levels might (at least simplistically) be associated with either a unique form of intoxication or a heightened propensity towards the development of tolerance and/or physical dependence with drinking. The TIQs and beta-carbolines have also been hypothesized to be capable of serving as false-neurotransmitters which might in turn affect the mode of intoxication.

These speculations are primarily of heuristic value. However, the TIQ and beta-carboline approach has some very indirect substantiation through the observation of high levels of salsolinol (the beta-carboline condensation product of AcH with serotonin) in the urine of alcoholics during detoxification (a study that did not use nonalcoholic intoxicated controls) (Collins et al, 1974). In a pilot study, our laboratory has examined urinary salsolinol after 0.75 ml of ethanol/kg body weight in FHP and FHN men, observing higher levels in the high-risk group. While the results are not statistically significant due to the small sample size and reflecting the pilot nature of the investigation, they are intriguing and point to the need for further evaluation of blood AcH and urinary salsolinols or TIQs after an ethanol load as possible biochemical markers for an alcoholic predisposition.

In summary, AcH levels have both direct and indirect potential importance as possible biological markers of a predisposition towards alcoholism. No solid conclusions can be reached because of differences in AcH methodology in different laboratories and the unreliability of most, if not all, of the analytic procedures. However, a number of studies have demonstrated a possible elevation in AcH levels after drinking in alcoholics or their relatives when compared to controls, and potential condensation products between AcH and monoamines do appear (through preliminary data) to be elevated in relatives of alcoholics when compared to controls. These may prove to be useful leads for the identification of biological markers in the future.

The results also question the possible mechanism responsible for the elevated AcH. While differences between higher and lower risk groups on the distribution or binding of AcH are possible, higher levels of this substance could also result from enhanced AcH production through ADH or decreased destruction through ALDH. These speculations form the basis for the next two subsections in this chapter.

Alcohol dehydrogenase (ADH)

As shown in Figure 2.1, the first and rate limiting step in the major ethanol metabolic pathway involves the oxidation to AcH by ADH (alcohol: NAD^+ oxidoreductase, EC 1.1.1.1). While other enzyme systems and nonenzymatic pathways are involved at higher BACs, ADH functions as almost the sole mechanism of ethanol destruction with BACs less than 20 mmol/l (approximately 100 mg/dl) (Li, 1977).

80–90 per cent of the body's ADH activity is in the liver, but the enzyme is widespread and found, in decreasing quantities, in the intestines, lung, kidneys, stomach, retina, prostate, spleen, and brain (Moser et al, 1968). Brain ADH has similar kinetics to liver, but total tissue levels are exceedingly small, with the rate of ethanol oxidation approximately 2 μmol/g of brain/hour versus 9 mmol/g hour in liver (Moser et al, 1968; Tabakoff & von Wartburg, 1975; Raskin & Sokoloff, 1968). The study of ADH properties in humans has been limited by the need for liver tissue obtained through autopsy or needle biopsy. However, in recent years such approaches have been expanded by the observation of ADH in skin fibroblasts which can be obtained through punch biopsy (Peterson et al, 1980), use of hair root cells (Goedde et al, 1980) and the possibility of the development of serum assays of ADH (Shimasue et al, 1972; Griffiths & Schuckit, in press; Harada et al, 1982).

When the first human liver ADH preparation was studied in 1964 it soon became apparent that there are important isoenzyme fractions, including some which have unique patterns of distribution in human populations (von Wartburg, 1980; Blair & Vallee, 1966). All ADH isoenzyme forms emphasized here have a molecular weight of between 80 000 and 85 000 daltons, appear in dimeric form containing 4 gram-atoms of zinc per mole of protein and use NAD (H) as a co-enzyme in preference to NADP (H) (Bosron & Li, 1981; von Wartburg, 1980). Most have a broad substrate specificity which includes primary and secondary aliphatic alcohols, diols as well as cyclic and aromatic alcohols (Li, 1977; von Wartburg, 1980). I will not discuss in detail related enzymes which do not prefer ethanol as a substrate (e.g. sorbital dehydrogenase and chi ADH (Jornvall, 1982; Vallee, 1982). The combined effect of the relevant isoenzymes results in what appears to be a Km for ethanol in man of approximately 2 to 3 mmol/l at pH 10 and with a higher Km at pH 7 (Lundquist & Wolthers, 1958). An important controlling step in the rapidity of action is the reoxidation of NADH. Most isoenzyme forms are inhibited by pyrazole which results in an 85 per cent or more inhibition of total ethanol elimination at most BAC's (Li, 1977).

In spite of these generalities, there are differences in the apparent properties of ADH depending upon the pH conditions, the substrate used and the organ sampled. Even within the liver the isoenzyme pattern changes with the use of needle biopsy or fresh autopsy specimens following sudden death versus regular autopsy liver samples (Li & Magnes, 1975; Azevedo et al, 1975).

Our level of understanding of the ADH isoenzyme patterns has expanded in recent years. Most information has developed through the use of starch gel electrophoresis, isoelectric focusing on polyacrylamide gels and through ADH subunit biochemical confirmation by means of dissociation and recombination experiments with partially purified isoenzymes (Bosron & Li, 1981).

The importance of ADH isoenzyme forms to biological markers of a potential predisposition towards alcoholism rests in part with the relatively detailed knowledge of the genetic control of most forms. There are hypothesized to be a minimum of three gene loci, ADH_1, ADH_2, and ADH_3 each producing at least one polypeptide chain, α, β, and γ chains respectively (Smith et al, 1972; Smith et al, 1973). The three basic chains can combine into three homodimers (e.g. $\alpha\alpha$, $\beta\beta$, and $\gamma\gamma$) and three heterodimers (e.g. $\alpha\beta$, $\alpha\gamma$, and $\beta\gamma$). These change with level of maturity as, for example, the $\alpha\alpha$ form is the only ADH noted in the early fetus, $\alpha\alpha$ and $\alpha\beta$ are seen in later fetus with an expansion to $\alpha\alpha$, $\alpha\beta$ and $\beta\beta$ in the neonate and the development of γ chains only after birth (von Wartburg, 1980; Li, 1977). In addition, two of the three gene loci can appear to have alleles which increase the number of potential homodimeric and heterodimeric forms considerably, with a resulting minimum of seven to nine up to a potential of 20 or more bands of human ADH on most properly prepared starch gel electrophoreses, though there is a good deal of variability between individuals (Blair & Vallee, 1966; Li, 1977).

Different investigators have proposed different schemes for naming the gene loci, polypeptide chains, and homodimeric or heterodimeric combinations. As noted in one approach, the second allele at the ADH_2 gene locus results in a B^2 chain which has been called atypical ADH by most investigators and ADH_{Bern} or $ADH_{Honolulu}$ by others (von Wartburg, 1980; Bosrow et al, 1980). These can exist as a homodimer (ADH_2 2–1) or a heterodimer (Harada et al, 1980a). Some other potential ADH phenotypes, especially those hypothesized to be located at the ADH_2 gene locus, have only recently been described but their validity has not yet been established (e.g. ADH_{Brazil} and ADH_{China}).

An additional scheme, discussed by Bosron and Li (1981), names the ADH phenotype for the polypeptide chain observed. As stated by those authors, when only the γ^1 chains are found for the ADH^3 locus, the phenotype is ADH^3 1–1, when γ^2 chains are observed the phenotype is ADH^3 2–2 and when γ^1 and γ^2 chains are seen, the phenotype is ADH_3 2–1. Despite the validity of most of these different approaches, in the present chapter subunits will be named as atypical ADH (also called ADH_{Bern}, $ADH_{Honolulu}$, ADH_2 2–2 or 2–1, etc.), $ADH_{Indianapolis}$, etc.

The development of knowledge of ADH isoenzymes has progressed from the recognition of homodimers and heterodimers of the α and β chains through the development of knowledge of ADH_2 alleles resulting in the identification of the atypical ADH and the γ chains from the ADH_3 locus (Bosron & Li, 1981; von Wartburg, 1965). Recent discoveries of a $_{\pi}$ADH and $_{Chi}$ADH ($_{\chi}$ADH) have required revision of the gene locus/polypeptide framework as these last two phenotypes have not been shown to adequately fit into the three ADH gene loci and their alleles. Indeed, it has been hypothesized that these two latter ADH forms may be unique and should each be placed in separate categories (Vallee, 1982).

A brief description of the more recently observed ADH phenotypes (i.e. dimeric polypeptide chains) is worthwhile. The first, atypical ADH, probably representing an allele at the ADH_2 position, was discussed in the 1960s by von Wartburg and coworkers (von Wartburg, 1980). This variant is found in 20 per cent of Swiss, up to 90 per cent of Orientals, and 5 to 10 per cent of American and English populations (Stomatoyamopolous et al, 1965; Li & Magnes, 1975; Smith et al, 1973; von Wartburg & Schurch, 1968; Harada et al, 1980b). The atypical ADH shows a pH optimum of 8.5 (versus 10.0 or higher for the more typical ADH forms) making it potentially more active at physiological conditions.

Another allele probably located at the ADH_2 locus is hypothetically responsible for an ADH phenotype noted in up to 25 per cent of Black American men (Bosron & Li, 1981; Li, 1982). This $ADH_{Indianapolis}$ has a dual optimum pH of 7.0 and 10.0 and a band which migrates cathodal to the β1β1 on starch gel electrophoresis. The Km for ethanol is about 50 mmol/l. In reality, $ADH_{Indianapolis}$ probably exists in three or four forms, one homodimer (pH optimum 7.0) and at least two heterodimers (pH optima 7.0 and 10.0) (Li, 1981; Bosron & Li, 1980).

An additional ADH phenotype has come from the demonstration of a very anodic band on starch gel electrophoresis found in fresh samples but not autopsy specimens or after chronic disease. This $_{\pi}$ADH form shares molecular weight, zinc content and many other ADH properties and has a pH optimum of 10.0 with a broad substrate specificity, but $_{\pi}$ADH differs from the other ADH isoenzymes in being more labile, poorly inhibited by pyrazole, showing a lack of ability to oxidize methanol or glycerol and a Km for ethanol which is from 20 to 60 or greater times higher than that seen for the most usual ADH forms (i.e. about 34 mmol/l) (Li, 1981; Bosron & Li, 1981; von Wartburg, 1980). The proposed phenotype $_{\chi}$ADH is also anodic on starch gel electrophoresis at pH 8.2, is not inhibited by pyrazole, and has been noted to oxidize ethanol poorly (there is no Km) with a preference for the longer chain alcohols (Bosron et al, 1980).

To place these findings in prospective, there may be 20 or more ADH isoenzyme forms, each with different properties and each under genetic control. The different Kms for atypical ADH, $_{\pi}$ADH, $_{\chi}$ADH, etc. their divergent distributions in various populations, and their high level of genetic control could all indicate that genetic factors expressed through ADH phenotypes could explain some population subgroup differences in the rate of ethanol metabolism and/or rapidity of formation and absolute level of AcH. These speculations are even more interesting with in vitro observation of possible more rapid ethanol metabolism by atypical ADH at physiological pHs (Stomatoyannopoulos et al, 1975; Wolff, 1973; Ewing et al, 1974).

The more intense flushing associated with higher AcH levels in Orientals could, at least theoretically, be the result of the 80 per cent prevalence of atypical ADH in those populations compared to as low as a 5 to 10 per cent prevalence in Caucasian groups (most groups, however, feel this flushing is related to ALDH as discussed below). The clinical impact of this theory, however, is dampened by the lack of data supporting actual faster metabolism in vivo with atypical ADH (von Wartburg, 1980; Edwards & Evans, 1967), the inconsistency of results indicating that Orientals or native Americans have faster rates of ethanol metabolism when compared to Caucasians (Benion & Li, 1970; Hanna, 1978), and the demonstration of no differences in the rate of ethanol metabolism in Oriental flushers versus nonflushers (Mizoi et al, 1968). However, it is possible that alcoholics when compared to controls demonstrate higher levels of atypical ADH (Ugarte et al, 1970; Kamaryt & Martinek, 1979; von Wartburg, 1980) and these speculations are worthy of future investigation.

In summary, the first major step in the breakdown of ethanol involves ADH, an enzyme whose basic structure and kinetic properties are being actively studied. ADH is a series of isoenzymes produced under genetic control through a minimum of three and possibly five or more gene loci resulting in 15 or more hypothesized isoenzyme forms of the resulting dimers. These would be of interest as possible biological markers of a predisposition towards alcoholism if different ADH isoenzyme patterns could be shown to correlate with the rate or type of ethanol metabolism in vivo. Atypical ADH is of potential significance to the development of alcoholism, as it (at least hypothetically) may be more active at physiological pH with resulting higher levels of AcH. This in turn could, theoretically, be responsible for an increased risk for alcoholism in some groups, and may decrease the risk for drinking in yet others. Despite the elegant research on ADH isoenzyme forms and their genetic control, the lack of pragmatic data to support the theoretical association between ADH isoenzyme patterns and the risk for alcoholism has encouraged investigators to look towards the second major enzyme in the usual pattern of ethanol metabolism, ALDH.

Aldehyde dehydrogenase (ALDH)

This set of enzymes has been most extensively studied in animal models with less information on humans than is true for ADH, a problem which may be important because of interspecies differences (Li, 1977). Classified as aldehyde: NAD^+ oxidoreductase (E C 1.2.1.3), ALDH metabolizes most aldehydes with a lack of specificity (Greenfield & Pietruszko, 1977). It is found in the liver, kidneys, intestine, heart, red blood cells, lung, brain, skeletal muscle, spleen and adipose tissues (Li, 1977). At least in rodent studies, the amount of ALDH present in brain tissue appears to be high enough to ensure that AcH values are quite low after drinking (Pietruszko et al, 1981).

These enzymes were first isolated from liver in 1968 with first evidence of isoenzyme forms in 1969 and subsequent purification in 1977 (Blair & Vallee, 1966; Kraemer & Dietrich, 1968; Pietruszko et al, 1972). The basic enzyme has a molecular weight of between 200 000 to 260 000 daltons, probably in the form of a tetramer (Bosron & Li, 1981; Li, 1977; von Wartburg, 1980). Relating to an increase in the number of active sites, changes in concentration, pH and cation-induced cleavage of the tetramer to a dimeric form functionably doubles the activity (Witner, 1982). The pH optimum is 9 or greater, with an activity at pH seven which is probably 25 per cent of that noted in pH9 (Li, 1977).

ALDH is responsible for the oxidation of aldehydes in divergent body areas, including the conversion of the vast majority of the AcH formed in the liver to acetate during ethanol metabolism. From the perspective of possible biochemical markers of a predisposition towards alcoholism, the possible existence of ALDH isoenzymes in the mitochondria, cytosol and microsomes in humans as determined from starch gel electrophoresis at pH 7 is of great interest. However, the specific number of human ALDH enzymes and their location has not been fully clarified.

Most authors agree there are a minimum of 2 to 4 human liver ALDH isoenzymes. As described by Greenfield & Pietruszko (1977) form 1, probably located in the cytosol, is slower migrating on electrophoresis, has a higher Km for AcH, about 0.1 mmol/l, and is strongly inhibited by disulfiram. Form 2, probably from mitochondria, is faster migrating, has a low Km for AcH (about 2–3 μmol/l at pH 9.5) and is relatively insensitive to disulfiram. Harada and coworkers (1978 & 1979a) and Goedde et al (1979) basically agree with the data on forms 1 and 2 which they have (unfortunately) labeled forms II and I, respectively. Those authors have also used isoelectric focusing to describe two additional liver ALDH isoenzymes (III and IV) active at neutral or alkaline pHs with Kms in the millimolar range. It has been suggested that these four enzymes forms may result from actions of at least two gene loci (Harada et al, 1978; Harada, 1980; Goedde et al, 1979 a & b).

Koivula (1975) has postulated at least three isoenzymes existing in the 3 cellular fractions in the human liver with 1 and perhaps 2 ALDH isoenzymes in mitochondria. The first and probably the most important mitochondrial form at the usual AcH levels (others feel this may be cytosolic), has a Km of approximately 1–3 μmol/l and has been hypothesized by some to be responsible for between 50 per cent and 80 per cent of the AcH metabolism, although a lesser role has been hypothesized by others (Peterson & Tabakoff, 1979; Koivula, 1975) and it may correlate with form 2 (or 1) described above. If the level of greater importance is true, this isoenzyme may be the rate limiting factor in AcH metabolism (Li, 1977). This low Km ALDH possibly residing in mitochondria shows faster electrophoretic mobility than the higher Km cytosolic form and demonstrates only one third of the sensitivity of disulfiram (von Wartburg, 1980; Greenfield & Pietruszko, 1977; Harada et al, 1980 b & C). It has also been hypothesized that there may be a cytosolic form similar to 1 or II above and an additional mitochondrial form with a Km of approximately 2 mM which is bound to the outer mitochondrial membrane and which would be expected to show physiological importance at only higher AcH levels (Li, 1977; Kowula, 1975).

It should be emphasized that while some investigators believe that the majority of AcH oxidation occurs in the mitochondria as a result of actions of the low Km (approximately μmol/l) ALDH form (Li, 1977) others argue that the higher Km cytosolic fraction appears to be more active at physiological pHs and (considering its sensitivity to inhibition by disulfiram) may be the more physiologically important ALDH (Jenkins & Peters, 1980). The picture is complicated even further by the possibility that there may be an additional low Km cytosolic form, although it is probable that this represents a contamination of samples with mitochondrial material (Harada et al, 1978; Koivula, 1975). Some of the disagreement in the literature probably results from the use of different substrate concentrations and pHs when testing ALDH (Pietruszko, 1982).

While most of these studies have been carried out with liver ALDH in humans, it is possible that different isoenzyme patterns might be seen in different organ systems, including the stomach and RBC's (Teng, 1981; Harada et al, 1980 c; Inoue et al, 1978; Pietruszko & Vallari, 1978). The RBC form is especially important as, if it resembles liver ALDH, it would offer the benefit of greater ease of sampling for study (i,e, it is much easier to draw blood than to do a liver biopsy). Studies to date indicate that there may be at least 2 RBC isoenzymes which, while demonstrating lower overall concentrations in RBC than in liver, might resemble liver ALDH kinetics (Inoue et al, 1979; Inoue et al, 1978; Inoue et al, 1980). While some authors disagree and feel there may only be one RBC enzyme form (Harada et al, 1978), the single or more predominant form appears to resemble the high Km cytosolic liver ALDH in it's tetrameric structure, molecular weight, and level of sensitivity to disulfiram (Inoue et al, 1979). Of even greater importance to the possibility of outlining biochemical markers for a predisposition towards alcoholism, Inoue et al (1980) have demonstrated a significant correlation between RBC ALDH activity and flushing with alcohol.

As has been discussed with ADH, different ALDH patterns in population subgroups could, theoretically, influence their AcH metabolism level and the level of flushing and/or their predisposition for alcoholism. For example, the low Km cytosolic ALDH is not equally distributed in all populations. While 100 per cent of a sample of Germans studied showed both the high and low Km forms of ALDH, the same was true for only 48 per cent of a Japanese population, with 52 per cent of that latter group demonstrating only the high Km form and not the most anodic, low Km ALDH (Harada et al, 1979 a & b; Goedde et al, 1976). A significantly higher percentage of Japanese alcoholics appear to have the low Km ALDH isoenzyme than the rest of the Japanese population (Harada, 1982). There is also at least a tentative correlation between the ALDH pattern (i.e. absence of the low Km ALDH) and flushing with less information supporting facial flush and atypical ADH (Goedde et al, 1980). These findings may have implications for some ethnic group differences in their response to ethanol, especially as related to the accumulation of AcH.

There are additional data supporting the possible role of ALDH in drinking choice. In animal studies, rats choosing to imbibe dilute ethanol solutions when they have access to water demonstrate increased ALDH mitochondrial activity (Koivula, 1975) while the opposite is true of the low drinking strains (Koivula & Lindros, 1975). In human studies, while there are no known differences between alcoholics and nonalcoholics in the distribution of high and low Km ALDH isoenzymes in the brain (Pietruszko et al, 1981), liver biopsies in noncirrhotic alcoholics versus controls showed decreased ALDH activity levels in the alcoholics (Jenkins & Peters, 1980). Because this latter study used alcoholics with basically normally functioning livers, this may indicate that there are differences in liver ALDH existing before the onset of alcoholism which, at least hypothetically, might in turn be responsible for the increased AcH which might be associated with either alcoholism or it's predisposition (Jenkins & Peters, 1980).

In summary, despite disagreement about the number and location of isoenzymes, the potential importance of ALDH as a biochemical marker in alcoholism rests with a variety of factors. First, almost all investigators agree there are different isoenzyme forms which are under probable genetic control. Second, these forms have different Kms and possible differential levels of activity at physiological pHs. Third, the end result is a possible explanation for different levels of AcH following drinking. If AcH levels have an influence on either the predisposition towards alcoholism or protection from this problem, then further studies of ALDH are warranted as a possible biological marker for the predisposition towards alcoholism.

Additional possible biochemical markers for a predisposition towards alcoholism

The possible biochemical markers for alcoholism discussed thus far have some coherence through the interaction of AcH, ADH, ALDH in the metabolism of ethanol. In most instances, possible differences between alcoholics and controls are paralleled by results from animal research or studies of relatives of alcoholics leaving a story which, while far from conclusive, is worthy of further work.

Numerous other biochemical differences between alcoholics and controls have also been noted. However, most of these additional potential biochemical markers must be considered even more heuristic and of less practical use than those discussed above, because there is an even greater paucity of data demonstrating that the differences do not just reflect the consequences of years of heavy drinking. This section briefly reviews a variety of such potential markers.

Monoamine oxidase (MAO)

MAO is a mitochondrial enzyme which catalyzes the oxidative deamination of primary amines, including naturally occurring catecholamines and indoleamines as well as synthetic amines (Murphy & Donnelly 1974; Sullivan et al, 1979). In humans and other primates a variety of behavioural traits may be related to MAO functioning. Thus, decreased platelet MAO activity is associated with higher levels of sensation-seeking behavior, more contact with mental health workers, and increased family rates of psychiatric disturbances (Coursey et al, 1979; Murphy et al, 1977; Buchsbaum et al, 1976). A relationship between MAO activity and specific psychiatric diagnosis is less certain with some hypothesized association between low platelet MAO and affective disorder (Davidson et al, 1980).

Another problem which may demonstrate an association with MAO activity is alcoholism, with a consensus of the literature supporting the notion of low platelet MAO activity in this disorder (Belmaker et al, 1980). Thus, low MAO activity has been shown in brains of alcoholic suicides and in platelets of living alcoholics (Schildkraut et al, 1975). Data from recovering alcoholics are less clear, with some investigations showing a trend towards return to 'normal' MAO activity within weeks or months of abstinence (Brown, 1977) and others showing what appears to be low MAO levels maintained over a 12 month period of nondrinking (Sullivan, 1978). Some of the discordant results may reflect heterogeneity in studied samples (Buchsbaum et al, 1976) or transitory changes in MAO activities (Alexopoulos et al, 1981).

Our laboratory has investigated platelet MAO activity levels at baseline (before ethanol) and 180 minutes after ethanol in 30 individuals, half of whom had a family history of alcoholism and half of whom did not (Schuckit et al, in press). Following our usual paradigm, the men were matched on demography, height/weight ratio, and drinking history. There was a nonsignificant trend for lower platelet MAO activities in those individuals with family histories of alcoholism when compared to controls (5.06 ± 1.26 versus 5.60 ± 1.00 respectively) at baseline, with a similar trend noted after ethanol (5.17 ± 1.21 and 5.46 ± 0.95 respectively). Considering the small sample size and small percentage of future alcoholics in even the FHP group, the answer cannot be considered definitive.

In summary, low platelet MAO activity may represent a predisposition towards life problems, a general predisposition towards psychiatric disorders, or a specific propensity towards alcoholism. In any event, the phenomenon is difficult to study due to heterogeneity of studied samples, the wide range of 'normal' MAO activities, and limitations in study methods. Nonetheless, MAO activities might be part of a group of biochemical markers which might help identify individuals at elevated risk for the future development of alcoholism. The results to date would appear to warrant future study.

Genetic markers

One way to try to establish a possible role for genetic factors in a disorder is to determine whether the problem shows a significant level of association with a relatively easily identified second factor known to be genetically influenced (Schuckit, 1980). A related, but even more robust approach is to investigate the flow of the problem and the marker within specific families in an attempt to establish actual genetic linkage (Hill et al, 1975). The most commonly studied genetic markers are blood proteins.

A number of studies have utilized relatively large populations to investigate a possible association between alcoholism and color blindness, phenylthiocarbamide (PTC) tasting, secretor versus nonsecretor status, etc. (Glieberman et al, 1981; Schuckit, in press, b). While most of these investigations have generated positive results within one population, it is rare to produce the same findings in another study population. The end result is that the genetic marker studies looking at associations have not been very promising as possible means of identifying biochemical markers for predispositions to alcoholism.

The linkage studies, while more difficult to do, have given tentative but more potentially promising results. In one of the more extensive overviews of the problem, Hill and coworkers (1975) have demonstrated a decreased prevalence of the S antigen in nonalcoholic relatives of alcoholics and shown apparent linkage in repulsion between the D gene of the Rh system and alcoholism. They also demonstrated a possible linkage between alcoholism and the SS phenotype for complement C3 and alcoholism. The greater specificity of the linkage approach when compared to association studies makes these findings worthy of future follow-up.

Some additional possible biochemical markers

This subsection rapidly reviews a number of biochemical markers which have had only cursory evaluation.

1. The first is related to the reported increased production of *2, 3 butanediol* in alcoholics. Veech (1981) saw evidence of this substance in 90 per cent of a group of alcoholics, but due to the preliminary nature of their work, did not establish the presence or absence of the substance after drinking in nonalcoholics.

2. In another approach, a variety of investigators have reported *chromosomal abnormalities* in alcoholics when compared to controls. Thus, De Torok (1972) showed a high degree of chromosomal aberrations with normal diploid composition in only 25 per cent of examined cells of alcoholics. Obe & Herha (1975) also noted an increased exchange aberration of chromatid

and chromosome type in the lymphocytes of alcoholics although it is probable that there was a return towards normal after abstinence for both of these findings.

3. In another study more difficult to carry out due to the type of tissue sampled, a common variant of a human brain specific protein, *Pcl Duarte*, was seen in 62 per cent of alcoholics and only 31 per cent of normals — findings similar to those for other psychiatric problems including affective disorder (Comings, 1979).

4. Abnormal levels of additional enzymes, such as *superoxide dismutase* have been demonstrated in subsets of alcoholics although these might represent changes accruing with heavy drinking and not the original cause of alcoholism (Del Villano et al, 1980).

5. Similar to the superoxide dismutase is the demonstration of a microheterogeneity in *serum transferrin* found by isoelectric focusing and demonstrated in 81 per cent of alcoholics and 1 per cent of controls — although there tends to be a return towards normal with abstinence (Stibler et al, 1980).

6. An additional approach to this problem has been outlined elsewhere in this text. There are a variety of *blood markers* interacting in different body systems which increase with heavy drinking. These include γ-glutamyltransferase, aspartate transaminase, mean corpuscular volume, uric acid, and most of the usual liver function tests (Rosalki & Rau, 1972; Morse & Hurt, 1979; Barboriak et al, 1981; Ryback et al, 1980; Whitehead et al, 1978). In addition, some authors have reported an increased plasma ratio of α-amino-n-butyric acid to leucine (A/L ratio) in chronic heavy drinkers (Shaw et al, 1976), although other investigators have not been able to replicate the results especially as they may relate to differentiating between temporarily increased alcohol intake and alcoholism (Morgan et al, 1977; Jones et al, 1981). The importance of these findings is the possibility that an induction of these enzymes or changes after heavy drinking might (theoretically) be different in individuals predisposed towards alcoholism than controls. This idea is purely speculation, but should be kept in mind by investigators looking for possible biochemical markers of a predisposition towards alcoholism.

7. Even controlling for ethanol intake, not all alcoholics are equally predisposed towards specific *alcohol-related problems*. This may mean that one approach for searching for biochemical markers could focus on these yielding a predisposition towards alcohol related pathology but not necessarily related to the general problem of alcoholism itself. In one set of studies, Blass & Gibson (1977) have shown an abnormality in transketolase which might predispose only some heavy drinkers to the development of neurological problems, especially Wernicke-Korsakoff's disease. Similarly, there is evidence that alcoholic identical twins may be more similar on their rate of cirrhosis than alcoholic fraternal twins, indicating the possibility of genetic factors in the predisposition towards cirrhosis within alcoholic populations (Hrubeck & Omenn, 1981). Thus, genetic markers for a

predisposition towards alcoholism might center on individual factors mediating a predisposition towards specific alcohol related problems which in turn make up a heterogeneous population of alcoholics.

Placing the findings in perspective

This chapter was written from a genetic and clinical viewpoint and not by a biochemist. The reader looking for a modern day test to identify 'pre-alcoholics' must certainly be disappointed by the state of the art, as no such valid and reliable tests yet exist. However, the researcher looking for areas of work of potential importance and the clinician looking towards the future has, hopefully, found material of promise.

The first group of possible biological markers include those important in the most prominent pathway of ethanol metabolism:

1. *Acetaldehyde* has been noted to be elevated in alcoholics and their relatives when compared to controls. These findings must be viewed in light of the methodological problems in measuring AcH, although in each of the relevant studies the same analytic procedure was used for alcoholics or their relatives and controls. There are at least 3 possible mechanisms whereby increases in AcH could increase risk for alcoholism, but this substance remains only a potential biological marker due to restrictions in the data yet available.

2. Closely related to the AcH elevations are the hypothetical increases in the *TIQs and beta carbolines*. With this in mind, the elevated levels of salsolinol in the urine of alcoholics coming off a drinking episode is of interest as a marker which might be easier to measure than AcH and which might correlate closely with the AcH blood levels. However, neither TIQ nor beta carboline have been subjected to adequately controlled investigations comparing groups at higher and lower risk for the future development of alcoholism.

3. *Alcohol dehydrogenase* has been extensively studied in animals and humans. The isoenzyme patterns appear to be under genetic control with various forms demonstrating different Kms at physiological pHs. The predominance of less typical forms of ADH in population groups showing higher levels of AcH and associated skin flushing points to the need to carry out further studies of ADH patterns in higher and lower risk groups.

4. *Aldehyde dehydrogenase* has been less extensively studied in human populations but also appears to be under genetic control with anywhere between 2 and 9 isoenzymes. The predominance of a higher Km enzyme form in groups demonstrating higher levels of AcH and animals showing unique patterns of ethanol selection, again points to the need for further studies of this enzyme in the high risk and low risk groups, with the hope of identifying a marker which may be of importance in the biochemical predisposition towards alcoholism.

There are a variety of other potential markers with even less information supporting their relevance for alcoholism. These include:

1. *Monamine oxidase* — the platelet activity of which has been demonstrated to be low in individuals with a variety of behavioral difficulties, including alcoholism. The ease of measurement of this potential marker for an alcoholic predisposition is most attractive, but the low level of specificity and the high level of variability of results make it of limited use.

2. A variety of blood proteins have served as potential *genetic markers* for alcoholism in both association and linkage studies. The methodological superiority of the latter approach but the paucity of available data combine for the need for greater research on linkage studies in an attempt to develop potential markers for an alcoholic predisposition.

3. A variety of *other substances* which have been found to be elevated in the blood of alcoholics after heavy drinking also require further evaluation. These include 2, 3 butanediol Pcl Duarte, superoxide dismutase and serum transfferin, each of which has its own assets and liabilities and none of which have been demonstrated to be higher in alcoholics than controls in an abstinent state.

4. Considering the probability of a genetic link in alcoholism, there are *chromosomal* aberrations which have been demonstrated in alcoholics. Some of these abnormalities appear to revert towards normal with abstinence, and their specific role as markers for a predisposition towards alcoholism must be considered tentative.

5. A variety of *blood markers* have been shown to be elevated after heavy drinking and to return toward normal with abstinence. One possible approach for future study of genetic markers for a predisposition towards alcoholism could include an evaluation of whether the enzyme pattern response to ethanol differs in individuals with a predisposition towards alcoholism and controls. These markers include GGT, liver function tests, uric acid and triglycerides among others.

6. Finally, in light of the possibility that alcoholism represents a heterogeneous group of problems each with their own genetic predisposition, an additional approach to studying genetic markers towards a predisposition towards alcoholism must be considered. Unique characteristics of transketolase may halp explain why some alcoholics develop Wernicke-Korsakoff's disease and genetic factors within alcoholics may lead to a predisposition toward cirrhosis. This raises the possible importance of looking for separate biochemical markers of a predisposition towards a series of alcohol related pathologies (e.g. pancreatitis, alcohol related convulsions, alcoholic paranoia, etc.) in trying to identify individuals at high risk for alcoholism.

ACKNOWLEDGEMENTS

This work is supported by the Veterans Administration, the Mental Health Clinical Research Center grant 5 P50 MM309 14-04, and ADAMMA Grant PHSAA04353-03 and a grant from the Alcoholic Beverage Medical Research Foundation.

REFERENCES

Alexopoulos G S, Liebermann K W, Frances R, Stokes P E 1981 Platelet MAO during the alcohol withdrawal syndrome. American Journal of Psychiatry 138: 125–1255

Amit Z, Brown Z W, Rockman G E, Smith B, Amir S 1980 Acetaldehyde: a positive reinforcer mediating ethanol consumption. In: Regleiter H (ed) Biology effects of alcohol. Plenum, New York, p 413

Azevedo E S, DaSilva M C B O, Taveres-Neto J 1975 Human alcohol dehydrogenase ADH_1, ADH_2 and ADH_3 loci in a mixed population of Bahia, Brazil. Annals of Human Genetics 39: 321–327

Barboriak J J, Jacobson G R, Cushman P, Herrington R E, Lipo R F, Daley M E et al 1980 Chronic alcohol abuse and high density lipoprotein cholesterol. Alcoholism: Clinical and Experimental Research 4: 346–349

Belmaker R H, Bracha H S, Ebstein R P 1980 Platelet monoamine oxidase in affective illness and alcoholism. Schizophrenia Bulletin 9: 320–323

Bennion L J, Li T K 1976 Lack of racial differences in metabolic rate and liver alcohol dehydrogenase. The New England Journal of Medicine 294: 9–13

Blass J P, Gibson G E 1977 Abnormality of a thiamine-requiring enzyme in patients with Wernicke-Korsakoff syndrome. The New England Journal of Medicine 297: 1367–1370

Blair H A, Vallee B L 1966 Some catalytic properties of human liver alcohol dehydrogenase. Biochemistry 5: 2026–3034

Bohman M 1978 Some genetic aspects of alcoholism and criminality. Archives of General Psychiatry 35: 269–276

Bohman M, Sigvardsson S, Cloninger C R 1981 Maternal inheritance of alcohol abuse. Cross-fostering analysis of adopted women. Archives General Psychiatry 38: 965–969

Bosron W F, Li T K 1981 Genetic determinants of alcohol and aldehyde dehydrogenases and alcohol metabolism. Seminars in Liver Disease 1: 179–188

Bosron W F, Li T K, Vallee B L 1980 New molecular forms of human liver alcohol dehydrogenase: Isolation and characterization of ADH Indianapolis. Proceedings of the National Academy of Science, USA 77: 5784–5788

Brown J B 1977 Platelet MAO and alcoholism. Americal Journal of Psychiatry 134: 206–207

Buchsbaum M, Coursey R D, Murphy D L 1976 The biochemical high-risk paradigm: behavioral and familial correlates of low platelet monoamine oxidase activity. Science 194: 339

Cadoret R J, Cain C A, Grove W M 1980 Development of alcoholism in adoptees raised apart from alcoholic biologic relatives. Archives of General Psychiatry 37: 561–563

Collins M A, Num W P 1979 Dopamine-related tetrahydroisoquinolines: Significant urinary excretion by alcoholics after alcohol consumption. Science 206: 1184–1186

Comings D E 1979 Pc 1 Duarte, a common polymorphism of a human brain protein, and its relationship to depressive disease and multiple sclerosis. Nature 277: 28–32

Coursey M D, Buchsbaum M S, Murphy D L 1979 Platelet MAO activity and evoked potentials in the identification of subjects biologically at risk for psychiatric disorders. British Journal of Psychiatry 134: 372–381

Cotton N S The familial incidence of alcoholism: a review. Journal of Studies on Alcohol 40: 89–116

Davidson J R T, McLeod M N, Turnbull C D, White H L and Feuer E J 1980 Platelet monoamine oxidase activity and the classification of depression. Archives of General Psychiatry 37: 771–773

Del Villano B C, Miller S I, Schacter L P, Tischfield J A 1980 Elevated superoxide dismutase in black alcoholics. Science 207: 991–994

De Torok D 1972 Chromosomal irregularities in alcoholics. Annals New York Academy of Science 197: 90–100

Edwards J A, Evans D A P 1967 Ethanol metabolism in subjects possessing typical and atypical liver alcohol dehydrogenase. Clinical Pharmacology Therapy 8: 824–829

Eriksson C J P 1980 Elevated blood acetaldehyde levels in alcoholics and their relatives: A reevaluation. Science 207: 1383–1384

Eriksson K 1981 Ethanol as a mutagen in vivo. Alcoholism: Clinical and Experimental Research. Proceedings of the Conference on Genetic and Biochemical Variability in Response to Alcohol 5: 462

Ewing J A, Beatrice D P M Rouse A, Pellizzari E D 1974 Alcohol sensitivity and ethnic background. Americal Journal of Psychiatry 131: 206–209
Farris J J, Jones B E 1978 Ethanol metabolism in male american indians and whites. Alcoholism: Clinical and Experimental Research 2: 77–81
Fenna D, Mix L, Schaefer O, Gilber J A L 1971 Ethanol metabolism in various racial groups. Canadian Medical Association Journal 105: 472–475
Frances R J, Timm S, Bucky S 1980 Studies of familial and non-familial alcoholism. Archives of General Psychiatry 37: 564–566
Freund G, O'Hallaren P 1965 Acetaldehyde concentrations in alveolar air following a standard dose of ethanol in man. Journal of Lipid Research 6: 471–477
Gleibermann L, Gershowitz H, Harburg E, Kuusinen S 1981 Blood groups and alcohol use. Journal of Studies on Alcohol 42: 557–563
Goedde H W, Agarwal D P, Harada S 1979a Alcohol metabolizing enzymes: studies of isozymes in human biopsies and cultured fibroblasts. Clinical Genetics 16: 29–33
Goedde H W, Harada S, Agarwal D P 1979b Racial differences in alcohol sensitivity: a new hypothesis. Human Genetics 51: 331–334
Goedde H W, Agarwal D P, Harada S 1980 Genetic studies on alcohol-metabolizing enzymes: detection of isozymes in human hair roots. Enzyme 25: 281–286
Goodwin D W, Guze S B 1980 Psychiatric Diagnosis. New York, Oxford University Press
Goodwin D W, Schulsinger F, Moller N, Hermansen L, Winokur G, Guze S B 1974 Drinking problems in adopted and nonadopted sons of alcoholics. Archives of General Psychiatry 31: 164–169
Greenfield N J, Pietruszko R 1977 Two aldehyde dehydrogenases from human liver. Isolation via affinity chromatography and characterization of the isoenzymes. Biochemical Biophysical Acta 483: 35–45
Griffiths J, Schuckit M A, Millikan B in press Alcohol dehydrogenase activity in serum: preliminary results. Enzyme in press
Haglund R M J, Schuckit M A 1977 The epidemiology of alcoholism. In: Estes, Heinemann E (eds) Alcoholism: development, consequences and intervention. Mosby, St Louis, p 28
Hanna J M 1978 Metabolic responses of Chinese, Japanese and Europeans to alcohol. Alcoholism 2: 89–92
Harada S, Agarwal D P, Goedde H W 1978 Isoenzyme variations in acetaldehyde dehydrogenase (E.D. 1.2.1.3.) in human tissues. Human Genetics 44: 181–185
Harada S, Agarwal D P, Goedde H W 1979 Isoelectric focusing in cellulose acetate membrane and flatbed granulated GEL: application to the study of human aldehyde dehydrogenase isozymes. Electrophoresis 687–693
Harada S, Agarwal D P, Goedde H W 1980 Electrophoretic and biochemical studies of human aldehyde dehydrogenase isoenzymes in various tissues. Life Science 26: 1773–1780
Harada S, Agarwal P, Goedde H W 1982 Polymorphism of ADH in human tissues and sera from Japanese populations. Presented at the International Titisee Symposium on Alcohol metabolism in humans and its enzymes. January 21–24, 1982, Titisee, Germany
Harada S, Misawa S, Agarwal D P, Goedde H W 1979 Studies on liver alcohol and acetaldehyde dehydrogenase variants in Japanese. Hoppe-Seylers Z. Physiology Chemistry 360: 278–281
Harada S, Misawa S, Agarwal D P, Goedde H W 1980 Liver alcohol dehydrogenase and aldehyde dehydrogenase in the Japanese: isoenzyme variation and its possible role in alcohol intoxication. American Journal of Human Genetics 32: 8–15
Hill S Y, Goodwin D W, Cadoret R, Osterland C K, Doner S M 1975 Association and linkage between alcoholism and eleven serological markers. Journal of Studies on Alcohol 36: 981–992
Hrubec Z, Omenn G S 1981 Evidence of genetic predisposition to alcoholic cirrhosis and psychosis: twin concordances for alcoholism and its biological end points by zygosity among male veterans. Alcoholism: Clinical and Experimental Research 5: 207–214
Inoue K, Fukunaga M, Yamasdawa K 1980 Correlation between human erythrocyte aldehyde dehydrogenase activity and sensitivity to alcohol. Pharmacology Biochemistry & Behavior 13: 295–297
Inoue K, Nishimukai H, Yamasawa K 1979 Purification and partial characterization of aldehyde dehydrogenase from human erythrocytes. Biochemica et Biophysica Acta 569: 117–123

Inoue K, Ohbora Y, Yamasawa K 1978 Metabolism of acetaldehyde by human erythrocytes. Life Sciences 23: 179–184

Jenkins W J, Peters T J 1980 Selectively reduced hepatic acetaldehyde dehydrogenase in alcoholics. The Lancet 1: 628–630

Jones J D, Morse R M, Hurt R D 1981 Plasma α-amino-n-butyric acid/leucine ratio in alcoholics. Alcoholism: Clinical and Experimental Research 5: 363–365

Jornvall H, Jeffery J 1982 Two different types of alcohol dehydrogenase. Paper presented at the International Titisee Symposium on Alcohol metabolism in humans and its enzymes. January 21–24, 1982, Titisee, Germany

Kaij L 1960 Studies on the etiology and sequels of abuse of alcohol. Department of Psychiatry, University of Lund, Sweden

Kamaryt J, Martinek K 1979 Genetically determined alcohol dehydrogenase variants in subjects with liver diseases. Scripta Medica 52: 265–268

Knop J, Angelo H, Christensen J M 1981 Is role of acetaldehyde in alcoholism based on an analytical artifact? Lancet 2: 102–103

Koivula T 1975 Subcellular distribution and characterization of human liver aldehydedehydrogenase fractions. Life Science 16: 1563–1569

Koivula T, Lindros K O 1975 Effects of long-term ethanol treatment on aldehyde and alcohol dehydrogenase activities in rat liver. Biochemical Pharmacology 24: 1937–1942

Kopun M, Proping P 1977 The kinetics of ethanol absorption and elimination in twins and supplementary repetitive experiments in singleton subjects. European Journal of Clinical Pharmacology 11: 337–344

Korsten M A, Matsuzaki S, Feinman L, Lieber C S 1975 High blood acetaldehyde levels after ethanol administration. The New England Journal of Medicine 292: 386–389

Kraemer R J, Deitrich R A 1968 Isolation and characterization of human liver aldehyde dehydrogenase. Journal of Biological Chemistry 243: 6402–6408

Krebs H A, Perkins J R 1970 The physiological role of liver alcohol dehydrogenase. Biochemical Journal 118: 635–644

Li T K 1977 Enzymology of human alcohol metabolism In: Meister A (ed) Alcoholism. Wiley, New York, 19–56

Li T K 1981 Human alcohol dehydrogenase isoenzymes. Alcoholism: Clinical and Experimental Research 5: 451–459

Li T K 1982 Dissociation — recombination studies of $ADH_{Indianapolis}$. Presented at the International Titisee Symposium on Alcohol metabolism in humans and its enzymes. January 21–24, 1982, Titisee, Germany

Li T K, Magnes L J 1975 Identification of a distinctive molecular form of alcohol dehydrogenase in human livers with high activity. Biochemical and Biophysical Research Communications 63: 202–208

Lieber C S 1977 Metabolism of ethanol. In: Lieber C S (ed) Metabolic aspects of alcoholism. MTP, Lancaster, p 1

Lieber C A, DeCarli L M 1970 Hepatic microsomal ethanol-oxidizing system. Journal of Biological Chemistry 245: 2505–2512

Lindros K O 1978 Acetaldehyde — Its metabolism and role in the actions of alcohol. Research Advances in Alcohol and Drug Problems 4: 111–175

Lindros K O, Salaspuro M, Pikkarainen P 1979 Studies on the role of the ADH pathway in incrased ethanol elimination after chronic alcohol intake in the rat and man. Alcohol and Aldehyde Metabolizing Systems 3: 210–217

Lundquist F, Wolthers H 1958 The kinetics of alcohol elimination in man. Acta Pharm Tox 14: 265–289

Malila A 1978 Intoxicating effects of three aliphatic alcoholics and barbitol on two rats strains. Pharmacology, Biochemistry and Behavior 8: 197–201

McClearn G E 1979 Genetics and alcoholism simulacra. Alcoholism: Clinical and Experimental Research 3: 255–258

Mizoi Y, Ijiri I, Tatsumo Y, Kijima T, Fukiwara S et al 1978 Relationship between facial flushing and blood acetaldehyde levels after alcohol intake. Pharmacology Biochemistry & Behavior 10: 303–311

Mizoi Y, Kogama M, Aachi J, Okada T, Fukunaga T Polymorphism of alcohol-metabolizing enzymes. Presented at the International Titisee Symposium on Alcohol metabolism in humans and its enzymes. January 21–24, 1982, Titisee, Germany

Morgan M Y, Milsom J P, Sherlock S 1977 Ratio of plasma alpha amino-n butyric acid to leucine as an empirical marker of alcoholism: diagnostic value. Science 197: 1183–1185
Morse R M, Hurt R D 1979 Screening for alcoholism. Journal of the American Medical Association 242: 2688–2690
Moser K, Papenberg J, von Wartburg J P 1968 Organverteilung und heterogenitat der alkoholdehydrogenase bei verschiedenen spezies. Enzyme Biology Clinical 9: 447–458
Murphy D L, Donnelly C H 1974 Monoamine oxidase in man: enzyme characteristics in platelets, plasma, and other human tissues. In: E Usdin (ed) Neuropsychopharmacology of monoamines and their regulatory enzymes. Raven, New York, p 71–81
Murphy D L, Belmaker R H et al 1977 Biogenic amine-related enzymes and personality variations in normals. Pschol Med 7: 149
Obe G, Herha J 1975 Chromosomal damage in chronic alcohol users. Humangenetic 29: 191–200
Partanen J, Bruun K, Markkanen T 1966 Inheritance of drinking behavior. Kekuskirjopoino-Centraltryckeriet, Helsinki
Penick E C, Read M R, Crowley P A, Powell B J 1978 Differentiation of alcoholics by family history. Journal of Studies on Alcohol 39: 1944–1948
Petersen D R, Tabakoff B 1979 Characterization of brain acetaldehyde oxidizing systems in the mouse. Drug Alcohol Dependency 4: 137–144
Peterson B J, Cornell N W, Beech R L 1980 Alcohol dehydrogenase in cultured human skin fibroblasts: human fibroblast alcohol dehydrogenase. Advances in Experimental Biology 132: 533–541
Pietruszko R 1982 Chemical modification of human aldehyde dehydrogenase. Presented at the International Titisee Symposium on Alcohol metabolism in humans and its enzymes. January 21–24, 1982, Titisee, Germany
Pietruszko R, Vallari R C 1978 Aldehyde dehydrogenase in human blood. FEBS Letter 92: 89–91
Pietruszko R, Theorell H, and de Zalenski C 1972 Heterogeneity of alcohol dehydrogenase from human liver. Archives Biochemical Biophysics 153: 279–293
Pietruszko R, Reed D M, Vallari R C, Major L F, Saini N, Hawley R J 1981 Brain aldehyde dehydrogenase in human alcoholics and controls. Alcoholism (NY) 5: 78–84
Propping P 1977 Genetic control of ethanol action on the central nervous system. An EEG study in twins. Human Genetics 35: 309–334
Raskin H, Sokoloff L 1968 Brain alcohol dehydrogenase. Science 162: 131–132
Reed T E, Kalant H, Gibbins R J, Kapur M, Rankin J G 1976 Alcohol and acetaldehyde metabolism in Caucasians, Chinese and Amerinds. Canadian Medical Association Journal 115: 851–855
Robins L N 1978 Sturdy childhood predictors of adult antisocial behaviour: replications from longitudinal studies. Psychological Medicine 8: 611–622
Rosalki S B, Rau D 1972 Serum γ-glutamyl transpeptidase activity in alcoholism. Clinica Chimica Acta 39: 41–47
Ryback R S, Eckardt M J, Pautler C P 1980 Biochemical and hematological correlates of alcoholism. Research Communications in chemical pathology and pharmacology 27: 533–550
Schildkraut J J, Herzog J M, Edelman S E 1975 Platelet MAO activity in schizophrenic disorders. In: American Psychiatric Association Annual Meeting Program (New Research Abstracts), Washington DC. American Psychiatric Association: 15–23
Schuckit M A 1979 Drug and alcohol abuse: a clinical guide to diagnosis and treatment. Plenum, New York
Schuckit M A 1980 Biological markers: metabolism and acute reactions to alcohol in sons of alcoholics. Pharmacology Biochemistry and Behavior 13: 9–16
Schuckit M A 1981a Peak blood alcohol levels in men at high risk for the future development of alcoholism. Alcoholism: Clinical and Experimental Research 5: 64–66
Schuckit M A 1981b Twin studies on substance abuse. In: Gedda L, Parisi P, Nance W E (eds) Twin research 3. Liss, New York, p 61–70
Schuckit M A Acetaldehyde and alcoholism: methodology. In: Hesselbrock V, Shaskin E, Meyer R (eds) Biological and genetic markers of alcoholism, Washington DC: National Institute on Alcohol Abuse and Alcoholism, US Government Printing Office, in press A
Schuckit M A A prospective study of genetic markers in alcoholism. In: Hanin I, Usden E

(eds) Biological markers in psychiatry and neurology. Pergamon, Oxford, in press B
Schuckit M A, Duby J Alcohol related flushing and risk for alcoholism in sons of alcoholics. Journal of Clinical Psychiatry, in press
Schuckit M A, and Rayses V 1979 Ethanol ingestion: differences in blood acetaldehyde concentrations in relatives of alcoholics and controls. American Association for the Advancement of Science. 203: 54–55
Schuckit M A, Goodwin D A, Winokur G A 1972 A study of alcoholism in half siblings. American Journal of Psychiatry 128: 1132
Schuckit M A, Shaskan E, Duby J, Vega R, Moss M Platelet MAO activities in the relatives of alcoholics and controls. Biological Psychiatry in press
Shaw S, Stimmel B, Lieber C S 1976 Plasma alpha amino-n-butyric acid to leucine ratio: an empirical biochemical marker of alcoholism. Science 194: 1057–1058
Shimasue A, Murakami M, Tsubokura T 1972 A specific method for the assay of alcohol dehydrogenase in human liver and serum. Hiroshima Journal of Medical Sciences 21: 131–140
Smith M, Hopkinson D A, Harris H 1972 Alcohol dehydrogenase isoenzymes in adult human stomach and liver: evidence for activity of the ADH_3 locus. Annals of Human Genetics 35: 243–253
Smith M, Hopkinson D A, Harris H 1973 Studies on the subunit structure and molecular size of human alcohol dehydrogenase isoenzymes determined by the different loci, ADH_1, ADH_2, and ADH_3. Annals of Human Genetics 36: 401–414
Stibler H, Borg S, Allgulander C 1980 Abnormal microheterogeneity of transferrin — a new maker of alcoholism? Substance and Alcohol Actions/Misuse 1: 247–252
Sullivan J L et al 1978 Stability of low blood platelet monoamine oxidase activity in human alcoholics. Biological Psychiatry 13: 391–397
Sullivan J L, Cavenar J O, Maltbie A A, Lister P, Zung W W K 1979 Familial biochemical and clinical correlates of alcoholics with low platelet monoamine oxidase activity. Biological Psychiatry 14: 385–394
Tabakoff B, von Wartburg J P 1975 Separation of aldehyde reductases and alcohol dehydrogenase from brain by affinity chromatography: metabolism of succinic semialdehyde and ethanol. Biochemical Biophysical Research Communication 63: 957–966
Tabakoff B, Anderson R A, and Ritzman R F 1976 Brain acetaldehyde after ethanol administration. Biochemical Pharmacology 25: 1305–1307
Teng Y S 1981 Stomach aldehyde dehydrogenase: report of a new locus. Human Heredity 31: 74–77
Truitt E B 1971 Blood acetaldehyde levels after alcohol consumption by alcoholic and nonalcoholic subjects. Biological Aspects of Alcohol 3: 212–232
Ugarte G, Pino M E, Altschiller H, Pereda T 1970 Atypical alcohol dehydrogenase in Children alcohol addicts with and without hepatic damage. Quarterly Journal Studies in Alcoholism 31: 571–577
Utne H E, Hansen F V, Winkler K, and Schulsinger F 1977 Alcohol elimination rates in adoptees with and without alcoholic parents. Journal of Studies on Alcohol 38: 1219–1223

3 *Ronald C. Denney*

Measuring alcohol

INTRODUCTION

Public attention has been greatly focused on the need to carry out analyses for ethanol, mainly as a result of the legislation on drinking and driving. From a clinical point of view this need has existed for a very long time, not just for breath, blood or urine samples but for a much wider range of tissues, as ethanol is the most commonly encountered drug associated with sudden and unexpected death. Early methods of analysis were almost completely chemical in nature and frequently required preliminary treatment to remove interfering substances. However, the last twenty years have seen enormous developments in other procedures for studying ethanol levels, in some instances obviating the previous need for pretreatment (Holleyhead, 1980).

The great importance placed upon ethanol analysis undoubtedly rests on the fact that, as it is distributed around the body in proportion to the water content of the tissue, it is theoretically possible to ascertain the ethanol content of any part of the body from a tissue sample taken from another point when equilibrium of distribution has been reached. Equilibrium occurs between 30 and 60 minutes after drinking has ceased. The most

Table 3.1 Conversion factors for the distribution of ethanol between whole blood and other body fluids and tissues

Tissue	Factor
Whole blood	1.00
Cisternal spinal fluid	1.10
Ureteral urine	1.33
Saliva	1.18
Blood plasm or serum	1.15
Brain	0.85
Liver	0.90
Kidney	0.83
Alveolar breath*	0.000476

* One volume of blood contains the same amount of ethanol as does 2100 volumes of alveolar breath

important ethanol level medically is normally that of whole blood, because of its direct effect on the central nervous system. Many of the available methods of measurement have been designed to determine this (with certain limitations) from the analysis of other tissues and fluids. The ethanol content for whole blood is obtained by dividing the corresponding ethanol content of other parts of the body by appropriate factors (Muehlberger, 1959) as listed in Table 3.1).

Again, because of the drink-drive laws, the greatest controversy has arisen over the ratios employed for the urine and breath conversions. In the case of urine there is considerable doubt about the validity of the 1.33 factor, as this is an eliminated fluid and not one in constant dynamic equilibrium with the rest of the body. In many ways the factor for breath is even more important, and the argument revolves around whether the volume of breath equivalent to that of blood is 2000 or 2200 times. This can, of course, lead to a difference of at least 10 per cent in values obtained on evidential breath testing equipment (Jones, 1978a).

Such variations may not always be of importance in purely chemical studies but are obviously of greater concern in forensic investigations, particularly in establishing legal breath alcohol limits comparable to corresponding blood alcohol levels.

Special care must also be taken in the collection and storage of samples prior to analysis, particularly those for post-mortem investigations. Such samples must be collected before any embalming is carried out, as embalming fluids contain a wide range of volatile materials which may interfere with ethanol analyses. Refrigeration of samples as soon as is practicable is essential in order to minimise both enzymatic oxidation of the ethanol and putrefaction of the tissue.

Preservation of samples which have to be stored prior to analysis is essential, and great variations can occur in ethanol levels if this is not done (Corry, 1978). Some strains of yeast, however, are capable of increasing the concentration of ethanol even in the presence of preservatives (Corry, 1981).

The most common preservatives for blood samples are sodium fluoride and potassium oxalate, the former as the bacteriostat and the latter as an anticoagulant. The anticoagulant is not required for urine samples and these are preserved with either phenyl mercury nitrate or sodium fluoride alone. Confidence in the integrity of samples and the analytical values obtained can only be established if the essential features of preservation and refrigeration are adhered to. Failure to do this must inevitably open the door to speculation on the validity of the analytical results.

CLASSIFICATION OF METHODS FOR MEASURING ALCOHOL

A very wide range of methods has been employed for the quantitative analysis of ethanol. They vary from the relatively simple but time consuming procedures suitable for only a limited number of determinations, to the highly automated systems applicable to multiple samples. In some procedures the actual analysis is only possible after an initial extraction, distillation or other separative step has been carried out. The various methods can be grouped under the four main headings of:

1. chemical methods
2. biochemical methods
3. physico-chemical methods
4. instrumental methods.

It should, however, be emphasised that these are not mutually exclusive, particularly as all methods are now being extended and developed into automatic instrumental procedures suitable for multiple sample treatment wherever possible.

The selection of an appropriate method of analysis is usually dictated by a number of criteria, and there can be no 'best' method. The choice will depend upon the nature and size of the sample available, wherever a small or large number of analyses are to be made, and whether it is intended for screening or absolute analysis, the type of instrumentation at hand, and the time available in which to produce the results. Because of these, there is still a clear need for the established chemical and biochemical procedures, despite the advances that have been made and are still taking place in the instrumental techniques.

CHEMICAL METHODS OF ANALYSIS

By far the oldest methods used for the quantitative analysis of ethanol are those involving chemical reactions and colour changes. Their suitability for this purpose remained unchallenged until the introduction of first the enzymatic oxidation method and later the gas chromatographic procedures in the 1950s. Even now, chemical methods are still employed in some laboratories and act as the basis for the 'Breathalyser 1000' evidential breath testing instrument.

Most of the chemical methods are based upon the oxidation of the ethanol to one of the three possible stages indicated by the following chemical equations:

$$\text{(a)}\ CH_3CH_2OH + O \rightarrow CH_3CHO + H_2O$$
$$\text{(b)}\ CH_3CHO + O \rightarrow CH_3COOH$$
$$\text{(c)}\ CH_3COOH + 4O \rightarrow 2CO_2 + 2H_2O$$

The procedures adopted are often dependent upon the volatility of the ethanol, and the extent of the oxidation is determined by the reaction conditions, particularly the temperature and concentration of reagents. Although a very wide range of oxidizing agents has been studied, including acidified and alkaline potassium permanganate, bromine and osmic acid, the only chemical method of real importance is that in which the oxidation is carried out by potassium dichromate in sulphuric acid. This was first introduced as a quantitative procedure by Bechamp (1865), the acetic acid produced being converted to sodium acetate which was isolated and weighed. However, most modern procedures are based upon determining the amount of unreacted potassium dichromate by titration and calculating the quantity used for the oxidation by difference, or, alternatively, upon the measurement of the intensity of the green coloration arising from the formation of the chromium (III) sulphate as the ethanol is oxidised:

$$\underset{\text{yellow}}{2K_2Cr_2O_7} + 8H_2SO_4 + 3CH_3CH_2OH \rightarrow 2Cr_2(SO_4)_3 + 2K_2SO_4 + 3CH_3COOH + 11H_2O$$

yellow — blue/green

The history of the development of the chemical oxidation methods has been discussed at length by Ward Smith (1965), and many modifications have taken place over the one hundred years in which they have been used.

The major developments in these analytical methods were carried out by Nicloux (1906, 1931) who devised several approaches over a period of about forty years. In most cases preliminary treatment of samples was necessary; blending in the case of tissues, and precipitation of proteins with tungstic acid for tissue and blood samples. This step was followed by distillation of the ethanol from the blood urine or tissue before an aliquot of the distillate was heated with the potassium dichromatic/sulphuric acid mixture which was intended to oxidise it to the acetic acid stage. Reproducibility within ±3 per cent was ultimately claimed to be possible using a sub-micro method.

Distillation of the ethanol from non-volatile components of the sample overcomes most of the problems involving interference due to preservatives, proteins or solid contaminants but also creates a rather time-consuming four-stage process of precipitation, distillation, oxidation and titration. Despite this, the general procedure was the basis of the Kozelka & Hine (1941) method recommended by the Royal Institute of Chemistry (Kent-Jones & Taylor, 1954) for the analysis of forensic blood and urine samples.

It was because of these disadvantages that Widmark (1922) had earlier considered methods applicable for cutting down the number of steps by carrying out a simultaneous distillation and oxidation. His general idea, which became widely adopted, involved suspending the sample in a small cup from the stopper of a closed 50 ml flask containing specified quantities of the potassium dichromate/sulphuric acid mixture. By heating the flask for 2 hours at 60 °C the volatile ethanol in the sample was progressively oxidized and at the end of the time the unreacted dichromate was determined by adding potassium iodide in order to release a corresponding amount of iodine that could be titrated with sodium thiosulphate.

The great value of Widmark's procedure lies in the fact that the separate distillation step is avoided and samples can just be left unattended for the specified period of time before being cooled and titrated. To enable large numbers of determinations to be carried out simultaneously on samples no

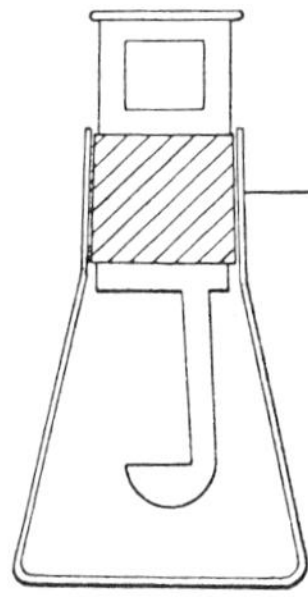

Fig. 3.1 Cavett flask.

larger than 0.1 ml, Cavett (1938) introduced a special flask (Fig. 3.1) in which a small cup is attached to the ground-glass stopper. This can be readily filled with the sample and removed after reaction which is carried out at 37 °C for 4 hours. Cavett's technique was the micro-method of analysis recommended by the Royal Institute of Chemistry in 1954, although reproducibility is limited to about ±10 per cent. The determination may similarly be carried out using a Conway diffusion apparatus.

The dichromate/sulphuric acid oxidation also serves as the basis for the roadside screening of ethanol in breath samples taken from motorists suspected of drinking before or whilst driving. For this purpose the reagent is deposited on the surface of silica gel granules and packed under controlled conditions into a short length of glass tubing, in which it is held in place by small pieces of wire mesh. When any ethanol is blown through the tube and over the granules there is a change of colour from the characteristic yellow of the dichromate ion to the deeper green colour of the chromium (III) ion. The measurement is made semi-quantitative by limiting the volume of breath blown through the tube by means of a fixed capacity plastic bag. Under these circumstances, the length of the green coloration produced in the tube is a measure of the ethanol content of the breath and can be directly related to the blood ethanol level. In the case of the roadside screening test a subject is considered to be over the legal limit if the extent of the green zone is beyond a line marked halfway along the length of the tube. The device is only of limited accuracy with a margin of error that can be as high as ±25 per cent. Because of this, the tube and bag has been frequently criticised and alternative screening instruments are now beginning to displace it.

The only real challenge to the use of potassium dichromate and sulphuric acid for chemical oxidation came from the use of either alkaline or acidified potassium permanganate. Several roadside screening devices were invented incorporating these (Denney, 1979), mainly for use in the USA. In all cases, the breath (and corresponding blood) ethanol level was shown to exceed a legal limit if there was complete loss of colour of a fixed amount of permanganate. Although studies have been made on the possibility of using permanganate in place of dichromate for the more accurate ethanol determinations on body fluids and tissues, investigators have frequently come to the conclusion that the Nicloux/Widmark methods are superior.

BIOCHEMICAL METHODS

Biochemical methods of ethanol analysis are almost completely limited to the enzymatic oxidation of ethanol to acetaldehyde (ethanol), first introduced by Bonnichsen & Theorell (1951). It uses yeast alcohol dehydrogenase (ADH) in conjunction with the coenzyme nicotinamide adenine dinucleotide (NAD^+) at pH 9 as shown in the following equation:

$$CH_3CH_2OH + NAD^+ \underset{}{\overset{ADH}{\rightleftharpoons}} CH_3CHO + NADH + H^+$$

The amount of reduced coenzyme NADH is proportional to the ethanol concentration in the sample and can be measured spectrophotometrically at 340 nm.

The procedure lends itself admirably to application on automatic analysers and is currently used extensively in Sweden as a confirmatory test for blood analyses. It has also been recommended (Poklis & MacKell, 1979) for routine confirmatory studies in post-mortem investigations. It is usual to deproteinise blood samples using trichloroacetic acid or perchloric acid prior to analysis (Mebs et al, 1979), although if samples are diluted by a factor of about 10 it is unnecessary to deproteinise before using the ADH procedure (Brown et al, 1971). It has been claimed that the ADH method is unsuitable for use with samples which have been preserved with sodium fluoride or mercurial type preservatives (Corry, 1978). Because of this, application to the analysis of saliva samples (Jones, 1979) has included a micro-distillation step to remove the ethanol from any preservative prior to mixing with the reagents. However, in general low levels of some preservatives are not considered to impair the determinations. The analyses can be carried out in the presence of up to at least 1 mg of sodium fluoride and 3 mg of potassium oxalate per ml of blood (Rosalki, 1971; Gulberg & Christian, 1981), and perfectly acceptable results are obtainable with preservative levels much higher than these (Rosalki, 1982). However, mercurial preservatives should be avoided, if possible, as the Hg^{2+} ion is actually used to inhibit enzyme activity (Davis et al, 1979).

Modifications of the standard ADH/NAD^+ approach have involved the use of phenazine methosulphate as an electron carrier with the ultimate formation of coloured formazan compounds which can be measured spectrophotometrically (Rosalki, 1971; Roos, 1971). But more recent advances in enzymatic oxidation studies have involved using immobilised ADH. Kuan et al (1978) treated blood samples with anticoagulant and deproteinised with trichloroacetic acid before buffering to pH 8.8 followed by an aqueous solution of NAD^+. The mixture was stirred in a fluorimeter cell with a stirrer on which the ADH had been immobilised on cellulose. The fluorescent intensity was measured at 465 nm after excitation at 370 nm.

An alternative approach (Attiyat & Christian, 1980) for ethanol in serum has been to immobilise the ADH on silanised glass beads and pass over it the sample mixed with $K_3Fe(CN)_6$, NAD^+ and dihydrolipoamide reductase buffered to pH 9. The NADH formed in the process leads to the production of $K_4Fe(CN)_6$ which is measured biamperometrically.

Further approaches to the ADH method for measuring ethanol have been in the construction of flow-through enzyme electrodes (Yro & Musha, 1979) in which a current is produced in proportion to the quantity of reacting ethanol. The main problems associated with these particular developments appear to be with the methods used for immobilising the ADH. Although not all the difficulties have yet been overcome in these continuous flow techniques the general approach looks very promising and may well lead to wider applications of enzymatic methods for ethanol analysis in the future. The ADH method is of particular value for this as it does not oxidise any methanol or acetone present although artificially high results are obtained if longer chain alcohols are present.

The only challenge to the preeminence of ADH has been the recent (Majkic & Berkes, 1980) oxidation of ethanol in serum by alcohol oxidase to produce hydrogen peroxide which in turn oxidises 2,2′-azino-di(3-ethyl benzthiazoline-6-sulphate) in the presence of peroxidase at 30 °C. After the reaction has been halted by hydrochloric acid the absorbance of the coloured solution is measured at either 410 or 650 nm. It is claimed that the method is more selective than is the earlier ADH procedure and may be applied to serum samples without deproteinization. In a comparison of procedures which have been tried Gulberg and Christian (1981) found that the highest activity of the enzyme was obtained when the alcohol oxidase was adsorbed onto controlled-pore silanized glass beads (45–80 mesh).

PHYSICO-CHEMICAL METHODS

Scientific literature abounds with papers dealing with various aspects of the application of gas chromatography (GC) to the analysis of ethanol in fluids and tissues. This is mainly because under carefully selected conditions it can not only be specific but also highly accurate, and at the same time can deal with a very high throughput of samples.

The one great difference that gas chromatography has over other analytical procedures is that the basic process involves separating the ethanol completely from the other volatile components. This occurs as the vaporised sample is transported in a continuous flow of an inert carrier gas through a narrow tube packed with an adsorbent or absorbent that acts as a molecular obstacle course. Individual substances in any mixture are separated from each other according to their molecular charactérisfics and are each detected as they leave the column. A signal from the detector is used to actuate a recorder which produces a peak on a chart which is in proportion to the quantity of substance separated and detected.

In early applications of GC to the analysis of ethanol in blood and urine for forensic purposes (Curry et al, 1966), the sample was injected directly into the gas stream at the head of the column. This created problems in that it led to the blocking of the column due to non-volatile substances and contamination due to pyrolysis of these substances. The problems were compounded by the fact that many of the samples analysed also contained inorganic preservatives that had been added to the samples.

Initially, these problems were overcome either by steam distilling the ethanol from the sample before carrying out the analysis or, in the case of blood samples, by preliminary treatment with a protein precipitant, such as dioxan, which could also act as a diluent (Davis, 1966).

The real advance in the use of gas chromatography for mass sample analysis came with the introduction of the head-space technique (Hachenberg & Schmidt, 1977). This has now become the standard form of forensic analysis for ethanol in blood, urine, serum and tissue extracts.

The procedure is based upon the concept that the vapour in equilibrium with a liquid possesses a composition which is representative (but not necessarily identical) with that of the liquid itself; so that by sampling and analysing the vapour it is possible to ascertain the original composition of the liquid by running the sample in parallel with a series of standards. One great advantage of the head-space procedure is that it can be applied equally as well to homogenized tissue as to liquid blood, urine or saliva (Mendenhall et al, 1980).

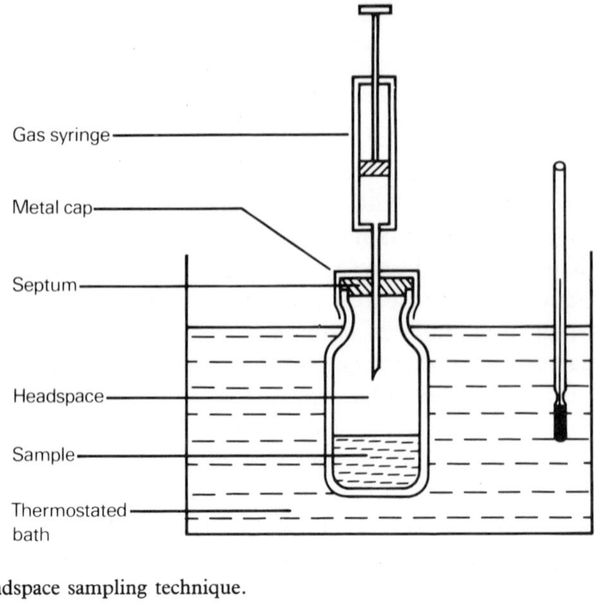

Fig. 3.2 Headspace sampling technique.

In practice, the head-space technique involves placing a measured amount of the sample to be analysed in a small container or vial fitted with a rubber septum cap. At the same time, to improve the accuracy of the procedure a measured volume of an internal standard (most frequently propanol or isopropanol) is added and the container then maintained between 40–60 °C for about 30 minutes (Fig. 3.2). The vapour above the liquid is then sampled with a syringe and injected onto the GC column.

Typical conditions for gas chromatography involve the use of a 2 m × 4 mm internal diameter stainless steel or glass column packed with Porapak Q 100–120 mesh, with the injection block and column temperatures at about 100 °C, and a helium carrier gas flow rate of 40 ml/min used in conjunction with a flame ionization detector.

The use of the internal standard means that the ethanol concentration of the sample is determined from a measurement of the ratio of the ethanol and propanol peak areas and comparison with a calibration plot obtained from known ratios of ethanol and the internal standard rather than from the absolute ethanol peak area by itself. This method compensates for any variations in the syringe injection volume, as these are reflected in both the ethanol and internal standard peaks (Denney, 1982).

With the highly automated head-space sampling and analysis systems used in many forensic laboratories, a high level of accuracy and reproducibility is attained, and this is checked at regular intervals with known ethanol concentrations. In many instances the standard deviation for determinations is better than 2 per cent. However, a wide range of potential errors need to be guarded against, particularly absorption of vapour by the septum (Drozd & Novak, 1979).

INSTRUMENTAL METHODS

Apart from the extensive use of gas chromatography, the highly sophisticated instrumental methods of ethanol analysis have been introduced almost exclusively for the purpose of measuring the amount of ethanol exhaled from the lungs of suspected drinking drivers. These instruments are now becoming used in medical research for a wide range of investigations involving ethanol and its physiological effects. Many of the developments that have been made in this field started in one form or another as roadside screening devices, and over the years have been modified and improved to the extent that they are now accurate and sensitive enough to be used for substantive or evidential purposes (Denney, 1981). This is possible as the margins of error obtained for the conversion of breath alcohol figures to the corresponding blood alcohol levels obtained from these instruments are at least comparable with those obtained from straightforward blood analyses. The absolute values obtained do, of course, depend upon the distribution ratio employed for the ethanol between blood and breath. Even though it is normally stated that deep alveolar breath should always be used, there is still debate over whether the ratio is a direct 1:2100 or a more variable figure, as previously mentioned. However, that variation in itself does not detract from the need to have some form of breath alcohol analysis that can replace the waste of time, money and effort that is attendant upon analysing thousands of blood samples.

There have been five major approaches to the problems of evidential breath testing, and each one has been adopted by police forces for use in law enforcement in different countries. The five are:

1. wet chemical methods
2. infrared absorption
3. portable gas chromatography
4. fuel cells
5. semiconductor detectors.

Instruments based upon the first three of these were the subject of comprehensive studies (Emerson et al, 1980; Isaacs et al, 1982) carried out for the United Kingdom Government to consider their suitability to take the place of the blood and urine tests. Similarly, fuel cells are the main working part of an instrument, the Alcolmeter, which has been used extensively for this purpose for several years within Northern Ireland (which has a slightly different drink-drive law from that in Great Britain). Instruments based upon the semiconductor detector have been used in Canada and in Japan.

The Breathalyser 1000 is the latest version of the most well-known wet chemical instrument that was first developed in the USA about 30 years ago. It operates on the previously discussed principle of the oxidation of ethanol by potassium dichromate in sulphuric acid. In early versions of the instrument the ethanol content of a breath sample was determined by the colour change occurring in an ampoule of reagent after a measured breath volume had been pumped through and compared with an unreacted reagent ampoule. In the model 1000, however, the reduction in the transmitted light due to the reaction taking place in the first ampoule is used to produce a current which moves the light source in order to rebalance the electrical output from the photocells sensing the transmitted light from the reacted ampoule and an unreacted blank. The movement of the source needed to balance the signals is proportional to the colour change that has taken place and hence to the amount of ethanol in the measured breath sample. The value obtained is presented on a digital display and printed onto a record card.

Several instruments have been developed in recent years using non-dispersive infrared light absorption for the quantitative measurement of ethanol in breath (Bonnichsen & Goldberg, 1981). Most of these measure the absorption of the infrared wavelength within the range 3.39–3.48 μm, as there are few other substances in breath which interfere by absorbing at that value. The most well established of these instruments is the CMI Intoxilyzer (Fig. 3.3) in which the overall volume of the gas cell is 600 ml and the radiation is provided by a tungsten-halogen lamp. Reflection of the light

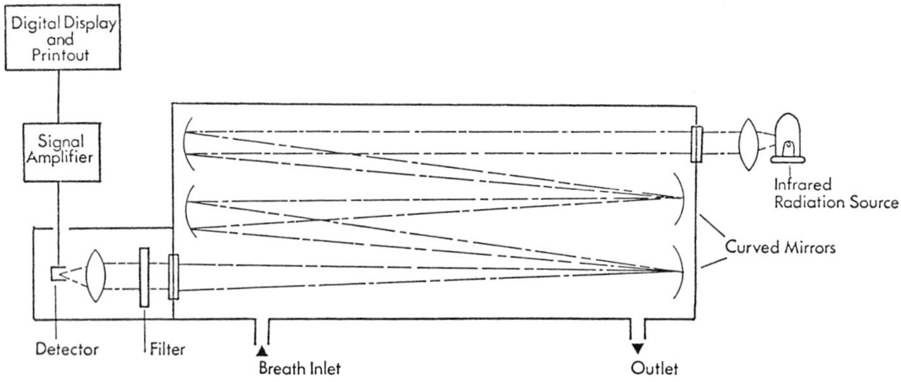

Fig. 3.3 Infrared breath testing instrument employment non-dispersion and multiple reflection.

within the cell enables a total path length of about 3 metres to be traversed before it passes through the interference filter at which the 3.42 μm wavelength is selected before continuing to the infrared-sensitive photocell. The output from this is proportional to the amount of ethanol in the cell, and is directly converted to the blood alcohol level for digital display and printing onto a record card.

Typical of the gas chromatographic instruments is the Gas Chromatograph Intoximeter Mark IV, in which the ethanol from a 0.25 ml volume of breath is separated out after being carried in a stream of nitrogen and hydrogen through a column of Porapak Q coated with 1 per cent Carbowax. The instrument uses a flame ionization detector and can be used to produce either a chart record and an integrated digital display or a print-out for the blood alcohol level corresponding to the breath alcohol value.

The main instrument based upon the use of fuel cells is the Alcolmeter (Jones et al, 1977), in which a 1.5 ml volume of breath blown through a tube is diverted into the cell housing where oxidation of any ethanol to acetic acid occurs on a platinum electrode (Fig. 3.4), producing a current in proportion to the concentration of ethanol in the breath sample. This

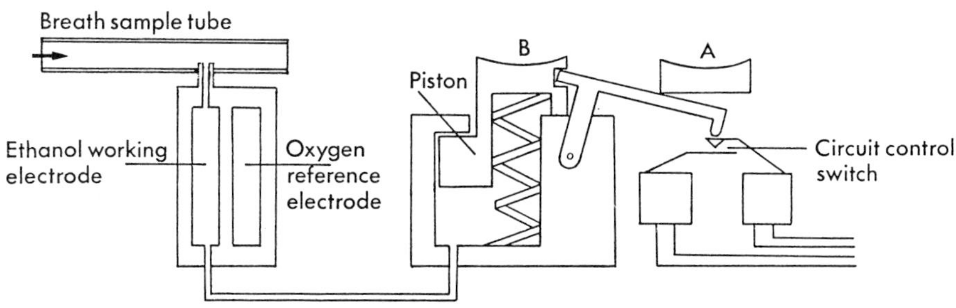

Fig. 3.4 Operating mechanism of the alcolmeter fuel cell breath testing instrument.

current is amplified and can be used to trigger a series of warning lights or to give a dial reading or a digital display and print-out of the corresponding blood alcohol level. An added advantage of the Alcolmeter is that its sampling system easily lends itself to being used for head-space analysis for tissues and fluids in general. For this purpose, it is only necessary to fit a hypodermic syringe in place of the normal breath alcohol tube and to recalibrate the sampling head with an appropriate set of standards. This procedure has been found to be comparable with gas chromatography and with ADH determination of ethanol carried out on saliva samples (Jones, 1978b). Because of its pronounced success, other fuel cells are being developed for both breath and head-space analysis.

Several instruments have been developed incorporating semiconductors as ethanol detectors. They depend upon the change of conductivity when any ethanol is absorbed on the surface; the resulting change in current being used to produce a metered signal corresponding to the breath or blood alcohol level (Tsukamoto, 1981). However, they do not appear to have met with the same wide acceptance as the other instruments. This is probably due to the fact that the semiconductor can not only respond to a fairly wide range of substances, but also does not give a totally linear response with concentration.

In general, instruments are suitable for establishing ethanol levels in blood from the values for breath, and hence for other tissue levels, so long as 5–10 per cent error is acceptable and the value obtained is well clear of a legislated or action value. In most cases in which the actual value is a critical one, either clinically or forensically, then recourse should normally be made to either gas chromatographic or enzymatic procedures carried out in duplicate for confirmation with a greater level of accuracy.

CONCLUSION

The large number of analytical methods available for ethanol measurement in medical and forensic laboratories means that a suitable procedure is available for all circumstances. Wet chemical and enzymatic analytical procedures and head-space gas chromatography require a certain amount of training and skill before reliable results can be expected. Reproducible results can usually be achieved with the instrumental breath analysers with very little instruction, and it is this factor that makes them of value in large scale studies.

REFERENCES

Attiyat S A, Christian G D 1980 Biamperometric determination of ethanol, lactate and glycerol using immobilised enzyme in flow streams. Analyst 105: 154–160

Bechamp M A 1865 On the fermentation of normal urine and the various organisms which are able to cause it. Compte Rendu Academie Science Paris 61: 374–377

Bonnichsen R, Goldberg L 1981 Large scale breath-blood comparisons under field conditions: methods evaluation techniques and results. In: Goldberg L (ed) Proceedings of the 8th International Conference on Alcohol Drugs and Traffic Safety, Stockholm, Sweden. Almquist & Wiksell, Stockholm, p 796–810

Bonnichsen R, Theorell H 1951 An enzymatic method for the microdetermination of ethanol. Scandinavian Journal of Clinical Laboratory Investigation 13: 58–62

Brown S S, Goenechea S, Gibson P F 1971 Automated assay of blood alcohol with an enzyme reaction rate monitor. Blutalkohol 8: 432–441

Cavett J W 1938 Determination of alcohol in blood and other body fluids. Journal of Laboratory and Clinical Medicine 23: 543–546

Corry J E L 1978 Possible sources of ethanol ante- and post-mortem: its relationship to the biochemistry and microbiology of decomposition. Journal of Applied Microbiology 44: 1–56

Corry J E L 1981 Methods of assessing the effects of microbes in blood and urine on ethanol levels. In: Goldberg L (ed) Proceedings of the 8th International Conference on Alcohol, Drugs and Traffic Safety, Stockholm, Sweden. Almquist & Wiksell, Stockholm, p 600–613

Curry A S, Walker G W, Simspon S 1966 Determination of ethanol in blood by gas chromatography. Analyst 91: 742–743

Davis G C, Holland K L, Kissinger P T 1979 Amperometric methods for oxide-reductase enzymes based on liquid chromatography with electrochemical detection. Alcohol dehydrogenase. Journal of Liquid Chromatography 2: 663–675

Davis R A 1966 Determination of ethanol in blood or tissue by gas chromatography. In: Borkenstein R (ed) Proceedings of the 4th International Conference on Alcohol and Traffic Safety. Indiana University, Bloomington, p 156–160

Denney R C 1979 Drinking and driving. Robert Hale, London

Denney R C 1981 Testing for drugs and alcohol in body fluids. Medical Laboratory World June: 25–27 & 50

Denney R C 1982 A dictionary of chromatography, 2nd edn. Macmillan, London, p 104–106

Drozd J, Novak J 1979 Headspace analysis by gas chromatography. Journal of Chromatography 165: 141–165

Emerson V J, Holleyhead R, Isaacs M D J, Fuller N A, Hunt D J 1980 The measurement of breath alcohol. Journal of the Forensic Science Society 20: 3–70

Gulberg E L, Christian G D 1981 The use of immobilized alcohol oxidase in the continuous flow determination of ethanol with an oxygen electrode. Analytica Chimica Acta 123: 125–133

Hachenberg H, Schmidt A P 1977 Gas chromatographic headspace analysis. Heyden, London

Holleyhead R 1980 A bibliography on ethyl alcohol for forensic science and medicine and the law. Forensic Science Society & Scottish Academic Press, Edinburgh

Isaacs M D J, Jacobs J M, Emerson V J, Broster C G, Hunt D J 1982 Field trial of three substantive breath alcohol testing instruments. Her Majesty's Stationery Office, London

Jones A W 1978a Variability of the blood: breath alcohol ratio in vivo. Journal of studies in alcohol 39: 1931–1939

Jones A W 1978b A rapid headspace method for ethyl alcohol determination in saliva samples. Analytical Biochemistry 86: 589–596

Jones A W 1979 Assessment of an automated enzymatic method for ethanol determination in microsamples of saliva. Scandinavian Journal of Clinical Laboratory Investigation 39: 199–203

Jones T P, Jones A W, Williams P M 1977 A new method for the rapid analysis of ethanol in breath, blood, urine and saliva using the alcolmeter evidential instrument. Proceedings of the 7th International Conference on Alcohol Drugs and Traffic Safety, Melbourne, 251–256

Kent-Jones D W, Taylor G 1954 Determination of alcohol in blood and urine. Analyst 79: 121–136

Kozelka F L, Hine C H 1941 Method for determination of ethyl alcohol for medicolegal purposes. Industrial and Engineering Chemistry Analytical Edition 13: 905–907

Kuan J W, Kuan S S, Guilbault G G 1978 The immobilised-enzyme stirrer. II Fluorimetric

determination of ethanol (in plasma) with use of immobilised alcohol dehydrogenase. Analytica Chimica Acta 100: 229–231
Majkic-Singh N, Berkes I 1980 Spectrophotometric determination of ethanol by an enzymatic method with 2,2′-azino-di-(3-ethylbenzthiazoline-6-sulphonate). Analytica Chimica Acta 115: 401–405
Mebs D, Schmidt K, Gerchon J 1979 Automated blood-alcohol determination (alcohol dehydrogenase method) with an LKB substrate analyzer. Blutalkohol 16: 29–35
Mendenhall C L, MacGee J, Green E S 1980 Simple rapid and sensitive method for the simultaneous quantitation of ethanol and acetaldehyde in biological materials using headspace gas chromatography. Journal of Chromatography 190: 197–200
Muehlberger C W 1959 The physiological action of alcohol. In: Heise H A (ed) Chemical tests for intoxication. American Medical Association, Chicago, p 6–10
Nicloux M 1906 Simplification de la methode de dosage de l'alcool dans le sang et dans les tissus. Compte Rendu des Séances de la Societé de Biologie, Paris 60: 1034–1037
Nicloux M 1931 Recherches sur l'alcool ethylique. Bulletin de la Societe de Chimie Biologique 13: 856–918
Poklis A, Mackell M A 1979 Use of gas chromatography and alcohol dehydrogenase in a routine procedure for the determination of ethanol in postmortem blood. Journal of Analytical Toxicology 3: 183–186
Rees K J 1971 Rapid sensitive and inexpensive method for estimating blood and urine alcohol concentration. Clinica Chimica Acta 31: 285–287
Rosalki S B 1971 A new colorimetric procedure for blood alcohol determination. Analytical Letters 4: 819–835
Rosalki S B 1982 Private communication
Tsukamoto S 1981 A new breath alcohol meter. In: Goldberg L (ed) Proceedings of the 8th International Conference on Alcohol Drugs and Traffic Safety, Stockholm, Sweden. Almquist & Wiksell, Stockholm, p 766–779
Ward Smith H 1965 Methods for determining alcohol. In: Curry A S (ed) Methods in forensic science, vol IV. Interscience, London, p 1–98
Widmark E M P 1922 Eine mikromethode zur bestimmung von aethylalkohol in blut. Biochemische Zeitschrift 131: 475–484
Yro T, Musha S 1979 Electrochemical enzymatic determination of ethanol and L-lactic acid with a carbon paste electrode modified chemically with nicotinamide adenine dinucleotide. Analytica Chimica Acta 110: 203–209

4 *Sidney B. Rosalki*

Identifying the alcoholic

INTRODUCTION

Alcoholics are reluctant to admit the extent of their drinking and the alcoholic origin of symptoms resulting therefrom. An estimated 50 per cent of subjects presenting with a definite clinical diagnosis of alcoholism deny excessive alcohol consumption (Bailey, Haberman & Steinberg, 1969).

Though the history, symptoms and signs of alcoholism listed in the tables in Chapter 1 may alert the physician, they may be absent, of late onset, or misinterpreted as of non-alcoholic origin. The cinical recognition of the alcoholic, therefore, remains a matter of difficulty. Biochemical changes can provide objective evidence of chronic alcohol excess and demonstrate any recent intake. Laboratory tests can facilitate the recognition of chronic excessive drinking, even when this is denied, and before the stage at which dependency or irreversible organ damage is established. They can monitor the progress and treatment of the alcoholic and can identify hepatic and non-hepatic complications. These tests can be used both to confirm a clinical suspicion or diagnosis of alcoholism or heavy drinking and to screen populations — high risk or otherwise. Test procedures can be divided into those designed to identify recent alcohol intake and those responsive mainly to chronic excess.

BIOCHEMICAL IDENTIFICATION OF RECENT ALCOHOL CONSUMPTION

Alcohol (ethanol) measurement

The demonstration of recent drinking, particularly when denied, may draw attention to possible chronic alcohol excess. Measurement of ethanol in blood, breath and urine has been investigated as a confirmatory test for alcohol excess in known alcoholics, and to identify drinking in selected population groups. In the known alcoholic, ethanol measurement in these, and in sweat (Philips, Vandervoort & Becker, 1980) can also be used to monitor compliance with abstinence.

Confirmation of alcoholism by ethanol measurement

Two groups of patients have been particularly studied: patients attending liver disease clinics and patients attending alcohol treatment centres.

Liver disease clinics. Random alcohol determinations are of only limited diagnostic value in patients attending clinics for liver disease. In patients attending a morning clinic only 18 per cent were found to show ethanol in their blood, whereas 36 per cent gave a history of heavy drinking (Hamlyn et al, 1975). At least three determinations were required in order to obtain a 50 per cent chance of detecting ethanol in the blood of patients with an alcoholic history.

Morning determinations appear both more sensitive and more specific than afternoon measurements. In alcoholics attending an afternoon liver clinic (Hamlyn, Hopper & Skillen, 1979), only 16 per cent of alcoholics showed increased blood ethanol, whereas ethanol was also present in blood in 18 per cent of patients with non-alcoholic liver disease and 8 per cent of controls ('social' drinkers only).

Alcohol measurement seems most valuable for monitoring claimed abstinence in the known alcoholic, where history may be very unreliable. Orrego and colleagues (1979) measured urine alcohol in patients with alcoholic liver disease followed daily for several months. Overall, 50 per cent of urines were found to contain alcohol. Patients with alcohol in their urine convincingly denied alcohol intake 52 per cent of the time they were questioned, and 25 per cent always denied drinking!

Alcohol treatment centres. About 50 per cent of patients attending a specialist clinic for problem drinkers had measurable levels of alcohol in their blood at initial examination (Pollak & Buckell, 1973). 25 (34 per cent) of 73 patients studied by the author on admission to an alcohol treatment centre (Fink, Marjot & Rosalki, 1979) showed an elevated blood alcohol.

Identification of drinking in selected population groups by ethanol measurement

Health surveys. 11 per cent of 422 males taking part in a health survey in Uppsala, Sweden, were found to have alcohol in their urine on the day of screening (Waern, Boberg & Hellsing, 1979). In one third of these there was other evidence of chronic excess alcohol intake, but in the remaining two thirds the alcohol ingestion was thought to be casual in nature.

General practitioner surgeries. Breath alcohol measurements have been used to identify alcohol consumption by patients attending general practitioners' surgeries (Wiseman et al, 1982). 3.5 per cent of just over 1000 randomly selected subjects showed the presence of alcohol in their breath, though in a significant proportion of these the measurement was at the lower limit of sensitivity of the detection instrument. Just under half of the patients with breath alcohol were thought to be problem drinkers (i.e. only 50 per cent true positives) and of these one third were known to the general practitioners. If an assessment is made of the likely number of problem drinkers in the practice population, the sensitivity of random breath alcohol measured as a test for problem drinking would lie between 20 and 40 per cent.

Accident and emergency departments. Blood alcohol measurements have been made in patients attending accident and casualty departments with trauma and head injury and some 50 per cent of such patients were found to show raised blood ethanol values (Galbraith et al, 1976; Rutherford, 1977). The majority had levels between 100 and 300 mg/dl (22 to 66 mmol/l). Clinical recognition of alcohol ingestion in such patients was found to show an error rate of around 12 per cent.

Breath alcohol measurements have also been made in patients attending an accident and emergency service during the evening hours (Holt et al, 1980). 40 per cent of such patients had consumed alcohol before attending, and 32 per cent had an equivalent blood alcohol level of above 80 mg/dl (17 mmol/l). Clinical assessment of intoxication yielded 19 per cent false negatives.

In drivers involved in road traffic accidents, with blood alcohol concentrations above 80 mg/dl (17 mmol/l), biochemical changes suggestive of chronic alcohol abuse have been observed in one quarter to one third (Weill et al, 1979; Tayside safe driving project, 1983). This indicates that the identification of a high blood alcohol in accident and trauma patients may reveal a significant percentage of those whose acute intake is associated with chronic alcohol excess.

Acute medical admissions. 7.3 per cent of 482 consecutive female acute medical admissions in Glasgow were shown by Northcote and colleagues (1983) to have alcohol in the blood. In 4.3 per cent of patients the level exceeded 80 mg/dl (17 mmol/l).

Significance of ethanol increase in body fluids in relation to alcoholism

The various quoted studies indicate that even at high blood ethanol concentrations (greater than 80 mg/dl, 17 mmol/l), alcohol ingestion may remain unrecognised clinically in approximately 20 per cent of subjects, and that in the absence of alcohol measurement, lesser degrees of ingestion would be unnoticed.

Ethanol measurements conclusively demonstrate recent alcohol intake, and it has been recommended (Annals of Internal Medicine, 1972), that a blood alcohol above 100 mg/dl (22 mmol/l) at routine medical examination, above 150 mg/dl (33 mmol/l) without intoxication or above 300 mg/dl (66 mmol/l) at any time should be considered as highly suggestive of alcoholism.

Alcohol analysis appears to be of only limited use for the detection of alcoholism since most alcoholics with an elevated value already admit to heavy drinking. When used to confirm alcoholism an abnormal level will be found in up to 50 per cent of known alcoholics, morning measurements being more frequently elevated than afternoon measurement and more specific. When used to screen for alcoholism an abnormal ethanol level is to be anticipated in only 20 to 50 per cent of alcoholics — whereas one half to two thirds of abnormal screening values result from casual drinking unassociated with alcoholism.

Probably the most valuable use of random alcohol measurements is in the follow-up of the known alcoholic, as an indicator of non-compliance with abstinence.

BIOCHEMICAL IDENTIFICATION OF CHRONIC EXCESSIVE ALCOHOL CONSUMPTION

The profound metabolic and toxic effects of alcohol on the liver are reflected by biochemical disturbances which although not specific for alcoholism, are nevertheless valuable for its identification. Abnormalities of plasma enzymes of hepatic origin have been the most useful, but other liver function test abnormalities, and alteration in the plasma level of various metabolites as a consequence of hepatic disturbance may also draw attention to alcohol excess. Additionally, the toxic effects of alcohol on other tissues, e.g. the erythrocyte have proved helpful for its recognition.

Test abnormalities from chronic excess alcohol consumption may be useful to confirm a clinical suspicion or, in the absence of clinical features, may suggest alcoholism as a diagnostic possibility to the attending physician. Whilst abnormal consumption is not synonymous with alcoholism, many biochemical abnormalities only appear in response to levels of alcohol intake where such a diagnosis is likely or when organ damage is established.

Abnormalities of plasma enzymes of hepatic origin

Serum γ-glutamyltransferase

Measurement of plasma or serum γ-glutamyltransferase activity (GGT, formerly known as γ-glutamyltranspeptidase) is the most valuable of all biochemical procedures for the detection of excess chronic alcohol intake (Rosalki et al, 1970; Rosalki & Rau, 1972). The enzyme originates from the liver, where alcohol may induce its synthesis (Rosalki, Tarlow & Rau, 1971; Rosalki et al, 1972; Ishii et al, 1976). This is an early effect of alcohol which precedes abnormal liver function, although with continuing alcohol excess, cholestasis and hepatocellular damage contribute to enzyme elevation. The enzyme is readily determined in the laboratory. The procedure is inexpensive and has been automated. The serum enzyme is stable for several months in frozen samples.

Increased serum GGT activity is observed in some 75 per cent of alcoholics. This high incidence is found in both in-patients and out-patients, even in the absence of clinical evidence of hepatic disease, and independent of recent exacerbation of drinking. In a personal series of 434 hospitalised

Table 4.1 γ-glutamyltransferase elevation in hospitalised alcoholics

	Incidence	Percentage
1. Spencer-Peet, Wood & Glatt, 1973	103/169	61
2. Boone, Routh & Schrantz, 1974	17/20	85
3. Fontan et al, 1975	51/68	75
4. Plaquet et al, 1975	83/86	95
5. Spencer-Peet et al, 1975	19/25	76
6. Patel & O'Gorman, 1975	32/67	48
7. Wu, Slavin & Levi, 1976	48/66	73
8. Baglin et al, 1976	167/282	59
9. Wietholtz & Colombo, 1976	79/90	88
10. See, Heffelfinger & Childers	85/135	63
11. Aron et al, 1977	80/120	67
12. Westwood, Cohen & McNamara, 1978	12/15	80
13. Levi & Chalmers, 1978	128/146	88
Total	903/1289	70

alcoholics (Rosalki, 1974, 1977 etc.) the serum enzyme was increased in 318 (73 per cent), and more frequently elevated than any other plasma enzyme. A review of 13 other published series (Table 4.1) shows 903 of 1289 patients (70 per cent) with raised serum GGT activity. Out-patient alcoholics show a similar incidence of raised values, 95 of 118 (81 per cent) of patients studied by the author and 122 of 183 (67 per cent) patients from 3 other published series (Pollak & Buckell, 1973; Levi et al, 1975; Hamlyn, Hopper & Skillen, 1979) having increased values.

In general, enzyme values average some two to three times the upper reference limit in hospitalised alcoholics and one and half times in alcoholic out-patients. However, values up to five times the upper reference limit are frequent in both groups, and levels up to 60 times the upper reference limit have been observed in alcoholics following recent exacerbation of drinking. Alcoholic females may show higher levels than males and a slightly higher incidence of GGT elevation (Rosalki, 1977; Levi & Chalmers, 1978).

Enzyme levels correlate with histological evidence of liver damage, inflammation and necrosis (Wu, Slavin & Levi, 1976). The highest levels being found with more advanced disease or hepatic inflammatory change. The *frequency* of elevation is however largely independent of hepatic histology (steatosis, hepatitis or cirrhosis) (Wu, Slavin & Levi, 1976; Van Waes & Lieber, 1977; Jenkins et al, 1982), though in alcoholics with normal liver histology, and without recent alcohol intake, GGT elevation is found in less than 30 per cent.

The incidence of GGT elevation in alcoholics is higher with regular daily drinking than with bout drinking (Wiseman & Spencer-Peet, 1977) and increases with the duration of the drinking bout prior to sampling (Wadstein & Skude, 1979a). In the advanced alcoholic with cirrhosis and drinking of many years standing (usually greater than 20 years) the incidence of GGT elevation may fall (Skude & Wadstein, 1977). Possible explanations for this include a reduction in the number of enzyme producing liver cells, the selective survival of alcohol-resistant individuals characterised by normal enzyme levels, or nutritional impairment (Rosalki, 1977), particularly vitamin and mineral deficiency, which may interfere with enzyme production.

Acute alcohol ingestion does not result in abnormal serum GGT levels in the normal subject, although it is possible it may do so in patients with pre-existing liver disease (Rosalki, 1975; Wietholtz & Colombo, 1976; See et al, 1976; Shaw & Marsh, 1981, Dunbar et al, 1982). Acute alcohol intakes simulating an evening's drinking, with alcohol ingestion ranging between 0.5 and 2.0 g of alcohol per kg body weight, produce insignificant or mild transient changes of GGT, generally with less than 10 per cent increase over base line levels on follow-up for up to 48 hours. Similarly, simulations of 3 consecutive evenings' drinking (Freer & Statland, 1977a) or 1 month's recurrent week-end drinking of 0.75 g per kg, produce minimal enzyme change (Freer & Statland, 1977b). A minimum of some 5 weeks' daily heavy drinking (more than 60 g a day) seems to be required before pathological serum GGT levels are observed (Belfrage et al, 1973).

In population surveys (vide infra) elevated GGT values are found in some 20 per cent of males and 15 per cent of females with admitted regular daily intakes of approximately 30 to 40 g, and some 40 per cent to 50 per cent of males and 30 per cent of females drinking 60 g or more daily (Rollason, Pincherle & Robinson, 1972; Whitfield et al, 1978).

When an alcoholic stops drinking, GGT values show a 50 per cent reduction within 2 weeks (mean 10 days) and near normal values within 5 weeks (Rosalki & Rau, 1972). More persistent elevation may be observed in the presence of underlying cirrhosis (Levi et al, 1975). The fall in GGT levels is generally exponential (Lamy et al, 1974). However, in some patients, especially when initial serum GGT levels are less than 5 times the upper limit, the fall may be delayed (Wadstein & Skude, 1979a). Sometimes a transient *increase* with hospitalisation has been noticed for serum GGT (Rosalki, 1974; Wadstein & Skude, 1979b), possibly from the effect of improved nutrition on hepatic GGT synthesis or release following admission. Serial measurements of GGT are of value in the known alcoholic for monitoring progress and therapy and claimed abstinence. Renewed drinking following normalisation from abstinence will be followed by rapid return of serum GGT activity to abnormal levels.

GGT abnormality is not specific for alcohol excess, since elevation may also result from long-standing therapeutic administration of enzyme-inducing drugs (e.g. phenobarbitone, phenytoin etc.; Rosalki, 1973), or from other hepatic disorders producing biliary statis or hepatocellular injury (Rosalki, 1975b). However, GGT elevation should always suggest the possibility of excess drinking, particularly if other evidence of liver disorder is lacking, and the rapid fall in serum GGT activity with abstinence provides useful confirmation (Lamy et al, 1976).

It should be noted that serum GGT activity normally declines during pregnancy (Rosalki, 1975) and that in patients receiving enzyme-inducing drugs, elevated GGT activity in the first trimester may revert to normal as pregnancy advances (Rosalki, 1973). A similar fall in GGT to normal with advancing pregnancy has been observed in heavy drinkers who continue to drink (Barrison et al, 1982). The recognition of excess alcohol intake in pregnancy is of special importance because of the danger to the developing fetus. GGT is only useful for this purpose if the determination is made in the first trimester.

It has been found valuable to combine GGT determination with measurement of the erythrocyte mean corpuscular volume (MCV), a measurement which can be readily carried out in the diagnostic haematology laboratory using modern automated cell counters. Chronic alcohol consumption damages the developing red cell and increases the erythrocyte volume and MCV (Herbert, Zalusky & Davidson, 1964; Wu, Chanarin & Levi, 1974). The prevalence of this abnormality (50 to 60 per cent) is lower than that of GGT, the degree of abnormality is smaller, and the response to abstinence less rapid, taking about two months to return towards normal after cessation of drinking (Baglin et al, 1976; Lamy et al, 1976). Many disorders other than alcoholism (e.g. folate or Vitamin B_{12} deficiency or non-alcohol liver disease etc.) can of course also increase MCV values (Davidson & Hamilton, 1978), though alcohol excess is now the most frequent cause of isolated MCV increase. Nevertheless, some patients with normal GGT may show MCV elevation, and in an unpublished personal study of 110 hospital in-patients and out-patients alcoholics, abnormality of one or other determination was observed in 85 per cent compared with 75 per cent for GGT alone and 50 per cent for MCV alone.

Serum transaminases and alkaline phosphatase

The activity of the serum transaminase enzymes aspartate transaminase (AST) and alanine transaminase (ALT) may be elevated as a consequence

Table 4.2 Hepatic effects of alcohol

	Clinical	Pathological
Steatosis	Hepatomegaly, tender liver	Fat infiltration
Alcoholic hepatitis	Anorexia, fever, pain, hepatomegaly ± jaundice	Cell necrosis, polymorph infiltration, alcoholic hyaline
Cirrhosis	Hepatomegaly, bleeding, jaundice, ascites, encephalopathy	Fibrosis, regeneration nodules

of hepatocellular injury, and serum alkaline phosphatase activity may be increased from cholestasis. Changes in these serum enzymes resulting from alcoholism are most conveniently considered in relation to the stage of the hepatic disorder. The clinical and histological features of each stage are summarised in Table 4.2 (see also Ch. 13).

Steatosis (*synonym: fatty liver*). This is the first stage of histologically identifiable hepatic injury from alcohol. It may be the sole histological abnormality in about 60 per cent of patients with minimal clinical liver disease (Eghaje & Juul, 1973; Carlon, Rugge & Zotti, 1976; Bruguera, Bordas & Rodes, 1977).

Hepatocellular injury from steatosis may give rise to mild elevation of serum aspartate and alanine transaminase (Bradus et al, 1963; Rosalki, 1976). On average, the incidence of elevation of these serum enzymes approximates to 40 and 20 per cent respectively. Both transaminases generally remain below four times the upper reference limit, with aspartate transaminase levels averaging twice the upper reference limit and characteristically higher than ALT (vide infra). Enzyme activity falls by approximately 50 per cent within one week of abstinence.

Cholestasis from steatosis may give rise to elevation of serum alkaline phosphatase in approximately 10 per cent of patients. In such subjects alkaline phosphatase levels remain below one and a half times the upper reference limits. The α-1 isoenzyme of alkaline phosphatase ('biliary' or kionozymic phosphatase) may be elevated in the serum even when total phosphatase levels are within normal limits (Brohult & Sunblad, 1973; Rosalki, 1974). It has been claimed that increase of the α-1-isoenzyme in serum is found in 60 per cent of alcoholics and is more sensitive than is GGT elevation (Brohult, Fridall & Sunblad), but in my experience this is not so, and it is found in only 20 per cent of alcoholic sera overall and a similar percentage in those with steatosis only (Nemesanszky et al, 1981).

Acute alcoholic hepatitis (*synonyms: alcoholic steatonecrosis, sclerosing hyaline necrosis*). This condition may follow a severe drinking bout in the pre-cirrhotic alcoholic. It occurs in approximately 30 per cent of alcoholics (Golambos, 1974; Lelbach, 1976). The biochemical features are those of cellular injury and biliary obstruction. Serum aspartate transaminase levels are raised in approximately 70 per cent and alanine transaminase in 50 per cent of patients. Aspartate transaminase levels are the higher, but both are below five times the upper reference limit.

Alkaline phosphatase levels are raised in about 40 per cent of patients. Levels are generally below two and a half times the upper reference limit though higher values are occasionally found with marked jaundice.

Alcohol cirrhosis. Approximately 10 per cent of chronic alcoholics with a history of 10 or more years daily ingestion of 160 ml (126 g) of ethanol show histological evidence of cirrhosis (Popper et al, 1974). Biochemical changes are predominantly those of chronic hepatocellular disorder.

Serum aspartate transaminase is increased in two-thirds to three-quarters of cirrhotics. Alanine transaminase is increased in 50 per cent (Rosalki, 1976; Hodgson & Thompson, 1976). Transaminase levels usually remain below five times the upper reference limit, with aspartate transaminase activity substantially higher than alanine transaminase.

Elevated alkaline phosphatase activity is found in about 50 per cent of patients overall and 75 per cent of patients with jaundice. Levels are usually below two and one-half times the upper reference limit of normal.

Effect of acute ethanol intake. Neither the transaminases nor alkaline phosphatase are significantly increased in healthy subjects with acute alcohol intakes between 0.5 and 2.0 g/kg body weight simulating social, evening or weekend drinking (Bang et al, 1958; Goldberg & Watts, 1965; Freer & Statland, 1977a,b; Shaw & Marsh, 1981) nor does modest ethanol administration (0.8 g/kg) have any significant effect on these enzymes in serum in alcoholics (Galambos, Asada & Shanks, 1963), though higher acute intake (1.5–2.0 g/kg) may cause transient increase (Bang et al, 1958).

More massive acute intakes (3–4 g/kg; Brohult et al, 1960) and more prolonged daily intakes of between 1 and 2 g/kg for two weeks (Rubin & Lieber, 1968) may double basal AST levels in healthy volunteers, and produce occasional pathological values.

Transaminase and alkaline phosphatase changes in alcoholic liver disease are summarised in Table 4.3 and compared with those for GGT. It can be seen that these enzymes are substantially less sensitive than GGT, particularly in early disease. However, since they are routinely included in liver function test profiles, are more sensitive than other procedures included therein (plasma proteins, bilirubin), and their determination may assist differentiation of alcoholic from non-alcoholic liver disease (vide infra) they remain of value for alcoholism identification.

Table 4.3 Approximate incidence of serum enzyme elevation in alcoholics

	GGT	AST	ALT	ALP
1. Steatosis	75%	40%	20%	10%
2. Alcoholic hepatitis	80%	70%	50%	40%
3. Cirrhosis (anicteric)	75%	70%	50%	50%

Enzyme ratios. The relative insensitivity of ALT and ALP when compared to AST and GGT respectively, has been used to facilitate the differentiation of alcoholic liver disease from other varieties of liver disorder with enzyme changes. One way of expressing such insensitivity has been to express enzyme values in the form of a ratio.

When AST values are moderately elevated (less than eight times are upper reference limit), AST: ALT ratios greater than 1 are found in some 80–90 per cent of patients with alcoholic steatosis, hepatitis and cirrhosis (Clermont & Chalmers, 1967; Rosalki, 1976). This may distinguish such AST elevation from that occuring in viral hepatitis, chronic active or chronic persistant hepatitis, surgical cholestatic jaundice and primary biliary cirrhosis, in which ALT greater than AST is the rule. AST: ALT ratios above 2 have been reported in approximately 70 per cent of patients with alcoholic hepatitis or active alcoholic cirrhosis (Cohen & Kaplan, 1979) whereas such ratios are infrequent (less than 30 per cent) in other chronic liver disorders.

It may be appropriate to mention also, that when AST elevation occurs in alcoholic liver disease there is a disproportionate increase in serum of the mitochondrial isoenzyme (Ishii et al, 1979) reflecting the special tendency of alcohol to cause mitochondrial damage (Lieber, 1973). Patients with mean values for total AST of approximately 1 and a half times the upper reference limit were found to have mean mitochrondrial AST approximately 4 times the upper reference limit for this isoenzyme. The mitochondrial isoenzyme may occupy 20 per cent of total AST activity, a proportion higher than is usual in non-alcoholic hepatitis or cirrhosis.

GGT : ALP ratios have also been used to differentiate alcoholic from non-alcoholic liver disease. A ratio greater than 1.4 : 1 has been reported as permitting this distinction with an efficiency of nearly 80 per cent (Lai, Ng & Hok, 1982).

It should be pointed out that enzyme activity ratios are critically dependent on methodology. Transaminase determinations are well standardised and the ratios are widely applicable. This is not the case for GGT and ALP measurement, and it is preferable to express their ratio in terms of their respective upper reference limits. When this is done, the critical differential diagnostic GGT : ALP ratio would appear to approximate to 4 : 1.

Glutamate dehydrogenase

Glutamate dehydrogenase (GDH) is a mitochondrial enzyme whose serum level may be increased following hepatic mitochondrial injury or cholestasis. Because damage to liver mitochondria is an early consequence of alcoholism (Lieber, 1973), serum GDH levels have been studied as a potential indicator of alcohol abuse. Most series report a 50–60 per cent incidence of elevation, with values averaging about twice the upper reference limit and almost all values below 5 times (Van Waes & Lieber, 1977; Mills et al, 1981; Jenkins et al, 1982). Despite the claim that serum GDH levels correlate well with the presence and severity of alcoholic hepatitis (Van Waes & Lieber, 1977) this does not appear to be so, and a similar incidence of elevation and similar serum levels are observed independent of the presence of hepatic necrosis, and in each histological class of liver disease (Mills et al, 1981; Jenkins et al, 1982). Raised serum values in early alcoholism with minimal liver biopsy changes may, in fact, in part be a consequence of induction of the enzyme by alcohol in liver mitchondria (Jenkins et al, 1982) signifying that alcohol excess may result in serum enzyme changes from induction in both microsomes (GGT) or mitochondria (GDH).

In almost all comparative studies, GDH has been shown to be less frequently abnormal than GGT. This may, in part, be a consequence of the shorter plasma half-life of GDH, for when drinking ceases, serum GDH levels fall by some 50 per cent within 48 hours (Weill J, personal communication). This rapid fall may facilitate the recognition of alcoholism, rather than some other liver disorder, as a cause of the initial elevation, but a disadvantage is the much reduced incidence compared with GGT in the alcoholic when drinking has been reduced over the week preceding the investigation (Jenkins et al, 1982). A further disadvantage of GDH is that methodology is less satisfactory.

Biochemical abnormalities resulting from the metabolic effects of alcohol on the liver

Abnormalities resulting from hepatic enzyme induction

The enzyme-inducing action of ethanol enhances the synthesis of hepatic microsomal enzymes (Lieber & de Carli, 1968). One consequence previously mentioned is elevation in serum of the hepatic enzyme γ-glutamyltransferase. Enhanced microsomal enzyme activity can also be identified by the increased clearance rate of orally administered drugs (Vessel & Page, 1969), and by increased urinary excretion of D-glucaric acid, a metabolite of the glucuronic acid pathway in the liver (Hunter et al, 1971). These abnormalities may precede evidence of histological change visible by light microscopy.

Drug clearance. Enhanced microsomal enzyme activity consequent upon chronic alcohol ingestion can result in increased clearance rates of drugs which are metabolised by the liver microsomes.

Providing appropriate radio-isotope counting equipment is available, measurement of the aminopyrine clearance is a convenient, non-invasive means of assessing enzyme induction. In this procedure the rate of hepatic metabolism of orally administered ^{14}C-labelled aminopyrine is assessed by measurement of the output of $^{14}CO_2$ in the breath. The procedure has been used in the study of alcoholics, and when cholestasis was absent (as judged by a normal serum alkaline phosphatase), a significant correlation was observed between the aminopyrine clearance and serum GGT activity in non-cirrhotic alcoholics (Lewis et al, 1977).

Despite this, and despite other indications that enzyme induction is usual in early alcoholism, measurement of aminopyrine clearance seems insensitive for its detection, with only one third of non-cirrhotic alcoholics showing increased clearance values (Lewis et al, 1977; Galizzi et al, 1978). This poor sensitivity may be because *reduced* clearance may result from acute alcohol ingestion (Audetat, Preisig & Bircher, 1977) or may follow hepato-cellular damage from alcohol. Indeed, in the presence of cirrhosis *diminished* values have been observed in some three-quarters of alcoholics (Lewis et al, 1977). Such reduction is non-specific and may be observed also with non-alcoholic liver disease.

Urinary D-glucaric acid excretion. Enzyme inducing agents are known to increase the urinary excretion of the metabolites of glucuronic acid, especially D-glucaric acid (Hunter et al, 1971). Two studies have reported the results of the measurement of D-glucaric acid in the urine of alcoholics. Spencer-Peet et al (1975) found increased urinary excretion in 56 per cent of 25 alcoholics attending an alcohol treatment centre and drinking up to the day of admission. They did not observe any correlation between urinary D-glucaric acid and serum GGT activity, the latter being elevated in 75 per cent of their subjects. Subsequently, Mezey (1976) reported increased urinary D-glucaric acid excretion in 7 hospitalised alcoholics, all consuming massive amounts of ethanol (greater than 250 g daily) up to the day before admission. The raised values in these patients were unrelated to the presence of liver disease (which is known to increase D-glucaric acid excretion), occurred despite poor food intake (which may result in diminished excretion) and returned to normal within 8 days of stopping drinking, but after 5 days of subsequent ethanol challenge (122 g of ethanol per day) urinary excretion again became raised.

Spencer-Peet and colleagues (1975) used an ion-exchange chromotographic method for D-glucaric acid measurement, while Mezey (1976) converted the glucaric acid to the lactone and used this to inhibit glucuronidase activity. The author has studied the urinary excretion of D-glucaric acid determined by a sensitive gas-chromatographic method, and has demonstrated increased urinary excretion in 35 of 37 alcoholics (Fink R, Rosalki S B, Longland R & Galgolli S, unpublished). This incidence (95 per cent) exceeded that of GGT (81 per cent) in the subjects studied and the degree of abnormality expressed as a multiple of the upper reference limit (mean approximately four times) exceeded that of serum GGT (mean approximately twice).

Other glucuronic acid metabolites (L-gulonic acid and xylitol) were also increased in the urine but less frequently than D-glucaric acid. A significant ($P < 0.05$) correlation between glucaric acid excretion and serum GGT activity was observed, suggesting enzyme induction as a common mechanism for their elevation.

Glucaric acid can be determined on 24 hour urine collections or measured on random morning specimens and related to urine creatinine concentration. Despite the high incidence of abnormality in alcoholics the determination is too complex for routine laboratory use, and the highest incidence of abnormality is found with the most complex method. Additional disadvantages are non-specificity (elevated excretion from non-alcoholic liver disease or as a consequence of exposure to other enzyme-inducing agents) and the transitory elevation following ethanol consumption.

Nevertheless, with simplified methodology the measurement might have some useful confirmatory role in detecting recent heavy alcohol intake.

α-amino-n-butyric acid: leucine ratio

In alcohol-fed experimental animals the plasma level of the amino-acid α-amino-n-butyric acid is elevated and the levels of branched-chain amino acids such as leucine are depressed. Both are diminished from poor nutrition. These observations led Shaw & colleagues (Shaw, Stimmel & Lieber, 1976) to study these amino acids in the plasma of alcoholics and use their ratio (A:L) to compensate for any nutritional abnormality. In 1976 they reported an elevated A:L ratio in 70 per cent of 42 alcoholic admissions. Such elevation was independent of nutritional state or accompanying biochemical or morphological evidence of liver damage. When measured within the first week of abstinence 89 per cent of alcoholics had a raised A:L ratio compared to 54 per cent after this time, but the determination was otherwise independent of acute alcohol intake. No patient with non-alcoholic liver disease showed an increased ratio.

In a subsequent study of 100 alcoholics within 7 days of drinking (Shaw, Lue & Lieber, 1978) the incidence of a raised A:L ratio was found to be 57 per cent. In these patients GGT elevation was observed in 74 per cent. In controls, and, in contrast to GGT, in non-alcoholic subjects with liver disease, the incidence of A:L increase was low. It was considered that the two determinations in combination could provide greater than 81 per cent sensitivity for alcoholism and that the A:L ratio was highly specific for the disorder.

The suggestions from these studies that measurement of the A:L ratio might be a sensitive and specific marker of alcoholism was promptly challenged by the work of Morgan, Milson & Sherlock (1977) who found the ratio to be both insensitive and non-specific for alcoholism. Abnormal values were found to correlate with liver damage irrespective of aetiology. Similar observations of poor sensitivity and non-specificity were subsequently reported by at least 5 other groups of workers (Dienstag et al, 1978; Ellingboe et al, 1978; Hildebrand et al, 1979; Moyer et al, 1979; Yudkoff et al, 1979). These studies showed that the increased A:L ratio occasionally observed in alcoholics results from disturbed hepatocellular function, and reported a variety of genetic, metabolic and infective disorders in which the ratio might also be raised.

Because of this poor sensitivity and specificity, quite apart from determination complexity, measurement of the A:L ratio cannot be recommended as of value in identifying the alcoholic.

Plasma protein abnormalities

Reduction in serum albumin levels is uncommon in alcoholism in the absence of cirrhosis (Pollak & Buckell, 1973; Patel & O'Gorman, 1975). In cirrhosis it is found as a non-specific abnormality in approximately 50 per cent of alcoholics (Hodgson & Thompson, 1976). Other non-specific protein changes include depression of orosomucoid, haptoglobin and transferrin levels and increased plasma concentrations of alpha-2 macroglobulin, caeruloplasmin and Immunoglubulins G, A and M (Agostoni et al, 1969; Murray-Lyon et al, 1972; Akdamar et al, 1972). Orosomucoid increase together with transferrin decrease may be found in the early stages of hepato-cellular deficiency but orosomucoid plasma concentration falls with advancing cirrhosis (Perler et al, 1983).

In contrast to other varieties of chronic liver disease, patients with alcoholic cirrhosis may show marked IgA elevation (Hobbs, 1967; Agostoni et al, 1969) with levels averaging 3 times the upper reference limit. This is found in about 60 per cent of cirrhotic alcoholics (Bailey et al, 1976). Elevation may persist for many months despite abstinence (Akdamar et al, 1972). In the non-cirrhotic alcoholic, IgA elevation is infrequent, being found in less than 30 per cent of patients, and levels remain below twice the upper reference limit (Bailey et al, 1976; Morgan et al, 1980). The combination of an increased IgA and a reduced transferrin level is particularly characteristic of alcoholic cirrhosis (Aron et al, 1971) being found in two-thirds of such patients. It is also found in one third of non-cirrhotic alcoholics and heavy drinkers (Fontan et al, 1975). The combination of modest transaminase elevation with AST greater than ALT and marked IgA elevation is also a feature of alcoholics cirrhosis. Such findings in a patient with suspect liver disorder may serve to identify alcoholism as its cause.

Plasma urate

Alcohol ingestion may increase urate synthesis (Faller & Fox, 1982), lactate formed from altered redox state resulting from alcohol intake may compete with renal tubular urate excretion (Lieber et al, 1962) and beer drinking may contribute to hyperuricaemia through its purine content (Gibson et al, 1983).

A progressive increase in plasma urate levels with alcohol consumption has been noted in males (Whitehead, Clarke & Whitfield, 1978; Whitfield et al, 1978a). In alcoholics the incidence of hyperuricaemia approximates to 40 per cent in males (Olin, Deveny & Weldon, 1973; Pollak & Buckell, 1973; Drum, Goldman & Jankowski, 1981) and a similar incidence is observed in male, but not female drinkers consuming nine or more drinks (approximately 70 g ethanol) per day (Whitfield et al, 1978a). In female alcoholics, hyperuricaemia is found in about 25 per cent. With abstinence, raised plasma urate levels may persist for several weeks (Olin, Devenyi & Weldon, 1973) or may fall more rapidly. Changes are inconstant and poorly reflect current drinking. Hyperuricaemia is not specific for alcoholism for it may result from renal disorder, drug therapy, gout etc. However, in combination with other clinical abnormalities (e.g. hypertension, Ramsay,

1979) or biochemical disturbance (e.g. increased serum enzymes) hyp uricaemia may be very suggestive of alcohol excess, and its inclusion in test profiles and discriminant functions (Whitfield et al, 1981) may enhance its diagnostic value.

Lipid abnormalities (see also Ch. 8)

The regular daily intake of more than 60 g ethanol by healthy volunteers will produce increasing levels of triglycerides and high density lipoprotein (HDL) — cholesterol and apolipoprotein A (Belfrage et al, 1973). Triglycerides start to rise within one week and HDL lipoproteins within 3–5 weeks. Single acute intakes of 3 g ethanol/kg (Brohult, Carlson & Reichard, 1960) may also produce a statistically significant increase in triglyceride levels within 3 to 10 days, and lesser intakes (1 g/kg) may increase HDL-cholesterol (Gorman & Small, 1981).

In population studies, triglyceride, HDL-cholesterol and apolipoprotein A, all correlate significantly with alcohol intake, with correlation coefficients between 0.16 and 0.3 (Castelli et al, 1973; Kreiss & Zack, 1981; Whitfield et al, 1981; Fex, Kristenson & Trell, 1982). Hypertriglyceridaemia is found in some 20 per cent of subjects regularly consuming nine or more drinks per day (Whitfield et al, 1978a).

In the recently drinking alcoholic, hypertriglyceridaemia and/or raised HDL (Danielson et al, 1978) may be found in some 60 per cent of patients, but with the development of liver disease the incidence of elevation falls (Losowsky, 1976; Kapur et al, 1980), so that overall only 30 per cent of alcoholics show plasma lipid abnormalities (Eisenbeth & Raab, 1960; Kallio, Saarimaa & Saarimaa, 1969, Morse & Hunt, 1979), generally hypertriglyceridaemia and increased HDL-cholesterol of modest degree with lipid levels below twice the upper reference limit. With abstinence, elevated triglyceride levels fall to normal within one to two weeks (Chait et al, 1972) though they may increase within a few hours of relapse. HDL levels also usually return to normal within one to two weeks (Johansson & Medhus, 1974).

The fact that lipid abnormalities are short-lived, show only a moderate incidence of elevation in alcoholics, and are non-specific, being elevated in both primary hyperlipidaemia and other secondary hyperlipidaemias (e.g. from diabetes, oral contraceptive therapy etc.), detracts from their value for alcoholism detection. However, triglyceride measurements are readily performed and routinely carried out for the investigation of suspect hyperlipidaemia. HDL-cholesterol is increasingly measured as a risk factor for coronary artery disease. Since alcohol ingestion is one of the most frequent causes of secondary hyperlipidaemia (Chait et al, 1972) alcohol excess should be suspected whenever lipid abnormality (especially a raised triglyceride) is found on medical examination. Again, the combination of lipid abnormality with other biochemical disturbance, e.g. enzyme changes, hyperuricaemia etc., increases the likelihood of alcohol excess, and the inclusion of lipid tests may improve the diagnostic performance of biochemical discriminant functions for alcohol diagnosis.

Biochemical abnormalities mainly independent of the hepatic effects of alcohol

Erythrocyte δ-amino-laevulinic acid dehydratase

The erythrocyte enzyme δ-amino-laevulinic acid dehydratase (DALD) catalyses the formation of porpho-bilinogen from δ-amino laevulinic acid in the porphyrin biosynthetic pathway. In intoxicated males attending a casualty department, Moore et al (1971) observed the activity of this enzyme to be inversely correlated (correlation coefficient r = 0.86) with blood ethanol concentration, significant depression of erythrocyte DALD activity being observed at a mean blood ethanol level of 225 mg/dl (49 mmol/l). In two healthy volunteers, acute ethanol administration resulted in rapid depression of erythrocyte DALD with a trough at two hours, coinciding with a peak of blood ethanol of 150 mg/dl (33 mmol/l) and returning to normal at 10 hours, by which time ethanol had disappeared from the blood.

In a subsequent study of 37 alcoholics examined within 48 hours of admission and with no alcohol in their blood at the time, these workers observed the erythrocyte enzyme to be reduced in 95 per cent (Moore & Goldberg, 1975). One week later none of the subjects studied showed subnormal erythrocyte DALD activity. In alcoholics on treatment, the erythrocyte enzyme activity was also noticed to increased with abstinence, but to diminish with relapse.

In contrast to this high incidence of subnormal levels, Hamlyn, Hopper & Skillen (1979) observed depression of erythrocyte DALD in only 38 per cent of chronic alcoholics with liver disease attending a liver clinic. Moore & Goldberg (1975) had reported the test to be more sensitive than GGT (95 per cent incidence of elevation of DALD compared with 63 per cent for GGT), but in the patients of Hamlyn and coworkers, GGT was the more sensitive (68 per cent elevation for GGT compared with 38 per cent for DALD). Unlike GGT, however, a change in erythrocyte enzyme activity was only occasionally seen in patients with non-alcoholic liver disease, nine per cent of whom showed reduced values.

The lability of erythrocyte DALD demands that special attention is paid to sample collection, and immediate examination of blood samples is required. Because of this, because of inconvenient methodology and because sensitivity to chronic alcohol ingestion has not been confirmed, the determination has so far found little application in the diagnostic laboratory for the recognition or confirmation of alcoholism. A further disadvantage is that exposure to toxic environmental compounds (e.g. lead) also may depress erythrocyte DALD activity.

Superoxide dismutase

Increased concentration of the erythrocyte enzyme cupro-zinc superoxide dismutase determined by radioimmunoassay has been reported in 13 of 19 (68 per cent) black alcoholics (Del Villano et al, 1979). It was suggested that the superoxide radical resulting from oxidation of acetaldehyde formed from ethanol induces the synthesis of the enzyme.

Since the enzyme was not found to be increased in the erythrocytes of white alcoholics and confirmatory reports are lacking, the determination appears to be of only limited value for the identification of alcoholism.

Minor haemoglobins

Erythrocyte hemolysates from alcoholics have been shown to have an increased concentration of a minor haemoglobin of rapid migration on cation exchange resin chromatography (Stevens et al, 1981). This increase in concentration of one of the components of the minor haemoglobins, haemoglobin A1 a–c, was observed in 8 out of 10 alcoholics and believed to be a consequence of adduct formation between haemoglobin and circulating acetaldehyde in these patients. Glycosylated haemoglobin was not elevated and haemoglobin Alc determined by immunoassay was reduced. The measurement of such haemoglobin adducts with acetaldehyde has been suggested as a marker of potential value in screening for alcoholism. However, its value for this purpose awaits confirmation.

Serum iso-transferrin

It has long been recognised that reduction in the serum protein transferrin occurs when alcoholism is complicated by hepatic cirrhosis (vide supra). More recently it has been claimed (Stibler, Borg & Allgulander, 1979) that a so-called micro-heterogenous component (iso-transferrin) of serum transferrin detectable by immuno-fixation following isoelectrophoretic focussing, and recognisable by its slightly more alkaline isoelectric point (pI 5.7) compared to the main transferrin component (pI 5.4), might be a marker of alcoholism. This component was observed in the serum of 81 per cent of patients with recent alcohol consumption (i.e. during the preceding three weeks) of greater than 60 g of ethanol per day. It was not seen in patients with liver disease of non-alcoholic origin, or in non-drinking controls. In the alcoholics, the serum transferrin pattern reverted to normal within 10 days of abstinence. The iso-transferrin was also observed to appear after the fifth day in volunteers consuming 0.6 g per kg body weight daily. It did not appear in response to acute heavy isolated ethanol consumption. Despite the obvious attraction of this investigation as a marker for drinking, i.e. high sensitivity and specificity indicated by this study, the laboratory technique required for its demonstration is complex and it also must be pointed out that independent confirmation is awaited.

Biochemical abnormalities in patient screening for alcoholism

In patients attending hospitals and alcohol treatment centres, alcoholism is likely to be associated with very high ethanol intakes and accompanied by organ damage. In consequence, a high incidence of biochemical abnormalities is to be anticipated and, as previously noted, has been observed. It is however, of importance to be able to assess the ability of test procedures to identify alcoholism in less severely affected individuals, e.g. those attending for general practitioner consultation, and to detect potentially harmful levels of drinking in the general population.

General practitioner attenders

In the author's original study (Rosalki et al, 1970), plasma enzymes and liver function tests were measured in a 'double-blind' study of 522 consecutive patients, the vast majority of whom were out-patients attending a London private general medical practice. The determination showing the highest incidence of abnormality, GGT, was able to detect 37 of the 50 known alcoholics in the patient population i.e. a test sensitivity (positivity in disease) of 74 per cent in a population with a prevalence of alcoholism of 9.6 per cent, and was abnormal in a further 56 non-alcoholics (i.e. specificity or negativity in non-disease, 88 per cent). For the patients showing a raised GGT, alcoholism was its cause in 40 per cent (i.e. predictive value of a positive test or PV + was 40 per cent) whereas alcoholism was absent from 97 per cent of patients with a normal GGT (i.e. predictive value of a negative test or PV – was 97 per cent).

In a subsequent 'double-blind' study (Baxter et al, 1981), serum enzymes, erythrocyte MCV and liver function tests were examined as potential screening tests for alcoholism in 200 randomly selected Health Service patients attending two London general practice surgeries. Patients were divided by questionnaire, sociologist's interview and physician consultation into two groups, with excessive alcohol intake (regular drinking of 80 g per day, or 40 g per day plus frequent binge drinking of 120 g per day) considered as 'likely' or 'unlikely'. In 52 of the 200 patients excessive drinking was considered likely. Abnormal raised values were observed in 44 per cent of such subjects for GGT, 16 per cent for MCV and 10 per cent for AST in the drinking likely group. The most sensitive test, GGT, showed a sensitivity of 44 per cent, a specificity of 84 per cent, a PV + of 50 per cent, and a PV – of 81 per cent. Exclusion of subjects with known non-alcohol-related disorders capable of yielding GGT increase (e.g. liver disease, enzyme-inducing drug therapy) increased the specificity from 81 per cent to 93 per cent and the PV + from 50 to 64 per cent.

The results of breath alcohol measurements in patients attending general practitioner surgeries (Wiseman et al, 1982) have been considered previously (vide supra). Sensitivity for problem drinking appears to approximate to 20 to 40 per cent, with a PV + of 50 per cent.

'Well-patient' screening

Using a computerised questionnaire to evaluate alcohol consumption in over 200 males attending a private health screening centre Rollason and colleagues (Rollason, Pincherle & Robinson, 1972) observed a significant correlation between GGT, AST, ALP and alcohol intake. The strongest correlation with alcohol consumption and the highest incidence of test abnormality was found with GGT, which was raised in 47 per cent of those regularly consuming more than six drinks a day (21 per cent of those screened) but in only 12 per cent of social drinkers.

A progressive increase in GGT, AST serum urate and MCV with increasing alcohol consumption in over 2000 healthy males was also observed by Whitehead and colleagues (Whitehead, Clarke & Whitfield, 1978). Once again GGT was the most frequently elevated enzyme being increased in 14.9 per cent of subjects compared with eight per cent for AST. In more than three quarters of subjects with a raised GGT this was believed to be related to alcohol consumption.

Whitfield and colleagues in Australia (Whitfield et al, 1978a; 1978b), reported results of a very extensive study of more than 4500 males, and 3300 women attending a multi-phasic health testing centre, and related laboratory results to answers to a questionnaire on the frequency of drinking and the number of drinks consumed per day. GGT, AST, triglyceride, urate and MCV levels were all correlated with drinking habits. For males consuming nine or more drinks daily (approximately 70 g alcohol), GGT was abnormal in 44 per cent, AST in 23 per cent, urate in 38 per cent, triglycerides in 20 per cent and MCV in 35 per cent. For females the corresponding figures were 28 per cent, 11 per cent, 0 per cent, 11 per cent and 16 per cent respectively. For a given frequency and degree of drinking, men showed more abnormality than women for each test studied. With increasing test abnormality, the probability of regular daily consumption of six or more drinks showed a steady increase, and the probability of admitting drinking at this level was 25 per cent for males with GGT values 87.5 per cent of the upper reference limit, compared with two per cent with values 12.5 per cent of the upper reference limit. In the population as a whole, 14 per cent of men and three per cent of women regularly consumed six or more drinks a day.

Bagrel and colleagues (Bagrel et al, 1979) examined GGT, ALT, urea, urate, iron and mean corpuscular volume in nearly 4000 men aged between 20 and 64 attending a Centre for Preventive Medicine in France. All the variables showed a significant correlation with alcohol consumption but this was greatest for GGT and MCV. The correlation for the former reaching 0.36 in subjects aged 30 to 49.

Correlation co-efficients between GGT and alcohol consumption similar to those reported by Bagrel were also observed by Chick and colleagues (Chick, Kreitman & Plant, 1981), from self-reporting of alcohol intake admitted at interview by 266 company directors and 222 manual workers involved in alcohol production. The correlation coefficient in the former group being 0.31 and in the latter 0.42. In subjects admitting to the consumption of more than 450 kg of alcohol per week (64 g per day) GGT had a sensitivity of approximately 50 per cent and a specificity averaging 85 per cent. The sensitivity of GGT was twice that of MCV. It may be noted that nearly 16 per cent of the combined population admitted to consuming more than 450 g of alcohol per week.

It is clear from these population screening studies that many biochemical variables show significant correlation with alcohol intake and an increasing incidence of abnormality and higher values with alcohol consumption.

Of the variables studied, GGT shows the greatest incidence of abnormality, and at levels of alcohol consumption at which an increased incidence of alcohol related disease commences (60 g or more per day) a sensitivity for alcohol excess of 40 to 50 per cent in males may be anticipated, with a specificity of more than 80 per cent, and with at least 50 per cent of abnormal screening values related to drinking. For females sensitivity is reduced by approximately 10 per cent.

Test combinations

The combination of several tests may yield a greater incidence of abnormality in alcoholics and heavy drinkers than each test individually. Mention has already been made of the value of using GGT and MCV in combination, resulting in abnormality of one or other in 85 per cent of 110 alcoholics studied by the author compared with 75 per cent for GGT alone, and 50 per cent for MCV alone.

In addition to increased sensitivity, tests used in combination can increase diagnostic specificity. For example, a raised GGT together with hypertriglyceridaemia and hyperuricemia would be very suggestive of alcoholism and (as previously described) increased AST : ALT ratios, especially with IgA elevation, or an increased GGT : ALP ratio, may serve to differentiate alcoholic from non-alcoholic liver disease, as may a raised plasma GGT:urea ratio (Bagrel et al, 1978), since hepatic urea synthesis may be reduced from ethanolic liver disease whilst GGT is elevated.

More sophisticated mathematical treatment of multiple laboratory test values has also been used to identify heavy drinking and to distinguish alcoholic from non-alcoholic disease. One technique has been to use discriminant function analysis, an allocation procedure which uses data from defined disease groups to produce weighting factors for tests and derive a discriminant which minimises within-group differences and maximises between-group differences. Chalmers and colleagues (1981) used discriminant function analysis of liver function tests, uric acid and MCV to distinguish between 265 male and female patients (mainly in-patients) with alcohol-related diseases drinking more than 80 g of alcohol a day, 133 gastroenterology out-patients drinking less than 20 g of alcohol a day and

104 patients with a variety of non-alcoholic liver diseases. The best discriminant was derived by combination of GGT, ALP and MCV. Using this discriminant, for women, 92 per cent of the high alcohol group, 100 per cent of the low alcohol group and 187 per cent of the non-alcoholic liver disease group were correctly allocated. For men, the corresponding figures were 80 per cent, 100 per cent and 71 per cent. Overall, more than 80 per cent of patients were correctly allocated.

Eckardt and colleagues (1981) used quadratic discriminant analysis to distinguish between 121 male alcoholic hospital in-patients and 130 male alcoholic out-patients. They studied 18 commonly requested biochemical tests measured on a multi-channel analyser, together with GGT and MCV. GGT and MCV in combination correctly categorised patients with 77 per cent accuracy, whereas the 10 other best tests (liver function tests, urea and electrolytes) used in combination resulted in greater than 95 per cent accuracy.

In a subsequent study these workers (Ryback et al, 1982) used quadratic discriminant analysis of a battery of 25 biochemical and haematological tests (but excluding GGT) to distinguish 51 hospitalised male patients with biopsy confirmed alcoholic liver disease from 57 males with non-alcoholic liver disease. Discriminant analysis correctly classified 96 per cent of patients in the former group and 89 per cent in the latter. These percentages reducing to 92 per cent and 80 per cent respectively using the nine best test variables (particularly liver function tests, urea, blood glucose and the erythrocyte and leucocyte count). A near identical accuracy of classification was obtained using the AST : ALT ratio alone. However, when used prospectively in 18 cases, approximately 80 per cent of patients in both alcoholic and non-alcoholic groups were correctly classified by the previously derived discriminant, whereas the AST : ALT ratio correctly identified only 75 per cent of the former and only 33 per cent of the latter.

Whitfield et al (1981) used multi-variate regression analysis of biochemical data from more than three and half thousand subjects attending their Australian multi-phasic health testing centre in order to assess alcohol consumption. They examined 16 biochemical tests together with MCV determination and confirmed their previous observations based on univariate analysis (Whitfield et al, 1975a,b) that GGT, AST, triglycerides, uric acid and MCV values were most closely correlated with consumption (highest for GGT, correlation 0.355 men and 0.203 for women, and MCV, 0.388 for men, 0.335 for women), but found an even greater relationship to heavy drinking when these tests were combined to form a multi-variate predictor. Using a multi-variate predictor derived from GGT, MCV and uric acid in males, and GGT and MCV in women the correlation improved to 0.476 and 0.364 respectively.

An assessment was made of the sensitivity and specificity of the various test procedures at test values giving a 50 per cent probability of heavy drinking, defined as the daily regular consumption of more than 90 ml (70 g) of ethanol in the male population. The prevalence of this being 9.5 per cent. GGT showed the highest sensitivity (80 per cent) and specificity (55 per cent) of all the individual tests examined. For comparison, the multi-variate predictor showed a sensitivity of 92 per cent and a specificity of 55 per cent.

Papoz and colleagues (1981) also applied multivariate analysis to 995 healthy subjects, (604 males and 391 females) attending at centres of preventive medicine for routine check-up. GGT and MCV values showed correlations with alcohol consumption of 0.35 and 0.34 respectively in males and 0.24 and 0.21 in females. Multiple regression analysis confirmed the superiority of GGT over MCV as a laboratory marker of alcohol intake and its superior performance in males, but also showed the advantage of using these tests in combination (multiple regression coefficient 0.45 for males and 0.30 for females). The lower sensitivity of GGT in females to modest levels of alcohol consumption in population studies may be due to depression of hepatic GGT enzyme induction from alcohol by female sex hormones, particularly estrogens. In alcoholics with higher levels of consumption, liver damage may result in an incidence of GGT abnormality in females which equals or exceeds that in males (vide supra).

CONCLUSIONS

This chapter has reviewed the biochemical procedures that have been used to identify chronic alcohol excess. The approximate incidence of abnormality of the more important of these is summarised in Table 4.4. Of the various diagnostic procedures serum γ-glutamyltransferase activity determination combines greatest convenience and sensitivity and is the most valuable individual procedure. Its diagnostic value is enhanced by its combination with other simple biochemical measurements routinely carried out by the diagnostic laboratory, particularly plasma enzymes included in routine liver function tests and uric acid and triglyceride determination. Measurement of ethanol in breath and MCV measurement by the haematology laboratory are simple determinations which are additionally helpful. Test combinations enhance both sensitivity and specificity and alcoholics

Table 4.4 Approximate incidence of biochemical test abnormalities in alcoholics

1. Enzymes	GGT (<75%); GGT: urea (<75%) AST (<70%); GDH (<70%) DALD (>40%)
2. Metabolites	Uric acid (<40%); TG/HDL (<30%) A : L (<70%); D-glucaric acid (>60%)
3. Proteins	IgA (<60%); IgA: transferrin (<60%) Isotransferrins (<80%); Haemoglobin adducts (<80%)
4. Ethanol	Blood/urine/breath (<50%)

No mention of osmolality

have been identified with an accuracy of greater than 80 per cent thereby. More complex and exotic measurements seem to add little to diagnosis.

REFERENCES

Agostoni A, Vergani C, Stabilini R, Marasini B 1969 Determination of seven serum proteins in alcoholic cirrhosis. Clinica Chimica Acta 26: 351–355

Akdamar K, Epps A C, Maumus L T, Sparks R D 1972 Immunoglobulin changes in liver disease. Annals of the New York Academy of Sciences 197: 101–107

Annals of Internal Medicine 1972 Criteria for the Diagnosis of Alcoholism 77: 249–258

Aron E, Baglin M C, Larmy J, Weill J 1977 Le depistage de la consommation alcoolique chronique excessive et le controle du sevrage. Semaine Hopital Paris 53: 1503–1509

Aron E, Lamy J N, Lamy L, Weill J D 1971 Presse Medicale 79: 8

Audetat V, Preisig R, Bircher R 1977 Der Aminopyrin-Atem test unter akuter Athanoleinwerkung. Schweizerische Medizinische Wochenschrift 107: 231–235

Baglin M D, Bernot J L, Bremond J L, Lamy J, Leroux M E, Weill J 1976 Efficacite comparée du volume globulaire moyen VGM et de la gammaglutamyltransferase (GT) sérique comme tests de triage des buveurs excessifs d'alcool. Clinica Chimica Acta 68: 321–326

Bagrel A, D'Houtaud A, Gueguen R, Siest G 1978 Rapport GGT/urée: indice de consommation alcoolique. Revue d'alcoolisme 24: 99–102

Bagrel A, Houtaud, Gueguen R, Siest G 1979 Relations between reported alcohol consumption and certain biological variables in an 'unselected' population. Clinical Chemistry 25: 1242–1246

Bailey M B, Haberman P W, Steinberg J 1969 Millbank Memorial Fund Quarterly 47: 235

Bailey R J, Krasner N, Eddleston A L W F, Williams R, Tee D E H, Doniach D, Kennedy L A, Batchelor J R 1976 Histocompatibility antigens, autoantibodies and immunoglobulins in alcoholic liver disease. British Medical Journal 2: 272–729

Bang W V, Iversen K, Jagt T, Madsen S 1958 Serum glutamic-oxaloacetate transaminase activity in acute and chronic alcoholism. Journal of the American Medical Association 168: 156–160

Barrison J G, Wright J T, Sampson B, Norris N F, Murray Lyon I M 1982 Screening for alcohol abuse in pregnancy. British Medical Journal 285: 1315

Baxter S, Fink R, Leader A R, Rosalki S B 1980 Laboratory tests for excessive alcohol consumption evaluated in general practice. British Journal on Alcohol and Alcoholism 15: 164–166

Belfrage P, Berg B, Cronholm T, Elmquist D, Hagerstrand I, Johansson B, Nilsson-Ehle P, Norden G, Sjovall J, Wiebe T 1973 Prolonged administration of ethanol to young healthy volunteers. Effects on biochemical, morphological and neurophysiological parameters. Acta Medica Scandinavica Supplement 552: 5–44

Boone D J, Routh J I, Schrantz R 1974 γ-glutamyltranspeptidase and 5′ nucleotidase. American Journal of Clinical Pathology 61: 321–327

Bradus S, Korn R J, Chomet B, West M, Zimmerman H J 1963 Hepatic function and serum enzyme levels in association with fatty metamorphosis of the liver. American Journal of Science 246: 69–75

Brohult J, Sundblad L 1973 Isoenzyme paterns of serum alkaline phosphatase in ethanol-induced liver injury. Acta Medica Scandinavica 195: 497

Brohult J, Carlson L A, Reichard H 1960 Serum enzyme activities, cholesterin and triglycerides after acute intake of alochol. Scandinavian Journal of Clinical and Laboratory Investigation, Supplement 92: 82–83

Brohult J, Fridell E, Sundbland L 1977 Studies on alkaline phosphatase isoenzymes, relation to γ-glutamyltransferase and lactate dehydrogenase isoenzymes. Clinica Chimica Acta 76: 205–211

Bruguera M, Bordas J, Rodes J 1977 Asymptomatic liver disease in alcoholics. Archives of Pathology and Laboratory Medicine 101: 644–647

Carlon G, Rugge M, Zotti S 1976 La epatite alcoolica minima. Lab III, 2: 195–211

Castelli W P, Doyle J T, Gordon T, Hames C G, Hjortland M L, Hulley S B, Kagan A, Zukel W J, 1977 Alcohol and Blood Lipids. Lancet 2: 153–155

Chait A, Mancini M, February A W, Lewis B 1972 Clinical and metabolic study of alcoholic hyperlipidaemia. Lancet 2: 62–64

Chalmers D M, Rinsler M G, MacDermott S, Spicer C C, Levi A J 1981 Biochemical and haematological indicator of excessive alcohol consumption. gut 22: 992–996

Chick J, Kreitman N, Plant M 1981 Mean cell volume and gamma-glutamyl-transpeptidase as markers of drinking in working men. Lancet 1: 1249–1251

Clermont R J, Chalmers T C 1967 The transaminase tests in liver disease. Medicine 46: 197–207

Cohen J A, Kaplan M M 1979 The SGOT/SGPT ratio — an indicator of alcoholic liver disease Digestive Diseases and Sciences 24: 835–838

Danielson B, Ekman R, Fex G, Johansson B G, Kristensson H, Nillsen-Ehle B, Wadstein J 1978 Changes in plasma high-density lipoproteins in chronic male alcoholics during and after abuse. Scandinavian Journal of Clinical and Laboratory Investigation 38: 113–119

Davidson R J L, Hamilton P J 1978 High mean red cell volume: its incidence and significance in routine haematology. Journal of Clinical Pathology 31: 493–498

Del Villano B C, Tischfield J A, Schacter L P Stilwil D, Miller S I 1979 Cupro-zinc superoxide dismutase: a possible biologic marker for alcoholism (studies in Black patients). Alcoholism Clinical and Experimental Research 3: 291–296

Dienstag J L, Carter E A, Wands J R, Isselbacher K J, Fischer J E 1978 Plasma α-amino-n-butyric acid to leucine ratio: nonspecificity as a marker for alcoholism. Gastroenterology 75: 561–565

Drum D E, Goldman P A, Jankowski C B 1981 Elevation of serum uric acid as a clue to alcohol abuse. Archives of Internal Medicine 141: 477–479

Dunbar J A, Hagart J, Martin B, Ogston S, Devgun M S 1982 Drivers, binge drinking and gammaglutamyltranspeptidase. British Medical Journal, 285: 1083

Eckardt M J, Ryback R S, Rawlings R R, Graubard B I 1981 Biochemical diagnosis of alcoholism: a test of the discriminatory capabilities of γ-glutamyltranspeptidase and mean corpuscular volume. Journal of the American Medical Association 246: 2707–2710

Eghoje K N, Juhl E 1973 Factors determining liver damage in chronic alcoholics. Scandinavian Journal of Gastroenterology 8: 505–512

Eisenbeth R, Raab J 1960 L'hyperlipidémies alcooliques. Archives des Maladies de l'appareil digestif et de la Nutrition 79: 572–579

Ellingboe J, Mendelson J H, Varanelli C C, Neuberger O, Borysow M 1978 Plasma alpha amino-n-butyric acid: leucine ratio. Normal values in alcoholics. Journal of Studies on Alcohol 39: 1467–1476

Faller J, Fox I H 1982 Ethanol-induced hyperuricemia: evidence for increased urate production by activation of adenine nucleotide turnover. New England Journal of Medicine 307: 1598–1602

Fex G, Kristenson H, Trell E 1982 Correlations of serum lipids and lipoptoteins with gamma-glutamyltransferase and attitude to alcohol consumption. Annals of Clinical Biochemistry 19: 345–349

Fink R, Marjot D H, Rosalki S B 1979 Detection of alcoholic cardiomyopathy by serum enzyme and isoenzyme determination. Annals of Clinical Biochemistry 16: 165–166

Fontan M, Caridroct M, Taine D, Miens C L, Weiss D, Nowaczy T H 1974 Approche biologique enzymatique en particulier du diagnostic precoce de l'alcoolisme chronique. Proceedings of the colloqium, Early diagnosis of alcoholism. Boehringer, Mannheim

Freer D E, Statland D E 1977a The effects of ethanol (0.75 g/kg body weight) on the activities of selected enzymes in sera of healthy young adults. 1. Intermediate-term effects. Clinical Chemistry 23: 830–834

Freer D E, Statland B E 1977b Effects of ethanol (0.75 g/kg body weight) on the activities of selected enzymes in sera of healthy young adults: 2. Inter-individual variations in response of γ-glutamyltransferase to repeated ethanol challenges. Clinical Chemistry 23: 2099–2101

Galambos J T 1974 Alcoholic hepatitis. In: Schaffner F, Sherlock S, Levy C M (eds) The liver and its diseases. Intercontinental Medical Book Co, New York, p 255–267

Galambos J T, Asada M, Shanks J Z 1963 The effect of intravenous ethanol on serum enzymes in patients with normal or diseased liver. Gastroenterology 44: 267–274

Galbraith S, Murray W R, Patel A R, Knill-Jones R 1976 The relationship between alcohol and head injury and its effect on the conscious level. British Journal of Surgery 63: 128–130

Galizzi J, Morgan M Y, Chitranakroh A, Sherlock S 1978 The detection of minimal alcoholic liver disease by three methods. Scandinavian Journal of Gastroenterology 13: 827–831
Gibson T, Rodgers A V, Simmonds H A, Court-Brown F, Todd E, Meilton V 1983 A controlled study of diet in patients with gout. Annals Rheumatic Diseases 42: 123–127
Goldberg D, Watts C 1965 Serum enzyme changes as evidence of liver reaction to oral alcohol. Gastroenterology 49: 256–261
Gorman L S, Small B 1981 Calculated risk factor changes using moderate ethanol ingestion. Clinical Chemistry 27: 1044
Hamlyn A N, Brown A J, Sherlock S, Baron D N 1975 Casual blood ethanol estimations in patients with chronic liver disease. Lancet 2i: 345–347
Hamlyn A N, Hopper J C, Skillen A W 1979 Assessment of erythrocyte γ-aminolaevulinate dehydratase for out-patient detection of alcoholic liver disease: comparison with γ-glutamyltransferase and casual blood ethanol. Clinica Chimica Acta 95: 453–459
Herbert V, Zalusky R, Davidson C S 1964 Correlation of folate deficiency with alcoholism and associated macrocytosis, anaemia and liver disease. Annals of Internal Medicine 58: 977–988
Hilderbrand R L, Hervig L K, Conway T L, Ward H W, Markland F S 1979 Alcohol intake, ratio of plasma alpha-amino-n-butyric acid to leucine and gamma glutamyl transpeptidase in non-alcoholics. Journal of Studies on Alcohol 40: 902–905
Hobbs J R 1967 Serum proteins in disease. Proceedings of the Royal Society of Medicine 60: 1250–1254
Hodgson H J F, Thompson R P H 1976 Cirrhosis in South London. Lancet 2i: 118–121
Holt S, Stewart I C, Dixon J M J, Elton R A, Taylor T V, Little K 1980 Alcohol and the emergency service patient. British Medical Journal 281: 638–640
Hunter J, Maxwell J D, Carella M, Stewart D A, Williams R 1971 Urinary D-glucaric acid excretion as a test for hepatic enzyme induction in man. Lancet 1: 572–575
Ishii H, Kanno T, Shigeta Y, Takagi S, Yasuraoka S Kano S, Takeshita E, Tsuchiya M 1976 Hepatic gamma glutamyl transpeptidase activity; Its activation by chronic ethanol administration. Gastroenterology 71: 913
Ishii H, Okuno F, Shigeta Y, Tsuchiya M 1979 Enhanced serum glutamic oxaloacetic transaminase activity of mitochondrial origin in chronic alcoholism. In: Galanter M (ed) Currents in alcoholism V. Grune & Stratton, New York, p 101–108
Jenkins W J, Rosalki S B, Foo Y, Scheuer P J, Nemesanszky E, Sherlock S 1982 Serum glutamate dehydrogenase is not a reliable marker of liver cell necrosis in alcoholism. Journal of Clinical Pathology 35: 207–210
Johansson B G, Medhus A 1974 Increase in plasma α lipoproteins in chronic alcoholics after acute abuse. Acta Medica Scandinavia 195: 273–277
Kallio V, Saarima H, Saarima A 1969 Serum lipids and postprandial lipaemia in alcoholics after a drinking bout. Quarterly Journal of Studies alcoholics after a drinking bout. Quarterly Journal of Studies of Alcohol 30: 565–569
Kapur B M, Holt S, Blake J, Orrego H 1980 HDL-cholesterol in alcoholics with liver disease. Clinical Chemistry 26: 966
Kreiss K, Zack M 1981 Alcohol consumption and high-density lipoprotein cholesterol. New England Journal of Medicine 304: 539
Lai C L, Ng R P, Lok A S F 1982 The diagnostic value of the ratio of serum gamma glutamyl transpeptidase to alkaline phosphatase in alcoholic liver disease. Scandinavian Journal of Gastroenterology 17: 41–47
Lamy J, Aron E, Bernot J L, Weill J 1976 GGTP activity as a test for the diagnosis of excessive alcohol intake. In: Siest G, Young D S (eds) Drug interference and drug measurement in clinical chemistry. Karger, Basel, p 42–47
Lamy J, Baglin M C, Ferrant J P, Weill J 1974 Diminution de la γ-glutamyltranspeptidase sérique des ethyliques a la suite du sevrage. Clinica Chimica Acta 56: 169–173
Lelbach W K 1976 Epidemiology of alcoholic liver disease. In: Popper H, Schaffner F (eds) Progress in liver disease 5. Grune & Stratton, New York, p 494–515
Levi A J, Chalmers D M 1978 Recognition of alcoholic liver disease in a district general hospital. Gut 19: 521–525
Levy A J, Chanarin I, Slavin G, Wu A 1975 Biochemical and haematological indices of excess alcohol consumption. Les Colloques de l'Institut National de la Santé et de la Recherche Médicale INSERM/MRC 54: 81–86

Lewis K O, Nicholson, G, Lance P, Paton A 1977 Aminopyrine breath test in alcoholic liver disease and in patients on enzyme-inducing drugs Journal of Clinical Pathology 30: 1040–1043
Lieber C S 1973 Hepatic and metabolic effect of alcohol (1966–1973) Gastroenterology 65: 821–846
Lieber C S, de Carli L M 1968 Ethanol oxidation by hepatic microcomes: adaptive increase after ethanol feeding. Science 162: 917–918
Lieber C S, Jones D P, Losowsky M S, Davidson C S 1962 Interrelation of uric acid and ethanol metabolism in man. Journal of Clinical Investigation 41: 1863–1870
Losowsky M S, Jones D P, Davidson C S, Lieber C S 1963 Studies of alcoholic hyperlipidemia and its mechanism. American Journal of Medicine 35: 794–803
Mayer E D, Caprioli J, Wiles J, McMenamy R H, Border J R, Cirra F B 1979 ABU/LEU as an indicator of liver function in sepsis. Clinical Chemistry 25: 114
Mezey E 1976 Increased excretion of D-glucaric acid in alcoholism. Research Communications in Chemical Pathology and Pharmacology 15: 735–742
Mills P R, Spooner R J, Russell R I, Boyle P, MacSween R N M 1981 Serum glutamate dehydrogenase as a marker of hepatocyte necrosis in alcoholic liver disease. British Medical Journal 283: 754–755
Moore M R, Beattie A D, Thompson G G, Goldberg A 1971 Depression of aminolaevulinic acid dehydrase activity by ethanol in man and rat. Clinical Science 40: 81–88
Moore M R, Goldberg A 1975 Some biochemical responses to ethanol in man. Anglo-French Symposium on Alcoholism IMSERM/MRC 54: 101–116
Morgan M Y, Milson J P, Sherlock S 1977 Ratio of plasma α-amino-n-butyric acid to leucine as an empirical marker of alcoholism. Science 197: 1183–1185
Morgan M Y, Ross M G R, Ng C M, Adams D M, Thomas H C, Sherlock S 1980 HLA-B8, immunoglobulins and antibody responses in alcohol-related liver disease. Journal of Clinical Pathology 33: 488–492
Morse R M, Hunt R D 1979 Screening for alcoholism. Journal of the American Medical Association 242: 2688–2690
Murray-Lyon I M, Clarke H G M, McPherson K, Williams R 1972 Quantitative immunoelectrophoresis of serum proteins in cryptogenic cirrhosis, alcoholic cirrhosis and active chronic hepatitis. Clinica Chimica Acta 39: 215–220
Nemesanszky E, Rosalki S B, Foo A Y, Jenkins W, Scheuer P J, Sherlock S 1981 Detection of organ injury due to ethanol by serum enzyme and isoenzyme examination. Journal of Clinical Chemistry and Clinical Biochemistry 19: 782
Northcote R J, Martin B J, Scullion H, Reilly D J 1983 Changing pattern of alcohol abuse in female acute medical admissions. British Medical Journal 286: 1702–1703
Olin J S, Derenyi P, Weldon K L 1973 Uric acid in alcoholics. Quarterly Journal of Studies of Alcohol 34: 1202–1207
Orrego H, Blendis L M, Blake J E, Kapur B M, Israel Y 1979 Reliability of assessment of alcohol intake based on personal interviews in a liver clinic. Lancet 2i: 1354–1376
Papoz L, Warnet J M, Pequignot G, Eschwege E, Claude J R, Schwartz D 1981 Alcohol consumption in a healthy population: Relationship to γ-glutamyltransferase activity and mean corpuscular volume. Journal of the American Medical Association 245: 1748–1751
Patel S, O'Gorman P 1975 Serum enzyme levels in alcoholism and drug dependency. Journal of Clinical Pathology 28: 414–417
Perler C, Chanson A, Engler R, Frey J 1983 Evolutionary changes in acute-phase proteins in alcoholic hepatocellular diseases. Clinical Chemistry 29: 45–47
Phillips M, Vandervoort R E, Becker C E 1980 A sweat test for alcohol consumption. In: Seixas F A (ed) Currents in alcohol 3. Grune & Stratton, New York, p 505–514
Plaquet R, Baillet J, Rogez J C, Hennin H 1974 La gamma-glutamyl-transpeptidase (GGT) dans le profil enzymatique de l'alcoolique chronique. Proceedings of colloquium, Early diagnosis of alcoholism, Paris. Boehringer, Mannheim
Pollak B,Buckell M 1973 Abnormal laboratory tests in the alcoholic patient. Journal of Alcoholism 9: 135–143
Popper H, Sherlock S, Leevy C M, Harris M L 1974 Nomenclature, diagnostic criteria and diagnostic methodology for diseases of the liver and biliary tract. Fogarty International Centre Proceedings 22
Ramsay L E 1979 Hyperuricaemia in hypertension: role of alcohol. British Medical Journal 1: 653–654

Rollason J G, Pincherle G, Robinson D 1972 Serum gamma glutamyl transpeptidase in relation to alcohol consumption. Clinica Chimica Acta 39: 75–80
Rosalki S B 1973 Gamma glutamyl transpeptidase in alcoholism and in patients receiving enzyme-inducing drugs. Proceedings of international colloqium γ GT, Paris. Boehringer, Mannheim, p 139–150
Rosalki S B 1974 Gamma glutamyl transpeptidase in alcoholics and heavy drinkers. Proceedings of colloqium, Early diagnosis of alcoholism, Paris. Boehringer, Mannheim
Rosalki S B 1975 Gamma glutamyl transpeptidase. In: Bodansky O, Latner A L (eds) Advances in clinical chemistry 17. Academic Press, New York, p 53–107
Rosalki S B 1976 Enzyme tests in diseases of the liver and hepatobiliary tract. In: Wilkinson J H (ed) The principles and practice of diagnosis enzymology. Edward Arnold, London, p 303–360
Rosalki S B 1977 Enzyme Tests for alcoholism. Revue Epidemiologie et de Santé Publique 25: 147–158
Rosalki S B, Rau D 1972 Serum γ-glutamyl transpeptidase activity in alcoholism. Clinica Chimica Acta 39: 41–47
Rosalki S B, Tarlow D, Rau D 1971 Plasma gamma-glutamyl transpeptidase elevation in patients receiving enzyme-inducing drugs. Lancet 2: 376
Rosalki S B, Rau D, Lehmann D, Prentice M 1970 Determination of Serum - glutamyltranspeptidase activity and its clinical applications. Annals of Clinical Biochemistry 7: 143–147
Rosalki S B, Rau D, Tarlow D, Baylis E M 1972 Gamma-glutamyl transpeptidase elevation in alcoholics and in patients receiving enzyme-inducing drugs. Scandinavian Journal of Clinical and Laboratory Investigation 29: suppl 126, abst 23.15
Rubin E, Lieber C S Alcohol-induced hepatic injury in non-alcoholic volunteers. New England Journal of Medicine 278: 869–876
Rutherford W H 1977 Diagnosis of alcohol ingestion in mild head injuries. Lancet i: 1021–1023
Ryback R S, Eckardt M J, Felsher B, Rawlings R R 1982 Biochemical and hematologic correlates of alcoholism and liver disease. Journal of the American Medical Association 248: 2261–2265
See J G S, Heffelfinger R, Childers D M 1976 Gamma-glutamyl transpeptidase and the alcoholics response to abstinence. Annals of Clinical Laboratory Science 6: 349
Shaw L M, Marsh E 1981 The effect of one evening of social drinking on serum γ glutamyltransfrase activity. Clinical Chemistry 27: 1036
Shaw S, Lue S L, Lieber C S 1978 Biochemical tests for the detection of alcoholism: Comparison of plasma alpha-amino-n-butyric acid with other available tests. Alcoholism: Clinical and Experimental Research 2: 3–7
Shaw S, Stimmel B, Lieber S C 1976 Plasma alpha-amino-n-butyric acid to leucine ratio: An experimental biochemical marker of alcoholism. Science 194: 1057–1058
Skude G, Wadstein J 1977 Amylase, hepatic enzymes and bilirubin in serum of chronic alcoholics. Acta Medica Scandinavica 201: 53–58
Spencer-Peet J, Wood D C F, Glatt M M 1973 Screening test for alcoholism. Lancet 2: 1089–1090
Spencer-Peet J, Wood D C F, Glatt M M, Wiseman S M 1975 Urinary D-glucaric acid excretion and serum gamma-glutamyl transpeptidase activity in alcoholism. British Journal of Addiction 70: 359–364
Stevens V J, Fantl W J, Newman C B, Sims R V, Cerami A, Peterson C M 1981 Acetaldehyde adducts with hemoglobin. Journal of Clinical Investigation 67: 361–369
Stibler H, Borg S, Allgulander C Clinical significance of abnormal heterogeneity of transferrin in relation to alcohol consumption. Acta Medica Scandinavica 206: 275–281
Tayside safe driving project, 1983 Problem drinking among drunk drivers. British Medical Journal 286: 1319–1322
Van Waes L, Lieber C S 1977 Glutamate dehydrogenase: a reliable marker of liver cell necrosis in the alcoholic. British Medical Journal 2: 1508
Vessell E S, Page J G 1969 Genetic control of phenobarbital induced shortening of plasma antipyrene half-lives in man. Journal of Clinical Investigation 48: 2202–2209
Wadstein J, Skude G 1979a Serum ethanol, hepatic enzymes and length of debauch in chronic alcoholics. Acta Medica Scandinavica 205: 317–318
Wadstein J, Skude G 1979b Changes in amylase, hepatic enzymes and bilirubin in serum

upon initiation of alcohol abstinence. Acta Medica Scandinavica 205: 313–316
Waern U, Boberg J, Hellsing K 1979 Evaluation of indices of alcohol intake in a population of 60 year old men in Uppsala, Sweden, Acta Medica Scandinavica 205: 353–360
Weill J, Murat J, Lamy J, Got C 1979 Les conducteurs a alcoolémie elevée, sont ils des buveurs chroniques ou aegus? La Nouvelle Presse Medicale 8: 1852
Westwood M, Cohen M I, McNamara H 1978 Serum γ-glutamyl transpeptidase activity: a chemical determinant of alcohol consumption during adolescence. Pediatrics 62: 560–562
Whitehead T P, Clarke C A, Whitfield A G W 1978 Biochemical and haematological markers of alcohol intake. Lancet 1: 978–981
Whitfield J B, Hensley W J, Bryden D, Gallagher H 1978a Some laboratory correlates of drinking habits. Annals of Clinical Biochemistry 15: 297–303
Whitfield J B, Hensley W J, Bryden D, Gallagher H 1978b Estimation of alcohol intake from laboratory results. Annals of Clinical Biochemistry 15: 304–306
Whitfield J B, Allen J K, Adena M, Gallagher H G, Hensley W J 1981 A multivariate assessment of alcohol consumption. International Journal of Epidemiology 10: 281–288
Wietholtz H, Colombo J P 1976 Das verhalten des γ-glutamyltranspeptidase und anderer Leberenzyme im plasma wahrend der Alkohol-Entziehungskur. Schweizerische Mediginische Wochenschrift 106: 981–987
Wiseman S M, Spencer-Peet J 1977 The effect of drinking patterns on enzyme screening tests for alcoholism. The Practitioner 219: 243–245
Wiseman S M, Tomson P V, Barnett J M, Jenkins M, Wilton J 1982 Use of an alcolmeter to detect problem drinkers. British Medical Journal 285: 1089–1090
Wu A, Chanarin I, Levi A J 1974 Macrocytosis of chronic alcoholism. Lancet 1: 829–830
Wu A, Slavin G, Levi A J 1976 Elevated serum gamma-glutamyl transferase (transpeptidase) and histological liver damage in alcoholism. American Journal Gastroenterology 65: 318–323
Yudkoff M, Blazer-Yost B, Cohn R, Segal S 1979 On the clinical significance of the plasma α-amino-n-butyric acid: leucine ratio. American Journal of Clinical Nutrition 32: 282–285

SECTION TWO

The hospitalised alcoholic

(i) Metabolic disturbances

5

Abdulla A-B. Badawy

Alcohol intoxication and withdrawal

INTRODUCTION

Alcohol (ethanol) is a toxic agent capable of disturbing a wide variety of functions, not only in the liver where it is largely metabolized, but also elsewhere in the body. The actions of alcohol can generally be classified into four major groups: (1) direct cytotoxic actions; (2) neurochemical and pharmacological actions leading to the physiological and psychological changes characteristic of acute alcohol intoxication, alcohol dependence and the alcohol-withdrawal states; (3) actions secondary to disturbed endocrine function; (4) actions resulting from ethanol's own metabolism. The disturbances caused by one or more of these four mechanisms and by any interaction(s) between them will determine the overall condition of the alcoholic patient upon admission to hospital, and, hence, the choice of appropriate treatment strategies and management investigations. Such choice is greatly facilitated by the rapid acquisition of knowledge of the biochemical and physiological status of the patient soon after admission. Such information is considered in detail elsewhere in this work, and can, therefore, be given only a brief discussion in the present article in relation to the management of acute alcohol intoxication and the alcohol-withdrawal syndrome.

It should, however, be pointed out that very few biochemical investigations have been carried out specifically in relation to alcohol withdrawal, and that interpretation of certain biochemical effects of chronic alcohol consumption is made difficult by the fact that studies performed in this respect were carried out on hospitalized patients who were abstinent; this suggests the need in future investigations to make a definite distinction between changes caused by chronic alcohol intake and those resulting from subsequent withdrawal.

It is important and perhaps inevitable that the alcoholic patients be classified initially upon admission into categories on the basis of their blood-ethanol concentrations (Table 5.1). Patients may then be expected to fall into three groups: (1) those with no alcohol in their blood; (2) those with no acute alcohol intoxication (blood-ethanol concentration below 80 mg/dl);

Table 5.1 Initial classification of alcoholic patients upon admission

Condition	Blood-ethanol	Action
Intoxication	>80 mg/dl	1. Treat coma urgently if present 2. Treat trauma if present 3. Assess biochemistry and behaviour simultaneously and correct abnormalities 4. Treat intoxication 5. Proceed later to treat withdrawal
No intoxication	<80 mg/dl	1. Assess behaviour and biochemistry
No intoxication	0	2. Assess concurrent illness and infection 3. Admit to withdrawal treatment 4. Take corrective and precautionary measures during withdrawal treatment

(3) those with acute alcohol intoxication (blood-ethanol concentration above 80 mg/dl). The determination of blood-ethanol concentration, which represents the most direct means of assessment of alcohol intake, is therefore the first biochemical test that should be performed once an admitted patient is confirmed or suspected as being an alcoholic or an alcohol-abuser.

BLOOD-ETHANOL CONCENTRATION

Blood-ethanol concentration can be determined accurately by either gas-liquid chromatography (GLC) or spectrophotometric assessment of the reduction of NAD^+ (oxidized nicotinamide-adenine dinucleotide) in the presence of ethanol and alcohol dehydrogenase (EC 1.1.1.1) (see Ch. 3). This latter technique is available in a commercial-kit form and can be automated and has been adapted (Rosalki, 1971) for colorimetric absorption purposes. If, however, these two techniques are not available in the hospital laboratory or are considered too slow in an emergency situation, then blood-ethanol concentration can be satisfactorily determined with a breathalyzer or an alcolmeter, whose principles and use have been described elsewhere in this publication (Ch. 3).

Plasma osmolality

Another useful, though indirect, test for the presence of alcohol in the blood is that involving the determination of serum (or plasma) osmolality. The latter, which should be determined by freezing-point depression, is known to be increased after oral ethanol consumption (Robinson & Loeb, 1971) or by the addition of the drug to plasma (Beard et al, 1974), and has been shown (Champion et al, 1975) in a large prospectively-studied group of acute-trauma patients to be directly related to blood-ethanol concentration. The following useful points have emerged from this latter study: (1) a serum osmolality value greater than 320 mmol/kg was observed in 90 per cent of patients in whose blood the concentration of ethanol was above 50 mg/dl;

(2) no patient with a blood-ethanol concentration above 150 mg/dl showed an osmolality value below that mentioned above; (3) no patient with a blood-ethanol concentration above 200 mg/dl had an osmolality below 340 mmol/kg. For calculation of osmolality and for the significance of the differences between calculated and determined values, the reader may wish to consult the article by Fink & Rosalki (1978). The advantages of this technique are its rapidity, simplicity, wide availability and its potential value to the management and clinical and legal interpretation, in a variety of clinical settings, of the condition of acutely-injured patients, the majority of whom (at least 60 per cent) sustain their injuries as a direct result of excessive alcohol intake. It should, however, be remembered that osmolality values can be influenced by many factors, such as ethanol metabolites (acetaldehyde and acetate), congeners in alcoholic beverages, dehydration, vomiting, renal impairment and diabetes mellitus (see Champion et al, 1975 and references cited therein).

ACUTE ALCOHOL INTOXICATION

Features

Although ethanol exerts both excitatory and inhibitory actions on behaviour and other physiological functions, it is certain that its depressant effects on the central nervous system (which may also involve disturbances at the cellular and molecular levels) are the major cause of acute alcohol intoxication. The characteristic signs of this condition are facial flushing, slurred speech and unsteady gait, accompanied by euphoria, hyperactivity, emotion and volubility. In severe intoxication, there is irrational thought, marked impairment of perception and gross loss of muscle control, with death following coma as a result of respiratory collapse. The effects of acute alcohol intoxication on human behaviour have been extensively studied and reviewed by many investigators (see e.g. Mello & Mendelson, 1978; Barry, 1979). The review by this latter author includes a useful Table providing an analysis of different behavioural disturbances as a function of changes in blood-ethanol concentration.

The post-intoxication phase, or hangover, is associated with: (1) physical symptoms, such as fatigue, headache, thirst, vertigo, gastric disorders, nausea, vomiting, insomnia, fine tremors of the hands, impaired liver function and raised or lowered blood pressure; (2) psychological symptoms, such as acute anxiety, guilt or remorse, depression and extreme sensitivity. Hangover usually lasts no more than 36 h after all traces of ethanol have disappeared from the blood.

Mechanism

Acute alcohol intoxication occurs when blood-ethanol concentration exceeds 80 mg/dl. Under these conditions, depression of the central nervous system occurs as a result of accumulation of ethanol in the blood at a rate far exceeding that of removal of the drug from the circulation. This latter rate in man is normally about 15 mg/dl/h and is determined mainly by the rate of ethanol metabolism, particularly in the liver, because metabolism represents about 95 per cent of the overall means of disposal of the drug, whereas the remaining 5 per cent can be accounted for by excretion via breath, sweat and urine. A person whose blood-ethanol concentration is 80 mg/dl will therefore require approximately 5 h before achieving total elimination of ethanol from the circulation. It follows therefore that the successful and rapid treatment of acute alcohol intoxication must involve either acceleration of the normal rate of elimination (pharmacokinetic antagonism) or reversal of the depressant effects of ethanol on the central nervous system (pharmacodynamic antagonism). Antagonists of acute alcohol intoxication acting by either mechanism have recently been described by Alkana & Noble (1979) as 'amethystic agents'.

Pharmacodynamic antagonism

Pharmacodynamic antagonism of acute alcohol intoxication can be achieved by a variety of drugs and chemicals that could be classified into six major categories: (1) catecholamines and related substances; (2) acetylcholine and related substances; (3) γ-aminobutyric acid and related substances; (4) analeptics; (5) cations; (6) other agents. A comprehensive list of these chemicals and the outcome of investigations of their antagonism of the various behavioural disturbances caused by acute alcohol intoxication in man and/or experimental animals can be seen in the review by Alkana & Noble (1979). Of the drugs tested in man, the following have been reported to be useful or promising as antagonists: aminophylline, *L*-dopa and ephedrine (Alkana et al, 1977), the analeptic agent pentylenetetrazol (Rosenbaum, 1942) and calcium chloride (Alha, 1951). It should, however, be emphasized that no systematic investigations of the possible clinical effectiveness of these latter drugs against a wide variety of behavioural disturbances have been performed, and, accordingly, further work is necessary to establish whether such drugs are effective pharmacodynamic antagonists of acute alcohol intoxication.

The opiate-receptor antagonist naloxone has also been reported to be capable of antagonizing acute alcohol intoxication and the associated disturbances in behaviour (Sørensen & Mattison, 1978; Jeffcoate et al, 1979; Jefferys et al, 1980; Kimball et al, 1980). The mechanism of action of naloxone in this condition is not clear, although it could be inferred that it may act on opiate receptors. However, recent work from this Laboratory in the rat suggests that naloxone may act as a pharmacokinetic antagonist of acute alcohol intoxication; this work will be discussed in the section on pharmacokinetic antagonism.

Alcohol metabolism

Alcohol metabolism has been extensively studied and reviewed by many workers (see e.g. Hawkins & Kalant, 1972; Badawy, 1978 and references cited in both). A brief account may, however, be useful here in relation to pharmacokinetic antagonism of acute alcohol intoxication.

Enzymes of alcohol metabolism

It is important to note that alcohol is metabolized mainly in the liver and that the major enzyme involved in this process in vivo is the NAD^+-dependent liver-cytosolic protein alcohol dehydrogenase, which catalyses the conversion of ethanol into acetaldehyde according to the following reaction.

$$CH_3CH_2OH + NAD^+ \longrightarrow CH_3CHO + NADH + H^+$$

The other two enzymes capable of oxidizing ethanol to acetaldehyde are catalase and the so-called microsomal ethanol-oxidizing system or MEOS, and the reactions involved are as follows.

$$CH_3CH_2OH + H_2O_2 \xrightarrow{\text{Catalase}} CH_3CHO + 2H_2O$$

$$CH_3CH_2OH + NADPH + H^+ + O_2 \xrightarrow{\text{Meos}} CH_3CHO + NADP^+ + 2H_2O$$

Under normal conditions, the contribution of catalase to the overall rate of ethanol metabolism in vivo is very moderate (2 per cent at best), but it is possible that this enzyme may play a more significant role under certain pathological conditions, such as those involving increased purine breakdown leading to an enhanced rate of generation of hydrogen peroxide, which is the most important factor determining catalase activity. On the other hand, MEOS appears to play a more active role in ethanol oxidation in vivo (estimates of its contribution vary between 5 per cent and 20 per cent). MEOS may also be of particular interest in relation to alcohol tolerance and alcohol-drug interactions (including cross-tolerance), in view of its inducibility by chronic consumption of alcohol and drugs, notably the barbiturates (for a detailed discussion, see Hawkins & Kalant, 1972; Badawy, 1978).

The acetaldehyde produced after ethanol oxidation by any of the above three enzyme systems is then converted into acetate by the action of a different enzyme, NAD^+-dependent mitochondrial aldehyde dehydrogenase, according to the following reaction.

$$CH_3CHO + NAD^+ + H_2O \longrightarrow CH_3COOH + NADH + H^+$$

Unlike alcohol dehydrogenase which is present mainly in the liver, aldehyde dehydrogenase has a widespread distribution in the body, and this raises the strong possibility that acetaldehyde produced by the hepatic oxidation of ethanol may be metabolized extrahepatically and can, thereby, cause disturbances in the redox state of the NAD couple (see below) outside the liver.

Disturbance of the redox state of the hepatic NAD couple by ethanol

In addition to the production of acetaldehyde, which is capable of exerting toxic effects of its own (see Badawy, 1980 and references cited therein), the other important result of ethanol oxidation by liver alcohol dehydrogenase is the formation in the hepatic cytosol of NADH at the expense of NAD^+, or, in other words, the disturbance of the redox state of the NAD couple. This disturbance has far-reaching implications for intermediary metabolism and other metabolic activities (Krebs, 1968); this is illustrated further in Chapters 7, 13 and 14

Limitation of ethanol metabolism by the redox disturbances

Of the many physiological factors (except genetic differences) influencing ethanol metabolism, the availability of NAD^+ and the rate of dissociation of the NADH-alcohol dehydrogenase complex are the most important, particularly in relation to acute alcohol intake and intoxication. When the rate of ethanol intake exceeds that of its metabolism, the oxidation of excessive amounts of the drug in the liver is impaired by the shortage of NAD^+ in the hepatic cytosol. Under these conditions, the liver can achieve a certain degree of success in the provision of NAD^+ by using the so-called substrate-shuttle systems. These overcome the impermeability of the mitochondrial membrane(s) to NAD^+(H) by effecting the intramitochondrial oxidation of cytosolic NADH after its indirect transfer into the former organelles. The most active of these systems is the malate-aspartate shuttle, which is illustrated in Figure 5.1. The presence of a suitable NAD^+-linked dehydro-

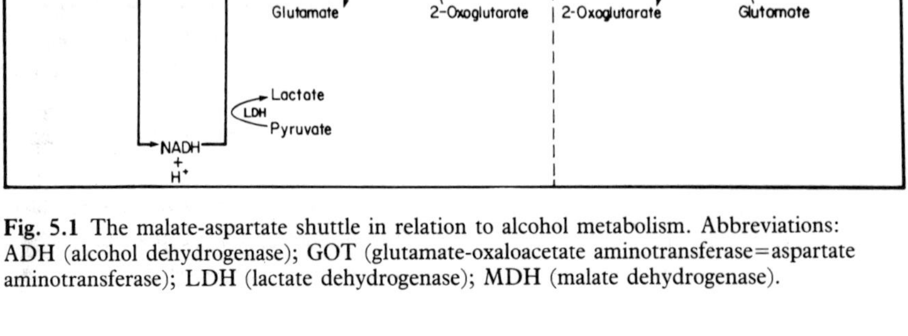

Fig. 5.1 The malate-aspartate shuttle in relation to alcohol metabolism. Abbreviations: ADH (alcohol dehydrogenase); GOT (glutamate-oxaloacetate aminotransferase=aspartate aminotransferase); LDH (lactate dehydrogenase); MDH (malate dehydrogenase).

genase in both cytosol and mitochondria is the vital requirement of a shuttle, and the whole process can be summarized by the following sequence of events using malate dehydrogenase as the relevant dehydrogenase: (1) the excess NADH in the cytosol (produced as a result of ethanol oxidation by alcohol dehydrogenase) activates cytosolic malate dehydrogenase in the direction of reduction of oxalo-acetate; (2) the malate produced by this latter reaction crosses into the mitochondria, where it is oxidized to oxaloacetate by mitochondrial malate dehydrogenase as part of the mitochondrial respiratory-chain activity; (3) because oxaloacetate cannot cross easily the mitochondrial membrane, it undergoes transamination with glutamate to produce aspartate (and 2-oxoglutarate); (4) aspartate leaves the mitochondria to the cytosol, where it is back-transaminated to oxaloacetate; (5) cytosolic malate dehydrogenase then converts oxaloacetate into malate and simultaneously converts NADH into NAD^+. In this manner, the availability of NAD^+ in the hepatic cytosol is increased and this leads to a resumption of ethanol oxidation by alcohol dehydrogenase. Ethanol metabolism can also be enhanced by the direct oxidation of NADH bound to alcohol dehydrogenase in the cytosol; a well known chemical capable of causing this direct oxidation of NADH is the fructose metabolite glyceraldehyde (see below).

Pharmacokinetic antagonism

Pharmacokinetic antagonism of acute alcohol intoxication can be achieved, at least theoretically, by a variety of procedures. However, those involving decreased ethanol absorption, altered ethanol distribution in body waters and enhanced ethanol excretion are ineffective. On the other hand, dialysis has proved successful in emergency situations in man (see e.g. Perey et al, 1965) and is indicated in patients with a blood-ethanol concentration of 500 mg/dl or above and in those with severe acidosis or with coma complicated by the presence of a dialysable drug (Sellers & Kalant, 1976). Dialysis is, however, considered too drastic in less severely-intoxicated cases.

Because, as mentioned earlier, ethanol metabolism represents 95 per cent of the overall means of disposal of the drug, the successful pharmacokinetic antagonism of acute alcohol intoxication must involve acceleration of ethanol metabolism, and, because of metabolic considerations, this can best be achieved by agents capable of regenerating cytosolic NAD^+ either indirectly or by direct oxidation of NADH bound to alcohol dehydrogenase. Three such agents have been examined in this context: arsenate, 2,4-dinitrophenol and fructose. The former two agents are, however, toxic in doses causing an effective acceleration of ethanol oxidation, and are thus of limited clinical value, whereas fructose, the least toxic of the three, appears to be the most effective pharmacokinetic antagonist of acute alcohol intoxication, with estimates of its efficacy varying between 15 per cent and 100 per cent (Lowenstein et al, 1970; Thieden et al, 1972; Damgaard et al, 1973). The mechanism(s) of action of fructose is complicated, but could involve a glyceraldehyde-mediated direct oxidation of NADH bound to alcohol dehydrogenase, a pyruvate-related oxidation of cytosolic NADH by the catalytic action of lactate dehydrogenase and an overall regeneration of NAD^+ as a consequence of fructose metabolism by various NAD^+-linked dehydrogenases involved in the fructose-metabolic sequence. In accelerating ethanol metabolism, however, fructose has been reported to be ineffective (Dundee et al, 1971) and inconsistent (Levy et al, 1977), and may cause unpleasant and even unwelcome side effects (Woods & Alberti, 1972; Cohen, 1972; Levy et al, 1977).

On the basis of the fact that mitochondrial oxidation of NADH must be coupled to ATP synthesis, Krebs & Stubbs (1975) found that ethanol oxidation by isolated hepatocytes can be accelerated by treatments known to enhance urea synthesis or gluconeogenesis and, hence, ATP production. Such treatments included a mixture of lactate, lysine, ornithine and ammonium chloride, and another combination of fructose, dihydroxyacetone, pyruvate and ammonium chloride, but the possible usefulness of such mixtures has not been assessed in intoxicated humans. It should, however, be pointed out that none of the above pharmacokinetic antagonists tested or suggested is likely to satisfy the important requirement of being able to accelerate ethanol metabolism by a tenfold factor (see Alkana & Noble, 1979) to achieve a rapid reversal of acute alcohol intoxication. The possibility that such a 'super-accelerator' of ethanol metabolism exists is suggested by the finding in the rat (Badawy & Evans, 1981) that naloxone, which has been shown to be valuable in rapidly antagonizing acute alcohol intoxication and the associated disturbance of behaviour in man (for references, see earlier), is capable of lowering blood-ethanol concentration from an intoxication value of 133 mg/dl to about 92 mg/dl within 30 min after administration (1 mg/kg body weight), and of causing a simultaneous reversal of the ethanol-induced disturbance of the redox states of the hepatic NAD(P) couples. This decrease in blood-ethanol concentration represents about 6-to-7-fold acceleration of ethanol metabolism, and it therefore remains to be seen whether naloxone reverses acute alcohol intoxication in man by the same mechanism. The above findings in the rat and the ability of naloxone to cause a very rapid arousal of alcohol-intoxicated patients strongly suggest that further clinical investigations of the actions of this opiate antagonist in this context may be fruitful.

Management

There are a number of scales currently in use for the assessment of intoxication of admitted patients. Hore & Rossall (1979) have suggested that, of these, the Glasgow coma scale appears to be the most simple and reliable, avoids indefinable terms used in the traditional scales and has met with wide acceptance both in specialized neurosurgical units and in accident departments. The Glasgow scale (Teasdale & Jennett, 1974) describes conscious level in terms of three behavioural responses: eye opening, verbal response and motor response, with each of these responses being divided into 4 or 5 sub-groups, ranging from no response through to spontaneous eye opening, orientated verbal response and obeying motor response respectively.

Concurrently with the above behavioural assessment, it must be recognized that coma due to respiratory failure is the most serious problem caused by acute alcohol intoxication. If present, coma must clearly receive urgent medical intervention. Immediate treatment must ensure an adequate airway and that the patient is positioned on his (her) side. If ventilatory insufficiency is present, mechanical ventilation should be performed. At the same time, blood glucose should be measured, and, if hypoglycaemia is present, intravenous injection of 50 ml of a 50 per cent solution of dextrose should be given immediately. Naloxone may also be useful in achieving a rapid arousal. Also as stated above, dialysis (haemo- or peritoneal) is indicated in patients with a blood-ethanol concentration of 500 mg/dl or above and in those with severe acidosis or with coma complicated by the presence of a dialysable drug.

Patients with acute alcohol intoxication are also at risk from possible injury to the head and other body parts, gastrointestinal bleeding, hepatic coma, water and electrolyte disturbances and acid-base imbalance, in addition to hypoglycaemia. Such complications must be recognized by physical examination and appropriate management investigations, including an assessment of liver functions and the determination (in blood, plasma or serum) of pH, P_{CO_2} and of concentrations of bicarbonate, ketones, glucose and electrolytes in addition to that of ethanol. Management may, therefore, involve correction of any water, electrolyte and/or acid-base disturbances and, as stated above, intravenous glucose therapy. Parenteral therapy with B vitamins (particularly thiamine) may also be useful, in relation to the risk of Wernicke's encephalopathy (see also Ch. 10).

Biochemical disturbances

Acute alcohol intoxication disturbs a great many variety of functions, the most important of which from the management viewpoint and in the context of the present discussion are: (1) water and electrolyte metabolism; (2) acid-base balance; (3) glucose metabolism; (4) endocrine function. The following is a brief account of the metabolic background of the disturbances of these functions by ethanol intoxication.

Water balance (see also Ch. 6)

For a detailed discussion of the effects of acute alcohol intoxication on water balance, the reader may wish to consult the recent review by Beard & Sargent (1979). Acute alcohol intoxication exerts a biphasic effect on water balance. Initially (during the phase of ascending blood-ethanol concentration), diuresis occurs as a result of inhibition of vasopressin release, and is characterized by an increase in renal free water clearance (Rubini et al, 1955; Ogata et al, 1968). The possibility that ethanol causes this initial increase in urine flow by altering the glomerular filtration rate has been excluded by the results of studies on creatinine and inulin clearance (for references, see Beard & Sargent, 1979). The mechanism by which ascending blood-ethanol concentration inhibits vasopressin release is not clearly understood at present, but it may involve an altered sensitivity or an increase in the set point of the vasopressin-releasing mechanism. By contrast with the above initial effect, the phase of descending blood-ethanol concentration is characterized by decreased water balance and, accordingly, there is fluid retention and an expansion of body fluid volumes (Nicholson & Taylor, 1938; Sargent et al, 1975). The fluid retention has been suggested by Beard & Sargent (1979) to be the result of a coordinated effort between fluid intake and fluid loss regulatory systems, and that the increased release of vasopressin during this phase may play an important role in this context.

Electrolyte metabolism (see also Ch. 6)

Beard & Sargent (1979) and Harris (1979) have recently reviewed the effects of acute alcohol intoxication on electrolyte balance. Monovalent cation excretion is either unaltered or slightly decreased during the phase of ascending blood-ethanol concentration (Strauss et al, 1950; Rubini et al, 1955), whereas subsequently (during the phase of descending blood-ethanol concentration) there is retention of sodium, potassium and chloride ions (Nicholson & Taylor, 1938). Na^+ retention during this latter phase has been studied in more detail and was found to involve enhanced sodium reabsorption (see Sargent et al, 1974).

Plasma zinc concentration is not altered, whereas urinary excretion of this cation is enhanced, probably by an intrarenal effect of ethanol, during the phase of ascending blood-ethanol concentration (Sargent et al, 1974). Acute alcohol intoxication appears to increase the urinary excretion of calcium and magnesium without altering their plasma concentrations (see Harris, 1979 and references cited therein). Further work is required to examine the mechanism(s) of these changes in divalent cation metabolism.

Acid-base balance

Most studies of the effects of acute alcohol intoxication on acid-base balance (reviewed recently by Sargent et al, 1979) have been concerned primarily with establishing the existence of abnormalities. It is, however, certain that a large dose of ethanol is capable of lowering blood pH and plasma bicarbonate concentration, and of increasing the concentrations of plasma lactate and ketone bodies (see e.g. Räiha & Mäenpää, 1964; Ylikahri et al, 1976).

These changes, which are indicative of respiratory and metabolic acidosis, can in general be explained by: (1) depression of the central nervous system leading to altered ventillation of blood gases; (2) increased production of reducing equivalents (hydrogen ions) secondarily to ethanol metabolism by hepatic alcohol dehydrogenase; (3) increased production of ketone bodies secondarily to hypermobilization of adipose-tissue fat coupled with enhanced fatty acid oxidation which is required for provision of energy in the presence of the so-called carbohydrate starvation.

Glucose metabolism (see also Ch. 7)

The complex effects of alcohol on glucose and carbohydrate metabolism have recently been reviewed by Marks (1978) and Reitz (1979) and are considered in detail elsewhere in this publication. The most important effect on glucose metabolism in relation to acute alcohol intoxication is, undoubtedly, hypoglycaemia, and it is generally thought that ethanol causes this effect mainly by inhibiting gluconeogenesis and that this inhibition applies largely to the pyruvate carboxylase reaction (Krebs et al, 1969), although other gluconeogenic enzymes are also altered.

Endocrine function (see also Ch. 14)

The complex effects of ethanol on endocrine function have been extensively studied and reviewed by many workers (see e.g. Wright, 1978; Kakihana & Butte, 1979; Ylikahri et al, 1981) and are considered in detail elsewhere in this publication. In relation to acute alcohol intoxication, it is known that the drug increases the release and, hence, the circulating and/or urinary concentrations of catecholamines (Perman, 1958; Anton, 1965), cortisol (Fazekas, 1966; Jenkins & Connolly, 1968), insulin (Marks, 1978 and references cited therein) and aldosterone and renin (Farmer & Fabre, 1975). The effects of acute alcohol intoxication on vasopressin release have already been described earlier, whereas those on growth hormone release are controversial, but most likely involve an inhibition during the early phase of intoxication and an enhancement during hangover (Ylikahri et al, 1981 and references cited therein). These actions of ethanol can, in general, be attributed to: (1) a direct effect on release and synthesis; (2) stress of the intoxication; (3) altered intermediary metabolism secondarily to ethanol oxidation by hepatic alcohol dehydrogenase.

Biochemical tests for investigating acute alcohol intoxication

Fink & Rosalki (1978) and Jones (1979) have reviewed the various biochemical disturbances caused by ethanol in relation to the clinical diagnosis of acute and chronic intake (see also Ch. 4). Tests related to acute intoxication are listed in Table 5.2, but the clinical biochemist should expect

Table 5.2 Biochemical tests for the management and investigation of acute alcohol intoxication

Type of test	Tests
Direct	1. *Blood ethanol 2. *Breath test 3. Urinary ethanol
Indirect a. secndary to alcohol metabolism	1. *Acidosis, 'anion gap', ketones 2. Lactate, uric acid 3. Lipids, free fatty acids, glycerol 4. Acetaldehyde, acetate
b. secondary to physiological effects of ethanol	1. *Blood glucose 2. *Serum osmolality 3. Urinary porphyrins 4. Pituitary-adrenal and pituitary-gonadal axes

* Tests of priority in urgent cases of intoxication

requests to perform only a few of them (blood ethanol, osmolality, glucose, ketoacidosis and acid-base balance and electrolytes) in relation to intoxicated patients requiring urgent treatment. The remainder of these tests may therefore be useful in less urgent situations, such as mildly-intoxicated individuals and experimental studies.

ALCOHOL WITHDRAWAL

Alcohol withdrawal has been the subject of much investigation and debate, and the reader may wish to consult the recent reviews by Shaw (1978) and Gessner (1979).

Aetiology and features

We owe much to the classical work of Victor & Adams (1953) who advanced the concept that cessation of alcohol intake by hospitalized patients with obvious alcoholic complications leads to the clinical symptoms of tremulousness, hallucinations, seizures and delerium tremens, and that these symptoms occur in a definite time sequence, with delirium tremens following seizures in 97 per cent of alcohol-withdrawn patients. It is now established from the chronological viewpoint that the milder symptoms of the tremulousness appear within a few hours of cessation of alcohol intake, whereas the severest, those of delirium tremens, develop later, usually after 72 h. However, although subsequent experimental studies by Isbell et al 1955) and Mendelson (1964) and many other workers have established that the various phenomena described above are related to cessation of alcohol intake, they failed to provide strong evidence in support of the notion that delirium tremens always follows convulsions. Although the work of Isbell et al (1955) and Mendelson (1964) also suggested that the severity of the withdrawal reaction(s) is a function of the amount and duration of alcohol intake, definite support to this relationship has subsequently been obtained from animal studies by Goldstein (1972) and Majchrowicz (1975). The withdrawal reaction or syndrome can also be influenced by other factors, such as concurrent illness or infection and extremely heavy drinking, which could induce an acute-withdrawal state (Mello & Mendelson, 1970; Gross et al, 1972; Feuerlein, 1974; Marjot, 1974) and by simultaneous withdrawal from other depressant drugs, such as the barbiturates, (Gessner, 1979 and references cited therein).

Tremulousness

This is the commonest and mildest of the alcohol-withdrawal symptoms, being experienced by every dependent alcoholic. In its mild form, tremors occur after a night of heavy drinking, and is rapid and regular, whereas in its severe form it becomes coarse and irregular and is accompanied by nausea and feelings of weakness, faintness, apprehension and irritability, with simple tasks such as dressing or drinking becoming major obstacles for the patient to overcome.

Hallucinations

Transitory hallucinations (auditory or visual) are not uncommon during alcohol withdrawal. Typical alcoholic hallucinosis occurs within 48 h of cessation of alcohol intake, and is characterized by hearing voices (usually of family members or friends) addressing the patient in a threatening or derogatory manner. The patient may then respond to such threats by experiencing fear and agitation, which may involve torment or suicidal behaviour. This illness is usually of a short duration, lasting about 6 days, but could occasionally persist for several weeks or a few months.

Convulsions

Alcohol-withdrawal fits, as opposed to fits of an epileptic caused by alcohol and precipitated during a drinking episode, usually occur 13–24 h after cessation of alcohol intake, and, as shown by Victor & Brausch (1967), between 7 and 48 h after withdrawal in 90 per cent of alcoholics. Fits occurring later than 48 h after withdrawal should be investigated for an alternative cause(s), such as benzodiazepine dependence. The alcohol-withdrawal fits are usually of the uncomplicated grand mal type (single or a few over a 1–2 h period), but rarely of the status epilepticus variety. In contrast with epileptic patients, those with alcohol withdrawal exhibit a basically normal EEG except during or soon after the occurrence of a fit.

Delirium tremens

This severest of the alcohol-withdrawal symptoms usually develops 3 days after withdrawal and is characterized by psychomotor, speech and autonomic hyperactivity, disorientation, confusion and a disordered sense of perception. In general, 5 per cent of a given population of alcohol-withdrawn patients will develop delirium tremens (Gross et al, 1974; Shaw, 1978). The syndrome could develop abruptly or may be preceded by fitful sleep broken by nightmares and transient hallucinosis by day, with feelings of restlessness and extreme anxiety. When fully manifest, delirium tremens is totally dominated by coarse persistent tremors of the hands, head and trunk, extreme restlessness and agitation, rapid pulse and perspiration. Mentally, the patient is totally disorientated and experiences visual hallucinations, with auditory hallucinations and delusions being often present. Such hallucinations are often accompanied by strong emotional experiences, usually of fear and apprehension, which lead to aggressive, destructive and suicidal behaviour. The syndrome usually lasts for 3–7 days after onset. The death rate from delirium tremens has fallen considerably and is currently rarely above 1 per cent, with death being usually the result of cardiovascular collapse, concurrent infection or hyperthermia.

Management

Behavioural-assessment

Of the various scales of behavioural-assessment of the withdrawal syndrome(s), those of Gross et al (1974) are the most comprehensive and the first to attempt to overcome the problem of quantification of the severity of withdrawal symptoms inherent in other scales. Gross et al (1974) have described two types of schedule: the total severity assessment (TSA) and the selective severity assessment (SSA) schedules. The TSA schedule consists of 30 clinical variables that are independently scored on a scale of between two and seven graduations (the scoring criteria being stipulated by the authors), and takes 30–45 min to complete. The SSA schedule is made up of 11 of the variables found in the TSA schedule, and is, therefore, a much shorter version and can accordingly be administered rapidly (10 min) by trained nursing staff. Gross et al (1974) also found that the scores obtained by using the SSA schedule can be highly significantly correlated (r=0.86) with those derived from the TSA schedule.

Physical and biochemical assessment

Before the start of specific therapy of the withdrawal syndrome(s), the clinical biochemist will have provided the clinician with rapid and valuable information on the biochemical and physiological status of the patient. The points listed in Table 5.3 summarize the various situations likely to be

Table 5.3 Possible clinical problems on alcohol withdrawal

Nature	Complication or disease
Direct	Acidosis, alkalosis, Cushing's-like syndrome, electrolyte disturbances, hypoglycaemia, hypertriglyceridaemia, hyperuricaemia, psychological disorders, trauma
Alcohol-related	Anaemia and other haematological disorders, cardiomyopathy, cardiovascular disorders, endocrine (including reproductive and fetal) abnormalities, kidney problems, liver disease, malabsorption, malnutrition, myopathies, neurological (and central nervous system) abnormalities, pancreatitis, porphyria
Concurrent	Various (e.g. diabetes, drug abuse and dependence, hypertension, infection, neoplasms, trauma)

encountered in this respect, and on the basis of the above biochemical information and physical examination, the clinician will take appropriate remedial and precautionary action concurrently with the treatment of alcohol withdrawal.

Treatment

Tremulousness. This can be treated by mild sedation with diazepam or chlormethiazole. Therapy with β-adrenoceptor blocking agents may also be useful in alleviating tremor and autonomic hyperactivity. Shaw (1978) suggested that, in general, no medication should be prescribed in this condition other than as part of a brief properly controlled withdrawal regimen.

Hallucinations. It is essential that alcoholic hallucinosis be treated in hospital and the patient is carefully observed to avoid harm to himself or others as a result of his actions. Accordingly, the behaviour of the patient must be observed at all times and adequate doses of an antipsychotic drug, such as chlorpromazine, are given.

Convulsions. A previous history of withdrawal fits or the occurrence of a fit or the observation of myoclonic twitchings are all indications for therapy with an anticonvulsant drug, such as phenytoin (diphenyl-hydantoin). If multiple fits develop, then intravenous valium (10 mg) should be given in addition to the oral phenytoin. The intravenous valium could, if necessary, be repeated.

Delirium tremens. This most serious of the alcohol-withdrawal reactions requires urgent medical attention. Thus in addition to monitoring the patient's blood pressure and heart rate, blood should be analysed for pH, Pa_{CO2}, bicarbonate, electrolytes and glucose, and appropriate corrective measures are taken. Intravenous injections must be avoided as much as possible, except if there is vomiting, diarrhoea or gross disturbances in electrolyte balance. It is at present generally recommended that fluid intake (orally) be encouraged (at least 6 litres per day). Recent work, however, suggests (see below) that alcohol withdrawal causes water intoxication in the brain; this finding is clearly important and could in due course lead to a reassessment of the above therapeutic recommendation of fluid intake (see also Ch. 6). As with acute alcohol intoxication and less-severe alcohol-withdrawal states, any concurrent illness or infection or trauma must be recognized and given appropriate medical and precautionary considerations. High-potency vitamin therapy for 5–7 days should be helpful, and adequate sedation (see below for drug therapy) should be given to prevent exhaustion and thereby facilitate proper nursing care. If fits are anticipated or if they occur despite drug therapy, then an anti-convulsant, such as phenytoin, should also be given.

Drug therapy of alcohol withdrawal. The most comprehensive account of drug therapy of the alcohol-withdrawal reactions to date is that of Gessner (1979). Drugs which have been used in this context could, in general, be classified into six major groups: (1) antipsychotic drugs (phenothiazines and haloperidol); (2) agents of the alcohol-barbiturate type (benzodiazepines, paraldehyde, barbiturates, ethanol and chlormethiazole); (3) other sedatives (benactyzine and hydroxyzine); (4) anticonvulsants (phenytoin, dipropylacetate or sodium valproate and others); (5) cations (magnesium sulphate and lithium carbonate); (6) other agents (propranolol). It is important to emphasize the following points in relation to choice of drug therapy of alcohol withdrawal: (a) antipsychotic drugs are dangerous to, and, therefore, contraindicated in, patients with delirium tremens and in those with less-severe withdrawal reactions, but may be useful in those with mild withdrawal symptoms such as tremulousness and also hallucinosis; (b) the most effective and safest group of drugs are those of the alcohol-barbiturate type (the two most popular are chlormethiazole and chlordiazepoxide in the UK and USA respectively); (c) there is, however, serious concern and evidence regarding the abuse potential of benzodiazepines (particularly diazepam) after long-term therapy or intake.

Biochemical disturbances

As stated in the introduction, very few clinical biochemical studies have been performed specifically in relation to alcohol withdrawal, and that interpretation of some findings attributed to chronic ethanol consumption is made difficult by the fact that the patients examined were abstinent following hospitalization and could therefore be considered to have been in a state of withdrawal, rather than dependence, and also by the presentation by some workers of data combining both abstinent and ethanol-drinking patients. It should be emphasized that the effects on a particular biochemical parameter of acute ethanol intake may not necessarily resemble those observed after chronic consumption, and that the latter effects may, upon subsequent withdrawal, disappear, become more pronounced or even replaced by new or opposite changes. Accordingly, it is important that future investigations must make a definite distinction between the above

Table 5.4 Biochemical changes during alcohol withdrawal in man

Type of change or effect	Parameter or effect
A. No or minimal change in parameter	Serum calcium, thyroid hormones
B. Return of parameter to normal	Liver function tests (without concurrent liver disease)
C. Chronic effect unchanged	Decreased plasma testosterone
D. New or different effect	Hypomagnesaemia, respiratory alkalosis, increased release of cortisol and catecholamines, disturbed biogenic amine metabolism, decreased TRH-dependent prolactin release

experimental conditions, and, as a first step aimed at stimulating such awareness, it may be useful to classify the effects of, or the changes observed during, alcohol withdrawal into the categories listed in Table 5.4. Only those changes given in the last category will be discussed briefly in this section, because they are the most relevant to the alcohol-withdrawal syndrome(s). To gain more detailed information on these changes and on the effects of chronic ethanol consumption on various biochemical systems, the reader may wish to consult the relevant reviews referred to earlier in this chapter in relation to acute alcohol intoxication, and also those presented elsewhere in this publication.

Water and electrolyte metabolism

Beard & Knott (1968) found that the increases in total body water, extracellular fluid volume and plasma volume and the associated electrolyte retention caused by chronic ethanol consumption were followed upon withdrawal by increases in water and solute excretion. More importantly is the finding by Knott & Beard (1969) that the severity of the withdrawal syndrome could be correlated with the extent of volume expansion during chronic alcohol intake. The above increases in water and solute excretion during alcohol withdrawal should not be interpreted to indicate a subsequent dehydration, because they merely represented a return to normal homeostasis. Recently, Besson et al (1981) reported by using data on brain images derived by the technique of nuclear magnetic resonance that alcohol withdrawal causes water intoxication in the brain, and suggested that this may be caused by the increase in vasopressin release during withdrawal (for this latter effect, see also Eisenhofer et al, 1982).

By contrast to the slight decrease or no change in serum calcium concentration, that of magnesium in serum, erythrocytes and skeletal muscle is known to be decreased in alcohol withdrawal (see e.g. Sullivan et al, 1969). The possibility that hypomagnesaemia is involved in the aetiology of the alcohol-withdrawal syndrome(s) is suggested by the findings that depletion of magnesium (and also calcium) causes similar symptoms (such as neuromuscular irritability, tetany, seizure sussceptibility and hallucinations) and that administration of salts of magnesium and calcium is capable of counteracting the effects of alcohol withdrawal, except delirium tremens (for references, see Harris, 1979). Of considerable interest in relation to the mechanism of the alcohol-withdrawal-induced hypomagnesaemia is the finding (Flink et al, 1979) that strongly suggests that the decrease in serum magnesium concentration is caused by binding of the cation to non-esterified fatty acids whose circulating concentration is elevated secondarily to enhanced lipolysis during alcohol withdrawal in dogs. Accordingly, these latter authors suggested that control of lipolysis may be a sound basis for therapy of alcohol withdrawal. The above finding is clearly important and thus merits further investigation, as does the magnesium therapy of the withdrawal syndrome(s).

Acid-base balance

Wolfe & Victor (1979) found that arterial pH is increased, whereas Pa_{CO2} is decreased during the period 8–5Oh following alcohol withdrawal. This is consistent with a predominantly respiratory alkalosis. In a subsequent study, Wolfe & Victor (1973) confirmed the above findings and also showed that at subsequent time intervals (60–80h after withdrawal) arterial pH has returned to normal, whereas Pa_{CO2} remained decreased. Although plasma bicarbonate concentration was not determined, these latter results suggest that this anion must have been decreased. Additionally, Brooks & Adams (1975) found that alcohol withdrawal increased lactate concentration in arterial blood and CSF and also that of bicarbonate in plasma. Further work on acid-base balance in alcohol withdrawal may be fruitful in view of evidence that the disturbance of this balance may be partially involved in the aetiology of the behavioural signs and symptoms of withdrawal.

Cortisol, biogenic amine metabolism and prolactin release

Alcohol withdrawal is associated with both increased cerebral dopaminergic activity and pituitary-adrenal activation. The former may explain the finding (Ylikahri et at, 1981) that the TRH-dependent release of prolactin is decreased in alcohol withdrawal, whereas pituitary-adrenal activation may be responsible for the reported elevation of plasma cortisol concentration (Merry & Marks, 1972) and of those of urinary catecholamines and their metabolites (Kissin et al, 1973; Ylikahri et al, 1981 and references cited therein). Kissin et al (1973) also reported that alcohol withdrawal decreases the urinary concentration of the indolylamine tryptamine and that this latter decrease (and to a lesser extent the increase in the urinary concentration of the catecholamine metabolite vanillomandelic acid) correlated with sleep disturbances. Although another indolylamine, 5-hydroxytryptamine, appears to play an important role in the regulation of sleep and mood, surprisingly little work has been done on its metabolism in alcohol withdrawal. Evidence obtained from experiments in the rat (see Badawy, 1981 and references cited therein) strongly suggests that brain 5-hydroxytryptamine synthesis is inhibited during alcohol withdrawal as a result of enhanced hepatic degradation of the tryptophan precursor secondarily to induction of liver tryptophan pyrrolase by the increased release of glucocorticoids. A detailed study of the metabolism of indolylamines and catecholamines in man during alcohol withdrawal may therefore throw light on mood changes and other behaviour associated with the alcohol-withdrawal syndrome(s).

ACKNOWLEDGEMENT

I thank Dr M. Evans for his interest and helpful comments.

REFERENCES

Alha A R 1951 Calcium chloride and alcohol: effect of therapeutic doses of calcium chloride on clinical stage of alcoholic intoxication and on blood alcohol. Annals of Medical and Experimental Biology (Fenn) 29: 125–136

Alkana R L, Noble E P 1979 Amethystic agents: reversal of acute ethanol intoxication in humans. In: Majchrowicz E, Noble E P (eds) Biochemistry and pharmacology of ethanol, vol 2. Plenum Press, New York, pp 349–374

Alkana R L, Parker E S, Cohen H B, Birch H, Noble E P 1977 Reversal of ethanol intoxication in humans: an assessment of the efficacy of L-dopa, aminophylline and ephedrine. Psychopharmacology 55: 203–212

Anton A H 1965 Ethanol and urinary catecholamines in man. Clinical Pharmacology and Therapeutics 6: 462–469

Badawy A A-B 1978 The metabolism of alcohol. Clinics in Endocrinology and Metabolism 7: 247–271

Badawy A A-B 1980 Biochemical mechanisms of the alcohol-induced liver injury. British Journal on Alcohol and Alcoholism 15: 28–44

Badawy A A-B 1981 Hepatic involvement in the effects of alcohol on brain serotonin synthesis. British Journal on Alcohol and Alcoholism 16: 161–163

Badawy A A-B, Evans M 1981 The mechanism of the antagonism by naloxone of acute alcohol intoxication. British Journal of Pharmacology 74: 514–516

Barry H III 1979 Behavioural manifestations of ethanol intoxication and physical dependence. In: Majchrowicz E, Noble E P (eds) Biochemistry and pharmacology of ethanol, vol 2. Plenum Press, New York, pp 511–531

Beard J D, Knott D H 1968 Fluid and electrolyte balance during acute withdrawal in chronic alcoholic patients. Journal of the American Medical Association 204: 135–139

Beard J D, Knott D H, Fink R D 1974 The use of plasma and urine osmolality in evaluating the acute phase of alcohol abuse. Southern Medical Journal 67: 271–273

Beard J D, Sargent W Q 1979 Water and electrolyte metabolism following ethanol intake and during acute withdrawal from ethanol. In: Majchrowicz E, Noble E P (eds) Biochemistry and pharmacology of ethanol, vol 2. Plenum Press, New York, pp 3–16

Besson J A O, Glen A I M, Foreman E A, MacDonald A, Smith F W, Hutchison J M S et al 1981 Nuclear magnetic resonance observations in alcoholic cerebral disorders and the role of vasopressin. Lancet 2: 923–924

Brooks B R, Adams R D 1975 Cerebrospinal fluid acid-base and lactate changes after seizures in unanesthetized man II. alcohol withdrawal seizures. Neurology 25: 943–948

Champion H R, Baker S P, Bennett C, Fisher R, Caplan Y H, Long W B et al 1975 Alcohol intoxication and serum osmolality. Lancet 1: 1402–1404

Cohen R D 1972 Effect of fructose on blood-alcohol levels. Lancet 2: 1086
Damgaard S E, Lundquist F, Tonnesen K, Hansen F, Sestoft L 1973 Metabolism of ethanol and fructose in the isolated perfused pig liver. European Journal of Biochemistry 33: 87–97
Dundee J W, Bovill J G, Isaac M 1971 Failure to demonstrate an increased removal of alcohol from the blood stream by fructose. Medical Science Law 11: 146–148
Eisenhofer G, Whiteside E, Lambie D, Johnson R 1982 Brain water during alcohol withdrawal. Lancet 1: 50
Farmer R W, Fabre L F Jr. 1975 Some endocrine aspects of alcoholism. Advances in Experimental Medicine and Biology 56: 277–289
Fazekas G 1966 Hydrocortisone content of human blood and alcohol content of blood and urine after wine consumption. Quarterly Journal of Studies on Alcohol 27: 439–446
Feuerlein W 1974 The acute alcohol withdrawal syndrome: findings and problems. British Journal of Addiction 69: 141–148
Fink R, Rosalki S B 1978 Clinical biochemistry of alcoholism. Clinics in Endocrinology and Metabolism 7: 297–319
Flink E B, Shane S R, Scobbo R R, Blehschmidt N G, McDowell P 1979 Relationship of free fatty acids and magnesium in ethanol withdrawal in dogs. Metabolism 28: 858–865
Gessner P K 1979 Drug therapy of the alcohol withdrawal syndrome. In: Majchrowicz E, Noble E P (eds) Biochemistry and pharmacology of ethanol, vol 2. Plenum Press, New York, pp 375–435
Goldstein D B 1972 Relationship of alcohol dose to intensity of withdrawal signs in mice. Journal of Pharmacology and Experimental Therapeutics 180: 203–215
Gross M M, Goodenough D R, Hastey J M, Rosenblatt S M, Lewis E 1972 Sleep disturbances in alcoholic intoxication and withdrawal. In: Mello N K, Mendelson J H (eds) Recent advances in studies of alcoholism. United States Government Printing Office, Washington DC, pp 317–397
Gross M M, Lewis E, Hastey J 1974 Acute alcohol withdrawal syndrome. In: Kissin B, Begleiter H (eds) The biology of alcoholism, vol 3. Plenum Press, New York, pp 191–263
Harris R A 1979 Metabolism of calcium and magnesium during ethanol intoxication and withdrawal. In: Majchrowicz E, Noble E P (eds) Biochemistry and pharmacology of ethanol, vol 2. Plenum Press, New York, pp 27–41
Hawkins R D, Kalant H 1972 The metabolism of ethanol and its metabolic effects. Pharmacological Reviews 24: 67–157
Hore B D, Rossall C J 1979 Intoxication and withdrawal assessment scales. British Journal on Alcohol and Alcoholism 14: 2–6
Isbell H, Fraser H F, Wikler A, Bellville R E, Eisenman A J 1955 An experimental study on the aetiology of rumfits and delerium tremens. Quarterly Journal of Studies on Alcohol 16: 1–33
Jeffcoate W J, Herbert M, Cullen M H, Hastings A G, Walder C P 1979 Prevention of the effects of alcohol intoxication by naloxone. Lancet 2: 1157–1159
Jefferys D B, Flanagan R J, Volans G N 1980 Reversal of ethanol-induced coma with naloxone. Lancet 1: 308–309
Jenkins J S, Connolly J 1968 Adrenocortical response to ethanol in man. British Medical Journal 2: 804–805
Jones D P 1979 Biochemical abnormalities accompanying alcoholism: implications for the clinical diagnosis of acute and chronic intoxication with ethanol. In: Majchrowicz E, Noble E P (eds) Biochemistry and pharmacology of ethanol, vol 1. Plenum Press, New York, pp 677–691
Kakihana R, Butte J C 1979 Ethanol and endocrine function. In: Majchrowicz E, Noble E P (eds) Biochemistry and pharmacology of ethanol, vol 2. Plenum Press, New York, pp 147–164
Kimball C D, Huang S M, Torget C E, Houck J C 1980 Plasma ethanol, endorphin and glucose experiment. Lancet 2: 418–419
Kissin B, Gross M M, Schutz I 1973 Correlation of urinary biogenic amines with sleep stages in chronic alcoholization and withdrawal. Advances in Experimental Medicine and Biology 35: 281–289
Knott D H, Beard J D 1969 A diuretic approach to acute withdrawal from alcohol. Southern Medical Journal 62: 485–488

Krebs H A 1968 The effects of ethanol on the metabolic activities of the liver. Advances in Enzyme Regulation 6: 467–480
Krebs H A, Freedland R A, Hems R, Stubbs M 1969 Inhibition of hepatic gluconeogenesis by ethanol. Biochemical Journal 112: 117–124
Krebs H A, Stubbs M 1975 Factors controlling the rate of alcohol disposal by the liver. Advances in Experimental Medicine and Biology 59: 149–161
Levy R, Elo T, Hanenson I B 1977 Intravenous fructose treatment of acute alcohol intoxication: effects on alcohol metabolism. Archives of Internal Medicine 137: 1175–1177
Lowenstein L M, Simone R, Boulter P, Nathan P 1970 Effect of fructose on alcohol concentrations in the blood of man. Journal of the American Medical Association 213: 1899–1901
Majchrowicz E 1975 Induction of physical dependence upon ethanol and the associated behavioral changes in rats. Psychopharmacologia 43: 245–254
Marjot D H 1974 Has alcohol psychomimetic and convulsant properties. British Journal of Addiction 69: 295–304
Marks V 1978 Alcohol and carbohydrate metabolism. Clinics in Endocrinology and Metabolism 7: 333–349
Mello N K, Mendelson J H 1970 Experimentally induced intoxication in alcoholics: a comparison between programmed and spontaneous drinking. Journal of Pharmacology and Experimental Therapeutics 173: 101–116
Mello N K, Mendelson J H 1978 Alcohol and human behavior. Handbook of Psychopharmacology 12: 235–317
Mendelson J H (ed) 1964 Experimentally induced chronic intoxication and withdrawal in alcoholics. Quarterly Journal of Studies on Alcohol, supplement 2
Merry J, Marks V 1972 The effect of alcohol, barbiturate and diazepam on hypothalamic/pituitary/adrenal function in chronic alcoholics. Lancet 2: 990–991
Nicholson W M, Taylor M H 1938 The effect of alcohol on the water and electrolyte balance in man. Journal of Clinical Investigation 17: 279–285
Ogata M, Mendelson J H, Mello N K 1968 Electrolytes and osmolality in alcoholics during experimentally induced intoxication. Psychosomatic Medicine 30: 463–488
Perey B J, Helle S J, MacLean L D 1965 Acute alcoholic poisoning: a complication of gastric hypothermia. Canadian Journal of Surgery 8: 194–196
Perman E S 1958 The effect of ethyl alcohol on the secretion from the adrenal medulla in man. Acta Physiologica Scandinavica 44: 241–247
Räiha N, Mäenpää P 1964 The influence of ethanol on the acid-base balance of the blood in man and rat. Scandinavian Journal of Clinical and Laboratory Investigation 16: 267–272
Reitz R C 1979 Effects of ethanol on the intermediary metabolism of liver and brain. In: Majchrowicz E, Noble E P (eds) Biochemistry and pharmacology of ethanol, vol 1 Plenum Press, New York, pp 353–382
Robinson A G, Loeb J N 1971 Ethanol ingestion — commonest cause of elevated plasma osmolality. New England Journal of Medicine 284: 1253–1255
Rosalki S B 1971 A new colorimetric procedure for alcohol determination. Analytical Letters 4: 819–835
Rosenbaum M 1942 Adaptation of the central nervous system to varying concentrations of alcohol in the blood. Archives of Neurology and Psychiatry 48: 1010–1012
Rubini M E, Kleeman C R, Lamdin E 1955 Studies on alcohol diuresis 1. The effect of ethyl alcohol on water electrolyte and acid-base metabolism. Journal of Clinical Investigation 34: 439–447
Sargent W Q, Beard J D, Knott D H 1979 Acid-base balance following ethanol intake and during acute withdrawal from ethanol. In: Majchrowicz E, Noble E P (eds) Biochemistry and pharmacology of ethanol, vol 2. Plenum Press, New York, pp 17–25
Sargent W Q, Simpson J R, Beard J D 1974 The effect of acute and chronic alcohol administration on renal hemodynamics and monovalent ion excretion. Journal of Pharmacology and Experimental Therapeutics 188: 461–471
Sargent W Q, Simpson J R, Beard J D 1975 Extracellular volume expansion after ethanol in dogs. Journal of Studies on Alcohol 36: 1468–1479
Sellers E M, Kalant H 1976 Alcohol intoxication and withdrawal. New England Journal of Medicine 294: 757–762

Shaw G K 1978 Alcohol and the nervous system. Clinics in Endocrinology and Metabolism 7: 385–404
Sørensen S C, Mattisson K 1978 Naloxone as an antagonist in severe alcohol intoxication. Lancet 2: 688
Strauss M B, Rosenbaum J D, Nelson W P III 1950 Effect of alcohol on renal excretion of water and electrolyte. Journal of Clinical Investigation 29: 1053–1058
Sullivan J F, Wolpert P N, Williams R, Egan J D 1969 Serum magnesium in chronic alcoholics. Annals of New York Academy of Science 162: 947–962
Teasdale G, Jennett B 1974 Assessment of coma and impaired consciousness: a practical scale. Lancet 2: 81–84
Thieden H I, Grunnet N, Damgaard S, Sestoft L 1972 Effect of fructose and glyceraldehyde on ethanol metabolism in human liver and in rat liver. European Journal of Biochemistry 30: 250–261
Victor M, Adams R D 1953 The effect of alcohol on the nervous system. Research Publications — Association for Research in Nervous and Mental Disease 32: 526–573
Victor M, Brausch C 1967 The role of abstinence in the genesis of alcoholic epilepsy. Epilepsia 8: 1–20
Wolfe S M, Victor M 1969 The relationship of hypomagnesemia and alkalosis to alcohol withdrawal. Annals of New York Academy of Science 162: 973–984
Wolfe S M, Victor M 1973 In: Bourne P G, Fox R (eds) Causation and treatment of the alcohol withdrawal syndrome. Academic Press, New York, pp 137–169
Woods J F, Alberti K G M M 1972 Dangers of intravenous fructose. Lancet 2: 1254–1357
Wright J 1978 Endocrine effects of alcohol. Clinics in Endocrinology and Metabolism 7: 351–367
Ylikahri R H, Huttunen M O, Härkönen M 1981 Hormonal changes during alcohol intoxication and withdrawal. Pharmacology, Biochemistry and Behavior 13, supplement 1: 131–137
Ylikahri R H, Leino T, Huttunen M O, Posõ A R, Ericksson C J P, Nikkilä E A 1976 Effects of fructose and glucose on the ethanol-induced metabolic changes and on the intensity of alcohol intoxication and hangover. European Journal of Clinical Investigation 6: 93–102

6 *Neil McIntyre*

The effects of alcohol on water, electrolytes and minerals

INTRODUCTION

When a person drinks ethanol he may become drunk. The next morning he may have a 'hangover'. If he drinks a lot of ethanol for a long time he may develop cirrhosis, pancreatitis, brain damage, peripheral neuropathy, myopathy or cardiomyopathy. He may become physically dependent on ethanol, and if it is withdrawn suddenly may develop delirium tremens or other neurological abnormalities. The causes of these various manifestations of ethanol abuse are poorly understood. The proposed mechanisms include abnormalities of sodium, potassium and water metabolism, and changes in the body composition of other minerals and trace elements.

In this chapter I review the effects of alcohol on water, electrolyte and mineral metabolism. In reading the literature it is difficult to establish what effects can be attributed to ethanol per se, and whether various clinical manifestations of ethanol abuse can be attributed to those effects. There are several reasons for this. Many studies have been done on animals or on normal subjects; the results might differ from those which would be found in alcoholics. The results might depend on the initial fluid and electrolyte status of the subject and the fluids given during the course of the study. Most studies are short ones, and late compensatory changes are not then studied. Studies done in chronic alcoholics are difficult to interpret if the patients have developed cirrhosis, as cirrhosis itself may be associated with changes in fluid, electrolyte and mineral metabolism. Prolonged vomiting and/or diarrhoea, and inadequate nutrition may also complicate matters.

In each section of this chapter I shall, where possible, discuss the changes produced by acute ingestion of ethanol in normal subjects and in animals; the effect of chronic ingestion; changes found in chronic alcoholics, attempting to differentiate those attributable to ethanol from those which might be due to cirrhosis or poor nutritional state; and finally I shall describe changes associated with ethanol withdrawal.

ETHANOL AND BODY WATER

Following absorption of ethanol, its concentration in body fluids rises to a level which depends on the amount drunk, on the rate of ingestion and speed of absorption, on the volume of total body water, and on the rate at which ethanol is metabolised. Ethanol distributes throughout the body water and its concentration in cell water is similar to that of extracellular fluid. Because it diffuses easily, the urine concentration is a good measure of the extracellular ethanol concentration.

Ethanol is a better diuretic than water (Simanowsky, 1886) and the effect is dose related. In 1932 Murray showed that antidiuretic hormone reduced the diuretic effect and in 1951 Van Slyke & Ames showed that ethanol diuresis did not occur in dogs with diabetes insipidus. It now seems clear that ethanol works by inhibiting the release of antidiuretic hormone from the supraoptico-hypophyseal system.

The diuretic effect is not a simple function of the blood ethanol level. Plasma antidiuretic hormone appears to fall only when ethanol is increasing, and antidiuretic hormone may increase above control values even when the blood ethanol is at its peak. There may be a 'rebound' increase in antidiuretic hormone when ethanol levels are falling. This compensatory response has been attributed to a small rise in serum sodium (Andersson, 1977), to activation of the renin angiotensin system, to hypokalaemia and to hypotension (see Ponticelli & Montagnino, 1979).

The diuretic response is short lived; a further diuresis occurs with more ethanol but the response decreases with successive doses even if there is a cumulative increase in blood ethanol.

With chronic ingestion of ethanol, little or no tolerance develops to the antidiuretic effect of acute ethanol administration. In both animal and human experiments an enhanced diuresis has been found (Marquis et al, 1975; Ogata, 1963), possibly due to the excretion of water retained during the period of chronic ingestion (see next section).

The way in which ethanol affects the supra-optic nucleus is not known (Cicero, 1981). Several mechanisms have been suggested: a decrease of plasma factors, such as calcium, which are necessary for antidiuretic hormone secretion; an action on intravascular volume; an effect on renal haemodynamics. But these explanations ignore the classical observation of Van Slyke & Ames (1951) that the diuretic effect of intracarotid ethanol was several times greater than that of intravenous ethanol. There must be a direct effect somewhere within the cranium. Stimuli that normally cause ADH release, such as sodium chloride or direct application of acetylcholine to neurons in the supraoptic nucleus, can override the diuretic effect; thus the neuronal locus of action may be above the neurosecretory cells. But ethanol interferes with the histological changes induced by sodium chloride in the antidiuretic hormone- containing cells of the supraoptic nucleus, and it also inhibits electrically evoked discharges in the hypothalamic secretory cells (Cicero, 1981).

The diuresis following ethanol results from an increase in free water clearance; indeed sodium and potassium excretion fall (see later). The osmolality of body fluids should increase (osmolality ≡ osmoles per kg of water; osmolarity ≡ osmoles per litre of solution). The effects on plasma osmolality are complex because ethanol itself exerts an osmotic effect; a high blood ethanol is one reason for discrepancy between a measured plasma osmolality and osmolality calculated on the basis of the plasma concentration of sodium and potassium (Robinson & Loeb, 1971). Because ethanol is distributed throughout the body water, and because both intracellular and extracellular compartments contribute to free water loss, there should be no significant redistribution of fluid and electrolytes following ethanol ingestion, and only small changes in plasma sodium concentrations and plasma volume would be anticipated. It has been claimed, surprisingly, that plasma and interstitial fluid volumes increase after the acute administration of ethanol in animal and human experiments (Nicholson & Taylor, 1940; Rubini et al, 1955; Lolli et al, 1944). Such observations are difficult to interpret but they suggest a shift of water from the intracellular compartment (Lolli et al, 1944).

SODIUM, POTASSIUM AND CHLORIDE (Ponticelli & Montagnino, 1979; Wadstein & Ohlin, 1979)

The increase in urine volume following acute administration of ethanol is not accompanied by a corresponding increase in either sodium, potassium or chloride excretion. In animal studies the excretion of these monovalent ions has been found to be increased, decreased or unchanged. The response appears to depend on the amount of ethanol given, on the animal's state of hydration and on the duration of urine collection.

In studies in man, using relatively small doses of alcohol, variable results have also been seen but again experimental protocols have varied. Nicholson & Taylor, in 1938, gave ethanol orally to ambulant subjects over a period of 8 hours, and observed a reduction in sodium, potassium and chloride excretion over a prolonged period. Eggleton & Smith (1946) found a marked fall in chloride output for 2–3 hours after alcohol, similar to that seen with a water diuresis: *it occurred even when the diuretic response to ethanol was suppressed by the administration of nicotine*. Strauss and his colleagues (1950) studied sitting subjects given alcohol over 4–6 minutes, and collected urine for 2 hourly periods. The excretion of sodium, potassium and chloride over 6 hours was greater than that in subjects given only water, but this was due to a greater excretion during the last few hours of the 6 hour study period.

Rubini et al (1955) gave ethanol over 5–10 minutes to semirecumbent subjects and observed a prompt fall in sodium, potassium and chloride excretion, with an early increase in the urinary Na/K ratio. The fall in sodium preceded the rise in urinary flow and persisted after urine flow rose to prealcohol rates. They observed similar effects in a patient with Addison's disease on a constant intake of deoxycortone acetate (DOCA), and in another patient with diabetes insipidus.

From these and other studies we may conclude that ethanol causes a rapid fall in sodium, potassium and chloride excretion, but there are some conflicting reports (Kalbfleisch et al, 1963). In normal subjects the retained ions are rapidly excreted and normal fluid and electrolyte status is rapidly restored. The mechanism of the reduced monovalent ion excretion is not known.

Chronic ethanol ingestion

There appears to be no tolerance in chronic alcoholics to either the diuretic effect of acute alcohol ingestion (Ogata, 1963) or to its effect on monovalent ion excretion. Kissin et al (1964) showed that chronic alcoholics responded not only with an increase in urine flow but also with a fall in sodium, potassium and chloride excretion, although there was a greater initial loss of water and electrolytes (during the first hour) compared to non-alcoholic controls.

In normal subjects, the combination of an increased free water clearance and a reduction in sodium excretion would be expected to lead to an increase in plasma osmolality and hypernatraemia. Both of these changes tend to occur, but the increase in sodium concentration is small and is generally considered to be insignificant. With chronic alcohol ingestion we might expect more striking changes in body water and electrolytes. Beard & Knott (1963) studied well nourished chronic alcoholics and found a high total body water with an increase in the extracellular and intracellular spaces. As plasma electrolytes were normal they concluded that there had been chronic retention of salt and water; this explained the greater initial excretion of salt and water. The extra fluid and electrolytes were lost over several days following withdrawal. Although erythrocyte electrolytes were initially within normal limits, alcohol withdrawal was associated with a loss of red cell sodium and an increase in potassium. In these subjects there were abnormalities of liver function tests. Kissin et al (1964) found lower urinary sodium levels in alcoholics than in normal subjects and concluded that there was a chronic retention of salt and water; this explained the greater excretion of salt and water seen initially in alcoholics after ethanol administration. Clearly the interpretation of such studies must depend on accurate information on the prior dietary status of the subjects, and on the extent of liver damage, which Kissin et al considered to be a contributary factor in their sutdies. With early liver damage, the diuretic response to ethanol and water was unimpaired, but it was lost in more advanced liver disease when both salt and water were retained.

Ogata and his colleagues (1968) gave large amounts of ethanol over many days to alcoholics who had abstained from ethanol for several weeks. None of these subjects had evidence of liver disease. The serum sodium level rose during alcohol ingestion (although it did not account for the *corrected* increase in osmolality); serum potassium levels fell. There was an initial diuresis with alcohol, but urine volumes were subsequently quite variable depending in part on the volume of water ingested. There was a fall in urinary sodium and potassium excretion during alcohol ingestion, and a significant fall in haematocrit which persisted into the post alcohol phase. These observations fit with a prolonged retention of sodium and potassium in chronic alcoholics, as long as dietary intake is adequate and there are no abnormal losses due to vomiting or diarrhoea. In several studies an increase of exchangeable body sodium has been found. As hyponatraemia is more common than hypernatraemia in chronic alcoholics (Salum, 1972) the increase in body sodium is presumably due to an increase in intracellular sodium (Wadstein & Ohlin, 1979) and there appears to be no water deficit.

Potassium

There is good evidence that potassium metabolism is disturbed in chronic alcoholics (Wadstein & Ohlin, 1979). There are several reports of hypokalaemia in such patients, and in Salum's study (1972) it was particularly common in those who develop delirium tremens. Total body potassium was reduced in patients and in rats with chronic alcoholism (Pierson et al, 1977). Potassium deficiency has been attributed to poor nutrition and excessive gastrointestinal losses.

Low serum potassium levels during ethanol withdrawal have been attributed to respiratoty alkalosis which shifts potassium into cells. Wadstein & Skude (1978) studied chronic alcoholics on admission to hospital. All had normal serum potassium on admission but showed a transient hypokalaemia before and during delirium tremens. This was not due to losses in urine or from the gastrointestinal tract, nor was it associated with a fall in pCO_2, and they assumed a shift into cells for other reasons. To explain their findings they postulated that chronic ethanol ingestion increases the intracellular Na/K ratio by inhibiting Na, K — ATPase. During ethanol withdrawal the activity of this enzyme is stimulated by an increase in circulating catecholamines, which causes a relative hyperpolarization of the cell membranes and a shift of potassium into cells to replace intracellular sodium. The transient nature of the hypokalaemia after withdrawal has been interpreted as evidence against severe total body deficiency. Clearly this is an important area and more work is required to clarify the disturbances of potassium metabolism in alcoholics.

The fluid and electrolyte status of chronic alcoholics is clearly not just of academic interest. Intensive fluid therapy has been advocated in the management of ethanol withdrawal and delirium tremens. Several groups have studied fluid and electrolyte handling during withdrawal but the results have been conflicting. In controlled studies, Ogata et al (1969) found transient increases in urine volume on cessation of drinking, but there were variable changes in urinary electrolytes. In later studies (Mendelson et al, 1979) they observed sharp but transient falls in serum sodium and potassium. Beard & Knott (1968) observed a fall in body weight, a significant increase in urinary sodium and chloride, and a transient decrease in urinary potassium followed by an increase. Serum sodium and potassium levels four days after withdrawal showed little change from admission values but they may have missed the transient changes seen by Mendelson. By contrast other authors (Flink et al, 1954; Sereny et al, 1966) have observed further sodium and potassium retention and weight gain during alcohol withdrawal, postulating a rebound increase in antidiuretic hormone secretion, and an increase in aldosterone secretion (but this would not explain retention of potassium). In the study of Sereny et al, it was of interest that the patients with liver damage tended to lose weight on alcohol withdrawal and had either negative or less positive sodium balance.

In none of these studies was frank delirium tremens present and it is difficult to know what advice to give on fluid and electrolyte requirements in this condition. Certainly dehydration and renal failure can occur if inadequate fluid therapy is given to subjects who must control their own intake. But Balsano & Reynolds (1970), who found an increased plasma volume in delirium tremens, treated 10 patients with fluid restriction and 10 patients with generous fluid administration (6l/24 h). Satisfactory recovery was much quicker in the fluid restricted group and the authors argued that fluid restriction therapy, popular until a few decades ago, deserves re-evaluation in the treatment of ethanol withdrawal syndromes. Wadstein & Ohlin (1979) agreed with this recommendation, but pointed out the need for vigilance and for the correction of losses caused by complicating problems.

Fluid and electrolyte handling in alcoholics deserves further study using modern techniques, and reinterpretation in the light of our greater understanding of the pathophysiology of such disorders.

MAGNESIUM (Flink, 1981; Rude & Singer, 1981)

Magnesium (relative atomic mass 24.3) is the fourth most abundant cation of the human body and the second most abundant in the intracellular fluid. There are about 1000 mmol of magnesium in a 70 kg person. About 50–60 per cent is present in bone; most is incorporated in the mineral lattice but about a third is present in an exchangeable pool. About 45 per cent of the body's magnesium is in cells, where it serves many important functions. It is a cofactor for ATP and is necessary for many enzymatic reactions, particularly those involving high energy phosphate transfer. It plays a role in the reversible association of intra cellular particles and in the binding of macromolecules to subcellular organelles. The intracellular magnesium concentration varies from 2–15 mmol/kg, depending on the tissue. The concentration in extracellular fluids is 0.7–1.1 mmol/l; in plasma about two thirds in present as free cation and the remainder is bound to proteins. The level of magnesium in plasma appears to correlate best with the exchangeable magnesium of bone. Unfortynately, there is not a good correlation between plasma magnesium and intracellular magnesium; there may be low intracellular magnesium with normal plasma magnesium and vice versa. But as it is difficult to measure bone and intracellular magnesium it is the plasma magnesium which is normally used to assess the body's magnesium status.

The daily requirement for magnesium is about 15 mmol in adults and this amount is normally present in the diet. It can be absorbed by the whole of the small bowel, by an active transport system which is Vitamin D dependent like that for calcium. About a third of ingested magnesium is absorbed. Magnesium is excreted mainly by the kidney but well over 90 per cent of the filtered magnesium is reabsorbed in the proximal tubule. The body is very efficient at conserving magnesium when the intake is low and clinical magnesium deficiency is normally seen only when deficient intake is associated with factors increasing magnesium loss via the kidneys or intestine.

The effect of alcohol

Acute administration of ethanol to rats (Sargent et al, 1975) and to man (Kalbfleisch et al, 1963) increased urinary excretion of magnesium. In man the effect lasted about two hours. The effect was similar in normal and alcoholic subjects and was present in two alcoholics with low plasma magnesium levels at the time of the study. The mechanism is not clear. Mendleson, Ogata & Mello (1969) gave ethanol to alcoholics over a prolonged period. Urinary magnesium increased with increase in urine flow, and the authors concluded that increased urinary magnesium loss occurred only while blood alcohol levels were rising (as with the diuresis). Ethanol had little effect on serum magnesium. Urinary magnesium levels were normal with high, sustained levels of blood alcohol, and it is not surprising that Dunn & Walser (1966) found no increase in urinary magnesium when a magnesium-depleted subject was given alcohol over a period of eight days.

Alcoholism is the commonest cause of hypomagnesaemia, but the incidence of low magnesium levels has varied in different series. Devgun et al (1981) found no significant difference between the mean plasma magnesium level in alcoholics and in normal controls; only 9 out of 108 alcoholics had levels below the reference range. In other series the incidence of hypomagnesaemia has been greater (Sullivan et al, 1969; Bogden & Troiano, 1978; Flink et al, 1954; Heaton et al, 1962). Several observations suggest that hypomagnesaemia does reflect deficiency of total body magnesium in alcoholics (Jones et al, 1969): magnesium retention can be demonstrated with repletion in alcoholics; the urinary excretion of magnesium does not increase proportionally with intravenous (IV) magnesium; a low calculated exchangeable body pool has been found; and there are reports of low magnesium in muscle biopsies.

The magnesium deficiency of chronic ethanol ingestion has been attributed to urinary loss of magnesium but it is likely that other factors (such as inadequate diet, diarrhoea and vomiting), are contributory, and normal urinary conservation mechanisms may not be effective in chronic alcoholic patients.

Magnesium deficiency has several metabolic consequences (Rude & Singer, 1981; Flink, 1981). It appears to cause hypocalcaemia, possibly due to impaired secretion of parathyroid hormone (PTH) and end organ resistance to PTH. Serum PTH levels rose within minutes when IV magnesium was given to a hypocalcaemic, magnesium deficient patient. The hypocalcaemia of magnesium deficiency is resistant to the action of Vitamin D.

Hypokalaemia is also common in magnesium deficiency, and may respond only to magnesium therapy. It appears to be due to an impaired ability of the kidney to reabsorb potassium. This and the calcium effects may be linked to the role of magnesium in adenosine triphosphate (ATP) metabolism.

Magnesium deficiency has been held responsible for haemolytic anaemia, dysphagia, and for the development of ventricular arrhythmias, including ventricular fibrillation and sudden death. Other electrocardiographic (ECG) changes (prolonged P–R and Q–T intervals and flat broad T waves) are similar to those of potassium deficiency, and there is evidence of increased susceptibility to digitalis intoxication.

There has been considerable interest in the neuromuscular effects of magnesium deficiency. It causes hyperactivity, which can occur in the absence of hypocalcaemia, with muscle tremors, fasciculation, positive Chvostek's and Trousseau's signs, and frank tetany. Central nervous signs such as nystagmus, ataxia, vertigo, athetoid and choreiform movements and convulsions have all been attributed to magnesium deficiency.

Stendig-Lindberg et al (1977) studied 7 patients with hypomagnesaemia associated with chronic alcoholism. Their muscle magnesium content was significantly lower than that of healthy controls. The sodium, chloride and water content was increased, due largely to an increase in extracellular water, but muscle potassium content was not significantly different. These patients had a significant reduction in the maximum isometric voluntary contraction force of the quadriceps femoris muscle. It was suggested that magnesium deficiency per se might be a causative factor in alcoholic myopathy.

Alcohol withdrawal

Because of its known sedative effects, magnesium was used empirically to treat delirium tremens (Wacker & Vallee, 1958). Subsequently it was demonstrated that the neuromuscular abnormalities described above occurred with experimental and clinical magnesium deficiency. Several groups found lower serum magnesium levels in patients with delirium tremens than in patients who do not suffer this complication on withdrawal (Sullivan et al, 1969; Mendelson, Ogata & Mello, 1969; Salum, 1972); it has been found that serum magnesium levels fall during the first two or three days following alcohol withdrawal when neurological manifestations are most likely. The mechanism of this fall (and of the accompanying drop in sodium and potassium) is not known but it may be associated with redistribution of these ions due to acid base changes.

Although magnesium deficiency may cause neurological abnormalities, delirium tremens and other manifestations can can also occur with normal or high magnesium levels, and the serum level may rise to normal before the development of delirium, this increase can occur without any magnesium supplementation. If magnesium deficiency per se is the cause of these abnormalities it is surprising that they are not seen in chronic alcoholics who are magnesium deficient prior to alcohol withdrawal (Fankhusen et al, 1964). Patenteral magnesium has appeared to be of benefit in some patients with delirium tremens, but no convincing benefit has been shown in controlled studies (Heaton et al, 1963; Vallee, Wacker & Ulmer, 1960).

There is better evidence that a low serum magnesium causes the epilepsy of alcohol withdrawal ('rum fits') and alcoholic tremulousness (Wolfe & Victor, 1969). Patients with these problems were sensitive to photic stimulation, which induced myoclonic movements and seizures, and a good correlation was found between the serum magnesium level and the threshold for photomyclonus. The fall in serum magnesium after alcohol withdrawal was associated with a respiratory alkalosis, which may have contributed to the hypomagnesaemia, but intravenous magnesium per se raised the threshold or abolished the photomyoclonus response. Patients with seizures who went on to develop delirium tremens did not show a photomyoclonic response at the time of delirium but magnesium levels had risen to normal by that time.

Despite conflicting evidence on the role of magnesium deficiency in the genesis of neuromuscular abnormalities it would seem sensible to check serum magnesium levels following ethanol withdrawal, and to give magnesium when serum levels are obviously reduced. Magnesium sulphate, 0.5 mmol per kg (IV or intramuscularly) can be given during the first 24 hours, and about half that amount during the subsequent 3 or 4 days; great caution must be observed in patients with renal failure; they should receive much smaller doses. (Rude & Singer, 1981; Flink, 1981).

Although a good deal of work has been done on magnesium metabolism in alcoholics it is clear that many questions remain unanswered and it is a field which would repay further careful study.

CALCIUM (Stamp, 1978)

Calcium (relative atomic mass 40.08) is the most abundant cation in our bodies, which contain 1–2 kg (25–50 mol) of this element; over 98 per cent of it is the skeleton. Although only a fraction of this amount is present in the extra-cellular fluid its concentration there is critical; when plasma levels deviate outside the normal range (2.1–2.6 mmol/l) there may be serious consequences. Plasma calcium is present largely as free ions or bound to proteins, but a small amount is present in diffusible complexes. The ionized calcium concentration affects neuromuscular excitability, is a factor regulating the secretion of parathyroid hormone, and plays a key role in various stages of blood coagulation.

The concentration of calcium in the cytosol is extremely low (around 1 μmol/l) but larger amounts are present in mitochondria, the endoplasmic reticulum, and in the tubules of the sarcolemma. Calcium is important for many cellular processes, including muscle contraction, endocytosis and exocytosis, glycogen metabolism, and the release of neurotransmitters. When cells are stimulated, there is a rapid influx of calcium into the cytosol; it binds to calmodulin, or other calcium binding proteins, and this in turn causes the activation or inhibition of various enzymes. Calcium is thus an important intracellular messenger (Cheung, 1982). The average diet provides about 25 mmols of calcium daily, mainly in dairy products; about a half is absorbed. Most calcium is absorbed in the proximal small intestine and the absorptive mechanism is stimulated by vitamin D.

Some calcium is lost from the body via the gastrointestinal tract and this loss appears to be unregulated. Urinary calcium loss is normally between 2.5 and 7.5 mmol per day. When the calcium intake is low or when calcium absorption is reduced through vitamin D deficiency, urinary calcium falls, but its renal conservation is relatively inefficient and either of these factors will lead to calcium deficiency. Resorption from bone tends to prevent reduction in extracellular fluid calcium concentration but only at the expense of bone thinning.

Effects of ethanol (Ponticelli & Montagnino, 1979)

In animal studies, ethanol has no effect on the plasma calcium concentration in small doses (e.g. 0.5 g/kg), but with larger doses (2–8 g/kg) hypocalcaemia occurs rapidly. It is not due to renal excretion of calcium and is seen after nephrectomy. It occurs following removal of the thyroid and parathyroids. In man, urinary calcium loss increases after acute ethanol ingestion (Kalbfleisch et al, 1963); plasma parathormone and calcitonin levels also increase and this may explain why hypocalcaemia is not usually found in man, although an acute *rise* in calcium was reported in one study (Markkanen & Nanto, 1966).

Acute ethanol administration increased urinary calcium in alcoholics in one study (Kalbfleisch et al, 1963); there was little change or a fall in another (Ogata et al, 1968). There was no change in plasma calcium. Little information is available on plasma and urinary calcium in chronic alcoholics. Devgun and his colleagues (1981) found normal plasma calcium in all of 129 chronic alcoholics. 25-hydrovitamin D levels were low but not as low as in subjects with osteomalacia. Calcium absorption was low in alcoholic subjects, possibly due to the impaired vitamin D metabolism seen in liver disease (Dechavanne et al, 1974). Chronic ethanol ingestion appeared to inhibit intestinal calcium transport in rats, by a mechanism independent of hepatic and pancreatic dysfunction, and the effect was not reversed by vitamin D.

There are several reports of alcoholic patients presenting with low serum calcium, usually in association with low serum magnesium. When intravenous magnesium was given to such subjects Sullivan et al (1969) found an increase in urinary calcium and a fall in serum calcium. In subjects with tetany, and both hypocalcaemia and hypomagnesaemia, serum calcium levels returned gradually to normal while the low magnesium persisted for a longer period (Wallack & Dimich, 1969).

Fractures are more common in alcoholics than in normal subjects. This is not surprising as they are more likely to fall. But the bone density in alcoholics under the age of 45 is similar to that found in non-alcoholic subjects over the age of 70. Saville (1977) believed that decreased dietary calcium, decreased fractional absorption, and increased urinary calcium loss might all contribute to this bone thinning, together with a stimulation of parathyroid hormone activity. Hypomagnesaemia might also cause parathyroid stimulation with further bone resorption.

Rubin (1979) suggested that ethanol affects calcium uptake by the sarcoplasmic reticulum and that this may account for cardiac and skeletal muscle abnormalities in alcoholics. In dogs, ethanol impairs calcium uptake by cardiac sarcoplasmic reticulum, and in human volunteers a similar effect was seen in skeletal muscle after a month of ethanol ingestion. Interference with calcium transport may eventually impair the supply of calcium to the contractile elements and thus have a negative inotropic effect.

The role of ethanol in calcium metabolism is poorly understood. The potential implications of disturbances of calcium homeostasis are clearly very great. More work needs to be done in this area.

PHOSPHORUS

Laboratories with multichannel analysers provide clinicians automatically with the results of serum inorganic phosphate estimations. These may help in the assessment of patients with renal functional impairment, and may provide clues in the analysis of metabolic bone disease. But many results are ignored as the clinical implications of abnormal serum phosphorus levels are poorly understood. This neglect does not reflect the biological importance of phosphorus. The body of a 70 kg man contains about 700 g of phosphorus (about 23 000 mmol). 80–85 per cent is found in bone and about 9 per cent in skeletal muscle. Phosphorus is an important constituent of nucleic acids and phospholipids; phosphorylation and dephosphorylation is important in enzyme regulation, in the storage and release of energy (e.g. in ATP:ADP reactions), and in the metabolism of sugars such as glucose and fructose. Phosphorus compounds (e.g. 2:3 diphosphoglycerate;

2:3 DPG) regulate the release of oxygen from erythrocytes. Inorganic phosphate is a major intracellular anion, but measurement of its intracellular concentration is difficult because of the presence of phosphorylated intermediates. Its concentration in extracellular fluid is between 0.9 and 1.5 mmol/l. About 12 per cent of total serum phosphate is bound to protein, 75 per cent is present as HPO_2- or $NaHPO_4$- and 10 per cent as H_2PO_4-.

Serum phosphate, which should be measured on fasting samples, is higher in children (1.3–2, 3 mmol/1) than in adults, and it tends to rise after the menopause. Ingestion of carbohydrate or fat lowers serum phosphate but there is a diurnal variation even with prolonged fasting. Serum phosphate falls with alkalosis.

Phosphorus is abundant in all natural foods, and absorption of phosphate is very efficient unless phosphate-binding substances such as non-absorbable antacids are ingested. The major control of phosphate metabolism is via the kidney, and phosphate reabsorption is inversely proportional to the filtered load. Reabsorption, which is inhibited by parathyroid hormone, occurs mainly in the proximal tubule; increased urinary phosphate excretion also occurs if proximal tubular sodium absorption is decreased.

Acute and chronic effects of ethanol

There have been few studies on the acute effects of ethanol on phosphate metabolism. In 1963 Kalbfleisch and his colleagues gave ethanol, orally and intravenously, to normal and alcoholic subjects. They observed little change in urinary phosphate excretion and no change in plasma phosphate levels. Subsequently they found that urinary phosphate rose in chronic alcoholics ingesting large amounts of ethanol, but only when there was hypomagnesemia. Markannen & Nanto (1966) infused 50 ml of ethanol into normal subjects over 3 hours; they found an increase in serum calcium and phosphate, and phosphorus excretion rose as high as 300 mg/h.

The chronic effects of alcohol ingestion on plasma and urinary phosphate are complex. In most chronic alcoholics who eat a normal diet, plasma phosphate levels are in the normal range. In alcoholics admitted for drying out, and not for medical complications of alcoholism, hyperphosphataemia was found to be more common (10 per cent) than hypophosphataemia (2.5 per cent), while the latter was seen more commonly (30 per cent) in alcoholic patients on the medical ward (Ryback et al, 1980). Hypophosphataemia, which has been observed in several surveys, has been attributed to poor dietary intake, the use of antacids, diarrhoea and vomiting, respiratory alkalosis, ethanol per se, magnesium deficiency, alcoholic hypocalcaemia and ketoacidosis (Knochel, 1977) but the exact mechanism is still not clear.

In alcoholics, serum phosphorus may fall to very low levels during the first few days after admission, and this fall may have important clinical consequences. Even patients with normal plasma phosphorus may have a low muscle phosphorus content (Knochel et al, 1975; Anderson et al, 1980) possibly due to phosphaturia associated with chronic magnesium deficiency. Respiratory alkalosis, common during alcohol withdrawal, causes a fall in plasma phosphorus and in urinary phosphorus excretion. This may appear secondary to a fall in intracellular inorganic phosphate, as a rise in intracellular pH increases phosphorylated intermediates within the cell. Refeeding may also cause hypophosphataemia through the production of phosphorylated intermediates. In patients who have low muscle phosphorus levels initially, a further fall in serum inorganic phosphate may cause muscle damage. Rhabdomyolysis is a well recognised complication in alcoholics and Knochel found elevation of serum creatine kinase (CK) in alcoholics following the development of hypophosphataemia. Ryback and his colleagues (1980), however, found no relationship between CK and phosphate levels in serum. Other consequences attributed to phosphorus deficiency and hypophosphataemia include red cell dysfunction, due to low levels of 2:3 DPG, white cell and platelet abnormalities, myocardial failure, abnormal liver function and neurological disturbances; the last three of these abnormalities may be related to poor tissue oxygenation secondary to deficiency of red cell 2:3 DPG.

The evidence that phosphorus metabolism is affected in chronic alcoholics is good, but it is not yet clear that abnormal phosphorus metabolism plays an important role in many alcoholic subjects. This area will be a fruitful field of research using new techniques, such as nuclear magnetic resonance (NMR), for studying intracellular phosphate metabolism.

ZINC (Prasad & Oberleas, 1976; Burch et al, 1978)

Zinc (relative atomic mass 65.4) is present in relatively large amounts in the human body; about 25–45 mmol are present in a 70 kg person and of this about 98 per cent is intracellular where it is chelated with cytosol and microsomal apo-enzymes. Skin, bone, muscle, visceral organs and the prostate are relatively rich in zinc. Zinc is a key component of dozens of metallo-enzymes such as carbonic anhydrase, alkaline phosphatase, carboxypeptidase and collagenase. The pancreas is rich in zinc which appears to play a role in the storage and secretion of insulin. Zinc seems to be important in bone development, in growth and sexual maturation and in the secretion of retinol binding proteins. Its presence in alcohol dehydrogenase has been a particular stimulus to the study of zinc in alcoholism and alcohol-related disease.

The concentration of zinc in plasma is very low (11–19 μmol/l). 30–40 per cent is bound firmly to a specific α 2 macroglobulin and 60 per cent is loosely bound to albumin. About one per cent is associated with amino acids, particularly histidine and cysteine. Unfortunately, the plasma zinc concentration is not considered to be a reliable indicator of tissue zinc. The recommended daily intake for a 70 kg adult is 15 mg/day (about 0.23 mmol). Meat and fish are rich sources. Zinc from vegetable sources may be relatively unavailable as it is chelated by phytates which prevent absorption. 50–60 per cent of ingested zinc is absorbed in the small intestine. The mechanism is unknown but appears to involve zinc-binding proteins, with absorption inversely related to the zinc content of the mucosa. Peak levels of ingested radio-active zinc appear at about 4 hours. Zinc and copper appear to compete for absorption.

After absorption, zinc is taken up by the liver and other tissues and is incorporated in zinc-containing proteins. About 10 μmols of zinc are excreted daily in the urine, and sweat contains about 15 μmol/l. Around 200 μmols are excreted each day in bile; some of this reabsorbed but faecal loss is the major route of zinc excretion.

Effect of alcohol

There are conflicting data about the acute affects of alcohol on zinc metabolism (Russell, 1980). In some studies there has been no rise in urinary zinc excretion with alcohol, while Gudbjarnasan & Prasad (1969) found a fall in serum zinc and increased urinary zinc when vodka was given to normal subjects. In more prolonged studies by Giovetti & Russell (1979), urinary zinc excretion doubled during the drinking period and serum zinc fell; opposite effects were observed when ethanol was discontinued. In rats, urinary and faecal excretion of zinc was increased by alcohol, and tissue levels of zinc were lower after 4 weeks than in control animals.

Devgun et al (1981) found no reduction in serum levels in alcoholic patients (no details of liver function were given); other workers have found low serum zinc in alcoholic subjects with and without liver disease (Bogdon & Troiano, 1978; Sullivan & Lankford, 1965; Sullivan & Heaney, 1970; Halsted et al, 1968). It is difficult to sort out the effects of ethanol per se and of liver disease on zinc metabolism (Burch, Hahn & Sullivan, 1978). Patients with cirrhosis have hyperzincuria and low serum and liver zinc levels. Recently, Scholmerich et al (1982) suggested that this occurs due to shunting of portal blood past the liver; absorbed zinc therefore enters the general circulation in large amounts and is excreted by the kidney.

This is an attractive hypothesis, but in studies on rats with portal blood diversion for 3 months, Epstein et al (1982) found a high liver zinc concentration and normal zinc levels in the brain and kidney. They therefore questioned the role of portal diversion in the production of zinc deficiency in alcoholic cirrhosis. Reduced hepatocellular function might also impair the hepatic uptake of zinc; low serum zinc levels associated with hyperzincuria have been found in the acute phase of viral hepatitis. Transient hyperzincuria in alcoholics may thus be due not to alcohol but to acute alcoholic hepatitis. This question requires further study.

Clearly zinc deficiency may occur in alcoholic patients, but may be more important in patients with liver damage. Several problems have resulted from zinc deficiency in children in Iran and Egypt; affected children are dwarfed, with hypogonadism, rough skin, poor appetite and mental lethargy (Prasad, 1976). In adults zinc deficiency has been incriminated as a cause of taste and smell disturbance, poor wound healing and impaired pancreatic function. It has been suggested that zinc plays a role in hepatic drug metabolism, because of its key role in the functioning of many enzymes (Burch et al, 1978). It has also been incriminated as a cause of abnormalities in the babies of alcoholic women, whose plasma zinc levels during pregnancy were lower than those of non alcoholic women (Flynn et al, 1981).

CONCLUSION

In this review, which is necessarily incomplete, I have tried to summarise the effects of ethanol on the handling of water, electrolytes and certain minerals. It is clear that these effects are important. But it is striking that no light has been shed on the basic mechanisms underlying these actions of ethanol. There is no good explanation for its effect on ADH secretion, or on urinary sodium, potassium and chloride excretion, nor is there an explanation for the effects on magnesium, calcium, zinc or phosphate metabolism.

I suspect that until we understand how ethanol works it will not be possible to interpret many of the conflicting results which have been obtained. Goldstein & Chin (1981) have suggested that ethanol exerts its pharmacological action by interfering with the fluidity of cell membranes and, on the basis of animal experiments, have suggested that tolerance to ethanol may be acquired by adaptive changes in the chemical composition of membranes which make them less susceptible to physical perturbation by ethanol. Their results do not explain why the diuretic action of ethanol, and its action on sodium and chloride excretion, are preserved or even enhanced in chronic alcoholics. But their studies do suggest a new approach to a very difficult problem, and this field is badly in need of new ideas!

REFERENCES

Anderson R, Haller R, Elms J et al 1980 Skeletal muscle phosphorus and magnesium deficiency in alcoholic myopathy. Quoted by Knockel J P. Archives of Internal Medicine 140: 613–614

Andersson B 1977 Regulation of body fluids. American Review of Physiology 39: 185–200

Balsano N A, Reynolds B M 1970 Fluid restriction in the management of acute alcholic withdrawal. Surgery 68: 283–286

Beard J D, Knott D H 1968 Fluid and electrolyte balance during acute withdrawal in chronic alcoholic patients. Journal of the American Medical Association 204: 133–139

Bogden J D, Troiano R A 1978 Plasma calcium, copper, magnesium and zinc concentrations in patients with the alcohol withdrawal syndrome. Clinical Chemistry 24: 1553–1556

Burch R E, Hahn H K J, Sullivan J F 1978 Other metals and the liver, with particular reference to zinc. In: Powell L (ed) Metals and the liver. Dekker, New York, ch 9, p 333–361

Cheung W Y 1982 Calmodulin. Scientific American no 6, 246: 48–56

Cicero T J 1981 Neuroendocrinological effects of alcohol. Annual Review of Medicine 32: 123–142
Dechavanne M, Barbier Y, Prost G, Pehlivanian E, Tolot E 1974 Study of absorption of ^{47}calcium in alcoholic cirrhosis: action of 25-hydroxychole-calciferol, vol 3. Novelle Presse Medicale, Paris, p 2549–2551
Devgun M S, Fiabane A, Paterson C R, Zarembski P 1981 Vitamin and mineral nutrition in chronic alcoholics including patients with Korsakoff's psychosis. British Journal of Nutrition 45: 469–473
Dunn M J, Walker M 1966 Magnesium depletion in normal man. Metabolism 15: 884–895
Eggleton M G, Smith I G 1946 The effect of ethyl alcohol and some other diuretics on chloride excretion in man. Journal of Physiology 104: 435–442
Epstein O, Spisni R, Woods J, Parhboo S, Burroughs A K, Dormandy T L 1982 The effect of portasystemic shunting on liver, brain and kidney zinc concentrations in the rat. British Journal of Experimental Pathology 63: 203–206
Fankushen D, Raskin D, Dimich A, Wallach S 1964 Significance of hypomagnesemia in alcoholic patients. American Journal of Medicine 37: 802–812
Flink E B 1981 Magnesium deficiency: Etiology and clinical spectrum. Acta Medica Scandinavica Supp 647: 125–137
Flink E B, Stutzman F L, Anderson A R, Konig T, Fraser R 1954 Magnesium deficiency after prolonged parenteral fluid administration and after chronic alcoholism complicated by delirium tremens. Journal of Laboratory and Clinical Medicine 43: 169–183
Flynn A, Martier S S, Sokol R J, Miller S L, Golden N L, Del Villano B C 1981 Zinc status of pregnant alcoholic women: A determinant of fetal outcome. Lancet 1: 572–575
Giovetti A C, Russell R M 1979 Effect of ethanol ingestion on serum and urine zinc and serum copper levels in chronic alcoholics. Clinical Research 27: 232A
Goldstein D B, Chin J H 1981 Interaction of ethanol with biological membranes. Federation Proceedings 40: 2073–2076
Gudbjarnason S, Prasad A S 1969 Cardiac metabolism in experimental alcoholism. In: Sandesia V M (ed) Biochemical and clinical aspects of alcohol metabolism. Thomas, Springfield, p 266–272
Halstead J A, Hackley B, Rudzki C, Smith J C 1968 Plasma zinc concentration in liver disease. Gastroenterology 51: 1098–1105
Heaton F W, Pyrah L N, Beresford C, Bryson R W and Martin D F 1962 Hypomagnesemia in chronic alcoholism. Lancet 2: 802–805
Jones J E, Shane S R, Jacobs W H, Flink E B 1969 Magnesium balance studies in chronic alcoholism. Annals of the New York Academy of Sciences 162: 934–946
Kalbfleisch J M, Lindeman R D, Ginn H E, Smith W O 1963 The effects of ethanol administration on urinary excretion of magnesium and other electrolytes in alcoholic and normal subjects. Journal of Clinical Investigation 42: 1471–1475
Kissin B, Schenker V J, Schenker A C, Belanger I R, Stucker M, Woerner R 1964 Hyperdiuresis after ethanol in chronic alcoholics. American Journal of Medical Sciences 248: 660–669
Knochel J P 1977 The pathophysiology and clinical characteristics of severe hypophosphatemia. Archives of Internal Medicine 137: 203–220
Knochel J P, Bilbery G L, Fuller T J 1975 The muscle cell in chronic alcoholism. The possible role of phosphate depletion in alcoholic myopathy. Annals of the New York Academy of Science 252: 274–286
Lolli G, Rubin M, Greenberg L A 1944 Effect of ethyl alcohol on volume of extrecellular water. Quarterly Journal of Studies in Alcohol 5: 1–4
Markkanern T, Nanto V 1966 The effect of ethanol infusion on the calcium phosphorus balance in man. Experimentia 22: 753–754
Marquis C, Marchetti G, Burlet C, Boulangé M 1975 Sécrétion urinaire et hormone antidiurétique chez des rats soumis a une administration répétée d'ethanol. Comptes Rendus de la Societe de Biologie 169: 154–161
Mendleson J H, Ogata M, Mello N K 1969 Effects of alcohol ingestion and withdrawal on magnesium states of alcoholics: Clinical and experimental findings. Annals of the New York Academy of Sciences 162: 918–933
Murray M M 1932 The diuretic action of alcohol and its relation to pituitrin. Journal of Physiology 76: 379–386

Nicholson W M, Taylor H M 1938 The effect of alcohol on the water and electrolyte balance in man. Journal of Clinical Investigation 17: 279–285
Nicholson W M, Taylor H M 1940 Blood volume studies in acute alcoholism. Quarterly Journal of Studies in Alcohol 1: 472–482
Neilsen J 1963 Magnesium metabolism in acute alcoholics. Danish Medical Bulletin 10: 225–233
Ogata M 1963 Clinical and experimental studies on water metabolism in alcoholics. Quarterly Journal of Studies in Alcohol 24: 398–411
Ogata M, Mendelson J H, Mello N K 1968 Electrolytes and osmolality in alcoholics during experimentally induced intoxication. Psychosomatic Medicine 30: 463–488
Pierson R N, Wang J, Frank W, Awen G, Rayyes A 1977 Alcohol affects intracellular potassium, sodium and water distributions in rats and man. Currents in Alcoholism 1: 161–178
Ponticelli C, Montagnino G 1979 Direct renal effects of alcohol. In: Avogaro P, Sirtori C R, Tremoli E (eds) Metabolic effects of alcohol. Elsevier/North Holland, New York, p 365–375
Prasad A S 1976 Deficiency of zinc in man and toxicity. In: Prasad A S, Oberleas D (eds) Trace elements in human health and disease, vol I. Zinc and copper. Academic Press, New York, ch 1, p 1–20
Prasad A S, Oberleas D (eds) 1976 Trace elements in human health and disease, vol I. Zinc and copper. Academic Press, New York
Robinson A G, Loeb J N 1971 Ethanol ingestion — Commonest cause of elevated plasma osmolality. New England Journal of Medicine 284: 1253–1255
Rubin E 1979 Alcoholic myopathy in heart and skeletal muscle. New England Journal of Medicine 301: 28–33
Rubini M E, Kleeman C R, Lamdin E 1955 Studies on alcohol diuresis: 1) The effect of ethyl alcohol ingestion on water, electrolyte and acid-base metabolism. Journal of Clinical Investigation 34: 439–447
Rude R K, Singer F R 1981 Magnesium deficiency and excess. Annual Review of Medicine 32: 245–259
Russell R M 1980 Vitamin A and zinc metabolism in alcoholism. American Journal of Clinical Nutrition 33: 2741–2749
Ryback R S, Eckardt M J, Pautler C P 1980 Clinical relationships between serum phosphorus and other blood chemistry values in alcoholics. Archives of Internal Medicine 140: 673–677
Salum I, 1972 Delirium tremens and certain other acute sequels of alcohol abuse. Acta Psychiatrica Scandinavia Supp 235: 145
Sargent W Q, Simpson J R, Beard J D 1975 Renal hemodynamics and electrolyte excretion after reserpine and ethanol. Journal of Pharmacology and Experimental Therapeutics 193: 356–362
Saville P D 1977 Alcohol and skeletal disease. In: Lieber C S (ed) Metabolic aspects of alcoholism. MTP Press, Lancaster, p 135–347
Scholmerich J, Kottgen E, Rauch N, Lohle E, Vuilleumier J P, Gerok W 1982 Portasystemic shunting as reason of zinc and vitamin A deficiency in patients with liver disease. Hepatology 2: 148
Sereny G, Rapoport A, Husdan H 1966 The effect of alcohol withdrawal on electrolyte and acid base balance. Metabolism 15: 896–904
Simanowsky N P 1886 Über die Gesundheitsschädlichkeit hefetrüber Biere und über den ablauf der künstlichen Verdauung bei Bierzusatz. Archiv für Hygiene Munchen U Leipzig 4: 1
Stamp T C B 1978 Mineral metabolism. In: Dickerson J W T, Lee H A (eds) Nutrition in the clinical management of disease. Edward Arnold, London, p 246–286
Stendig-Lindberg G, Bergstrom J, Hultman E 1977 Hypomagnesaemia and muscle electrolytes and metabolites. Acta Medica Scandinavica 201: 272–280
Strauss M B, Rosenbaum J D, Nelson W P 1950 The effect of alcohol on the renal excretion of water and electrolyte. Journal of Clinical Investigation 29: 1053–1058
Sullivan J F, Heaney R P 1970 Zinc metabolism in alcoholic liver disease. American Journal of Clinical Nutrition 23: 170–177
Sullivan J F, Lankford H G 1965 Zinc metabolism and chronic alcoholism. American

Journal of Clinical Nutrition 17: 57–63
Sullivan J F, Wolpert P W, Williams R, Egan J D 1969 Serum magnesium in chronic alcoholism. Annals of the New York Academy of Science 162: 947–962
Vallee B L, Wacker W E C, Ulmer D D 1960 Magnesium deficiency tetany syndrome in man. New England Journal of Medicine 262: 155–161
Van Slyke H B, Ames R G 1951 Alcohol diuresis. Acta Endocrinologica 7: 110–121
Wacker W E C, Vallee B L 1958 Magnesium metabolism. New England Journal of Medicine 259: 431–438, 475–482
Wadstein J, Ohlin H 1979 Changes in water, serum electrolytes and basic acid balance in alcohol. In: Avogaro P, Sirtori C R, Tremoli E (eds) Metabolic effects of alcohol. Elsevier/North Holland, New York, p 357–364
Wadstein J, Skude G 1978 Does hypokalaemia precede delirium tremens? Lancet 2: 549–550
Wallach S, Dimich A, 1969 Radiomagnesium turnover in hypomagnesemic states. Annals of the New York Academy of Sciences 162: 963–972
Wolfe S M, Victor M 1969 The relationship of hypomagnesemia and alkalosis to alcohol withdrawal symptoms. Annals of New York Academy of Sciences 162: 974–984

7

John Wright   Vincent Marks

The effects of alcohol on carbohydrate metabolism

INTRODUCTION

Disturbances in carbohydrate metabolism result, inevitably, in either hyperglycaemia with carbohydrate intolerance, hypoglycaemia or, occasionally, a combination of both. Such is the multifactorial influence of alcohol on carbohydrate metabolism, it is not surprising that any, or all, of these patterns may be produced. The effects of alcohol are due not only to the biochemical changes resulting from the metabolism of the alcohol itself but also to the effects on insulin secretion and other endocrine functions, of liver disease and of alcohol abuse on general nutritional status. Although each will be considered separately, any combination of them can determine the net result.

Assessment of published data is complicated by wide variations in experimental protocols and by the difficulties of comparing results of animal with human studies and of studies on normal subjects with those on chronic alcoholics. In view of these complexities, it is understandable that, despite broad agreement in many areas, a number of inconsistencies and contradictions in the literature remain unexplained.

ALCOHOL METABOLISM

Only about 10 per cent of ingested alcohol is excreted unchanged in the urine and breath; the remainder is metabolised, almost exclusively in the liver. Three different enzyme systems are capable of metabolising alcohol. These are alcohol dehydrogenase (ADH), the microsomal ethanol oxidising system (MEOS) and catalase. In each of these systems, alcohol is initially metabolised to acetaldehyde but there are important differences in the cofactors involved:

$$CH_3CH_2OH + NAD^+ \xrightarrow{ADH} CH_3CHO + NADH + H^+$$

$$CH_3CH_2OH + NADPH + H^+ + O_2 \xrightarrow{MEOS} CH_3CHO + NADP^+ + 2H_2O$$

$$CH_3CH_2OH + H_2O_2 \xrightarrow{\text{Catalase}} CH_3CHO + 2H_2O$$

The acetaldehyde formed in each of these reactions is further metabolised to acetate by aldehyde dehydrogenase (ALDH):

$$CH_3CHO + NAD^+ + H_2O \longrightarrow CH_3COOH + NADH + H^+$$

The relative importance of the enzme systems responsible for initial oxidation of alcohol to acetaldehyde has been the subject of considerable investigation and debate. The most important pathway physiologically is that involving ADH. With a Km for ethanol of 0.5–2.0 mmol/l (2.3–9.2 mg/dl), this system is particularly active at relatively low concentrations of alcohol. The involvement of MEOS in alcohol metabolism in vivo is not clear. The activity of this system can be increased by inducers of drug-metabolising enzymes such as barbiturates, but alcohol itself does not appear to possess this property, and the ability of induced MEOS activity to increase ethanol oxidation in vivo has not been convincingly shown. Nevertheless, the Km of MEOS for ethanol (7–9 mmol/l) is considerably higher than that of ADH, and it may, therefore, play a significant role at high blood ethanol concentrations (above 10 mmol/l; 46 mg/dl). Even at this level, however, ADH still accounts for over 60 per cent of the alcohol metabolised. Catalase is almost certainly unimportant physiologically.

GLUCONEOGENESIS

Oxidation of alcohol by ADH (and of acetaldehyde by ALDH) results in the accumulation of NADH within the liver cells and a decrease in NAD^+:NADH ratio. Apart from tending to inhibit the further oxidation of ethanol to acetaldehyde, the alteration in redox state has a major inhibitory effect on gluconeogenesis. (This effect may, to some extent, be mitigated by participation of MEOS in alcohol metabolism in the presence of high alcohol concentrations and in chronic alcohol abuse.) The mechanism of the inhibitory effect of alcohol on gluconeogenesis was elucidated by Krebs (1968) who showed that whilst alcohol inhibited gluconeogenesis in the liver, it did not do so in the kidneys (which do not contain ADH), and that the degree of inhibition decreased as the ethanol concentration rose over 10 mmol/l, above which there is a decrease in ADH activity.

The fall in cytosolic NAD^+:NADH ratio produced by alcohol results in a rise in the lactate:pyruvate ratio mainly due to a fall in pyruvate concentration. This, in turn, decreases the activity of pyruvate carboxylase, a key enzyme early in the gluconeogenesis pathway. The inhibition of gluconeogenesis from precursors other than those involving pyruvate as an intermediary is probably also explicable on the basis of changes in the redox state of the NAD^+ couple (Krebs, 1968).

In prolonged starvation, the kidney assumes a more important role in gluconeogenesis, accounting for up to 50 per cent of the glucose synthesised.

Whether this also occurs in chronic alcoholic subjects, at risk from recurrent hypoglycaemia, is unknown.

Inhibition of gluconeogenesis as outlined above, is probably the main way that alcohol effects carbohydrate metabolism and the principal mechanism by which alcohol consumption predisposes to hypoglycaemia. Ethanol has no direct effect on glycogen metabolism although it may stimulate glycogenolysis indirectly by provoking secretion of catabolic hormones, particularly cortisol and the catecholamines, when it is taken in excessive amounts. This may prevent the development of hypoglycaemia in well-fed subjects and occasionally may even result in hyperglycaemia (see below). When, on the other hand, liver glycogen stores are limited or depleted, the inhibition of gluconeogenesis predominates and results in a fall in glucose production and consequently in hypoglycaemia.

INSULIN SECRETION

The precise influence of alcohol on insulin secretion is controversial. Although the administration of alcohol alone does not affect insulin secretion, the majority of studies carried out on man report enhanced insulin responses to glucose when given with, or after, alcohol (Kühl & Andersen, 1974; Nikkilä & Taskinen, 1975; McMonagle & Felig, 1975; Dornhorst & Ouyang, 1971; O'Keefe & Marks, 1977). Despite this consensus, there are occasional reports of alcohol having either no effect (Shanley, 1972) or a delaying effect on the insulin response to glucose (Wapnick, 1972). In contrast to those on humans, animal studies often suggest an impairment of the insulin response to glucose in vivo and in vitro (Shah, 1977; Singh, 1971), although this does appear to depend largely upon the species and doses of alcohol used.

More problematical than interpretation of plasma insulin levels in relation to insulin secretion is the assessment of their meaning in terms of carbohydrate metabolism. Thus, whilst most authors have demonstrated improved glucose tolerance (McMonagle & Felig, 1975), enhanced glucose disposal (Nikkilä & Taskinen, 1975) or even frank hypoglycaemia (O'Keefe & Marks, 1977) in response to the higher insulin levels provoked by a combination of alocohol and carbohydrate compared with carbohydrate alone, others have reported either impairment of glucose tolerance (Dornhorst & Ouyang, 1971) or unaltered glucose levels in the presence of increased plasma insulin levels (Kühl & Andersen, 1974), suggesting the production of a relative insulin resistance by alcohol.

Clearly, not only the species studied, but also the dose, timing and route of alcohol administration and its relation to glucose administration influence the effects of alcohol on insulin secretion. It seems unlikely that they can all be attributed to intermediate products of ethanol metabolism or to changes in calcium metabolism as has been suggested by Shah et al (1977). There is, however, no completely satisfactory explanation as to how alcohol influences insulin secretion. Alcohol, by mouth, has been shown to stimulate secretin release, possibly by reducing duodenal pH (Straus et al, 1975), but no data are available with regard to its effect on other gastrointestinal hormones, particularly those thought to play a major role in the enteroinsular axis. A dual effect of alcohol, i.e. an indirect stimulation of insulin secretion via gastrointestinal insulinotropic hormones and reflexes, and a direct inhibition of the β-cell, could explain some of the conflicting results from published studies. Against this is some evidence for a direct priming effect of alcohol on β-cells arising from the demonstration of an enhanced insulin respose to both high and low doses of glucagon in the presence of alcohol (Wright et al, 1979). This is at variance with the findings of Friedenberg et al (1971), who gave glucagon to their subjects following prolonged pre-exposure to alcohol and only after they had already received a number of glucose injections.

There is no evidence for an effect of alcohol on the catabolism of insulin itself independent of any effect exerted through alcohol-associated liver disease.

Alcohol abuse is an important cause of chronic pancreatitis, accounting for the majority of cases in some countries and at least 50 per cent of those occurring in the United Kingdom (Fink & Rosalki, 1978). Although exocrine pancreatic function tends to be more severely effected than endocrine function, a significant proportion of patients with chronic pancreatitis exhibit impaired glucose tolerance due to diminished insulin secretion and, occasionally, frank diabetes requiring treatment with insulin.

Pancreatic damage is also seen in association with haemosiderosis, a common complication of alcohol abuse in those parts of the world where the customary beverages (Bantu beers and red wine, for example) contain a high concentration of iron. It is, however, also common in the general alcoholic population, possibly due to enhanced absorption of iron. The massive insulin resistance occasionally see in patients with haemochromatosis and haemosiderosis, some of whom may require several thousand units of insulin daily (Dymock et al, 1972), suggests that the mechanism of carbohydrate intolerance in this condition is complex, and probably involves hepatic insensitivity to insulin as well as pancreatic insufficiency.

OTHER ENDOCRINE FUNCTIONS

Both acute and chronic alcohol consumption can influence the function of endocrine and neuroendocrine systems, with secondary effects on carbohydrate metabolism. The most important, in this respect, are effects upon pituitary secretion of ACTH and growth hormone (GH), and upon sympathetic nervous activity and the adreno-medullary secretion of catecholamines.

Acute, severe intoxication, particularly in the alcohol-naive subject, evokes a stress response, with stimulation of ACTH (and cortisol) secretion, and activation of the sympathetic neuroendocrine system. This is frequently associated with the appearance of transient hyperglycaemia followed by reactive hypoglycaemia some hours later (Forsander et al, 1975). In experimental animals, a sublethal dose of alcohol produces an acute increase in catecholamine secretion and hyperglycaemia (Klingman & Goodall, 1957). Prior adrenalectomy prevents development of the hyperglycaemia (Klingman, Bane & Haag, 1959) suggesting that it is due, not to a direct effect of alcohol, but indirectly to that of the catecholamines through their ability to stimulate glycogenolysis and gluconeogenesis, and to inhibit insulin secretion.

In man, a modest dose of alcohol, sufficient to raise blood alcohol levels above 22 mmol/l (100 mg/dl), results in stimulation of ACTH, cortisol and catecholamine secretion in most normal subjects. The GH response is less consistent, appears to require a higher dose of alcohol and may be influenced by other metabolites, particularly free fatty acids. The influence of these hormonal changes on carbohydrate metabolism is uncertain. In none of the studies of the effects of alcohol on glucose tolerance discussed above were measurements of cortisol, GH or catecholamines performed, but it is possible that changes in these catabolic hormones account for the apparent insulin resistance seen in some of these studies. Catecholamine secretion in response to modest intoxication has been shown to be higher in women than in men, probably due to their lesser degree of habituation (Myrsten et al, 1975). This fact may help to explain the impairment of glucose tolerance observed in the exclusively female group of healthy young volunteers studied by Dornhorst & Ouyang (1971) in contrast to most other studies in which glucose tolerance was improved or unaltered by the modest amounts of alcohol used.

In chronic alcoholism, not only the cortisol response to moderate, acute intoxication, but also the cortisol, catecholamine and GH response to insulin-induced hypoglycaemia are impaired or absent in about one quarter of the patients (Wright, 1978). This hypothalamic-pituitary unresponsiveness, which apparently recovers following prolonged periods of abstinence, predisposes to development of hypoglycaemia and, more importantly, impairs recovery from established hypoglycaemia.

Paradoxically, prolonged drinking by chronic alcoholics may result in sustained hypercortisolaemia (Mendelson, Ogata & Mello, 1971; Stokes et al, 1973) and occasionally in the development of 'alcohol-induced pseudo-Cushing's syndrome' which is difficult to distinguish, both clinically and biochemically, from idiopathic Cushing's syndrome (Smals et al, 1976; Rees et al, 1977; see also Ch. 14). This is often associated with hyperglycaemia and carbohydrate intolerance which resolve, along with the other stigmata of the syndrome, on cessation of drinking.

ALCOHOLIC LIVER DISEASE

The extent to which liver disease contributes to abnormalities of carbohydrate metabolism seen in association with alcohol abuse is uncertain. Overt liver disease is so relatively common, and can develop so rapidly, that it must be assumed that minor degrees of liver dysfunction are almost inevitable and probably occur without histological evidence of liver damage in any persistently heavy drinker. The enormous functional reserve of the liver generally mitigates the effects of damage but may not protect against the effects of alcohol which are evenly spread throughout the hepatic parenchyma.

The subject of carbohydrate metabolism in alcoholic liver disease has recently been comprehensively reviewed (Johnston & Alberti, 1976) and since a full discussion of it is beyond the scope of this chapter, only the major points will be summarised.

The liver is the major site of gluconeogenesis in the fasting state and of glucose disposal, under the influence of insulin, in the fed state. Inhibition of hepatic gluconeogenesis is the major, though probably not the only, factor in the development of alcohol-induced hypoglycaemia (see above). In contrast, renal gluconeogenesis is virtually unaffected by alcohol and assumes a more prominent role in the maintenance of blood glucose levels in patients with chronic liver disease. Although frank hypoglycaemia is an uncommon occurrence in liver disease (except in acute hepatic failure), fasting blood levels of gluconeogenic precursors are often elevated, particularly in patients with alcoholic cirrhosis, presumably due to their diminished clearance from the blood. This, together with the inhibition of gluconeogenesis by alcohol, predisposes to development of hyperlactataemia in association with hypoglycaemia. The reduction of glycogen stores in the liver, reflected in a diminished blood glucose response to glucagon stimulation, further exacerbates the tendency to hypoglycaemia.

In addition to its impaired ability to maintain blood glucose concentration in the fasted state, the damaged liver has a diminished capacity for the disposal of carbohydrate in the fed state, and alcoholic cirrhosis is characteristically associated with insulin resistance. The mechanism is unclear but there is almost certainly a peripheral as well as a hepatic component. Aggravating factors include poor dietary intake of carbohydrate, decreased insulin degradation, a reduced number of hepatic insulin receptors, portal-systemic shunting, and hypersecretion (and/or diminished degradation) of insulin antagonists such as glucagon, cortisol and catecholamines.

Whatever the mechanisms, the triad of glucose intolerance, hyperinsulinism and hyperglucagonaemia typifies alcoholic liver disease and, in combination with a reduced capacity for gluconeogenesis, predisposes to fasting hypoglycaemia, impaired glucose tolerance and reactive hypoglycaemia.

POOR NUTRITIONAL STATUS IN ALCOHOLISM

Nutritional deficiencies are commonly found in association with alcohol abuse (Thomson, 1978; see also Ch. 10) and may influence carbohydrate metabolism independently of their role in the pathogenesis of alcoholic liver disease. Alcohol itself is an important source of energy, supplying 7.1 KCal/g and accounting for an average of 6 per cent or more of dietary

Table 7.1 Enzymes of carbohydrate metabolism requiring cofactors potentially deficient in chronic alcoholism

Cofactor	Enzyme	Metabolic pathway
Thiamine pyrophosphate (TPP)	Pyruvate dehydrogenase	Conversion of pyruvate to acetyl CoA
	Transketolase	Pentose phosphate shunt
Zinc	Lactate dehydrogenase	Pyruvate ⇌ Lactate
	Pyruvate carboxylase	Gluconeogenesis
	Glyceraldehyde 3-P dehydrogenase	Glycolysis and gluconeogenesis
Magnesium	Hexokinase, glucokinase	Glycolysis
	Phosphoglucomutase	
	Phosphofructokinase	
	Phosphoglycerate kinase	
	Phosphoglyceromutase	Glycogenolysis
	Enolase	
	Pyruvate kinase	
	Glycogen phosphorlyase	
	Pyruvate carboxylase	Gluconeogenesis

energy in many countries. The carbohydrate content of alcoholic beverages is extremely variable, contributing as much as 80 per cent of total calories in some beers but totally absent from pure spirits. In view of the importance of an adequate dietary intake in maintaining carbohydrate tolerance, the results of 'glucose tolerance tests' must be interpreted with caution in alcoholics. In addition, an inadequate or irregular diet can lead to depletion of liver glycogen stores which may, in turn, be exacerbated by concomitant liver disease. This further increases the susceptibility of alcoholic subjects to hypoglycaemia and impairs the metabolic response to established hypoglycaemia.

The diet of chronic alcoholic patients is frequently deficient in a number of ingredients including vitamins and trace metals which act as cofactors for enzymes involved in carbohydrate metabolism (Table 7.1). Thiamine deficiency, for example, may be present as assessed by red cell transketolase measurement, in up to 40 per cent of untreated chronic alcoholics (Fink & Rosalki, 1978). The extent to which deficiencies of any of these factors results in demonstrable biochemical abnormalities is speculative, but some of the reactions involved clearly occupy key positions in a number of metabolic pathways. The particular susceptibility of important enzymes such as pyruvate carboxylase to dietary deficiencies is evident from Table 7.1.

CLINICAL PATTERNS OF HYPERGLYCAEMIA

Of the two clinical consequences of disturbances in carbohydrate metabolism caused by alcohol (i.e. hyper- and hypoglycaemia), hyperglycaemia is probably the less common and certainly has the less serious implications.

Hyperglycaemia is occasionally seen in subjects with severe intoxication or patients with ethanol poisoning, particularly if the alcohol was consumed with a large quantity of readily-absorbed carbohydrate. However, in this situation, it is imperative to monitor patients carefully during recovery in order to detect the early development of hypoglycaemia. Specific treatment for the hyperglycaemia is not usually required and in the absence of complicating factors such as obesity, the majority of patients investigated following recovery from the acute episode have normal glucose tolerance.

The incidence of carbohydrate intolerance in alcoholic subjects investigated by means of a formal glucose tolerance test varies considerably between published studies (Marks & Wright, 1976; Serenyi & Endrenyi, 1979). The reason for the high incidence in some studies is unclear but probably reflects differences in patient preparation or in underlying, subclinical liver disease. No long-term follow-up studies have been reported on patients in whom carbohydrate intolerance has been documented either following continued drinking or following a long period of abstention.

Occasional patients are reported in whom alcohol abuse has led to the development of frank clinical diabetes (Philips & Safrit, 1971). This is usually relatively mild but may be accompanied by gross hypertriglyceridaemia which resolves with control of the diabetes. This may be a manifestation of underlying liver disease and may precipitate pancreatitis, itself a potential cause of insulin deficiency. In view of the high prevalence of both diabetes and alcohol abuse in the population, it is important to demonstrate that carbohydrate tolerance improves following abstinence from alcohol before it can be implicated as the cause of diabetes in any individual subject. Dietary treatment, with or without oral hypoglycaemic agents, is usually adequate to control alcohol-induced diabetes when it does occur.

CLINICAL PATTERNS OF HYPOGLYCAEMIA

First described over 40 years ago, hypoglycaemia is one of the most serious and potentially fatal metabolic complications of alcohol abuse, with a mortality of around 10 per cent in adults. A number of distinct clinical patterns can be recognised, reflecting the different pathophysiological mechanisms by which the hypoglycaemia is caused.

Alcohol-induced fasting hypoglycaemia

Once liver glycogen stores have been depleted, maintenance of blood glucose concentration during fasting is dependendent upon gluconeogenesis. Inhibition of hepatic gluconeogenesis by alcohol is largely responsible for its ability to cause hypoglycaemia in fasting subjects. This can be reliably reproduced in normal subjects by giving them alcohol either orally or intravenously after a fast of 36 hours or more (prior to which, presumably, mobilisation of glycogen, which is not inhibited by alcohol, prevents the development of hypoglycaemia). The fall in blood glucose is accompanied by a rise in plasma cortisol but not of growth hormone (which appears to be suppressed by the concurrent elevation in free fatty acid levels) and by appropriate suppression of insulin and C-peptide secretion, though this has been disputed (Joffe et al, 1977). Plasma glucagon levels rise above fasting levels during alcohol-induced hypoglycaemia (Palmer & Ensinck, 1974; Joffe et al, 1977) probably due to the reduction in insulin secretion. The suggestion that increased peripheral utilisation of glucose contributes towards the development of alcohol-induced fasting hypoglycaemia (Searle et al, 1974) was not supported by a recent study which confirmed inhibition of gluconeogenesis as the dominant factor (Wilson et al, 1981).

Clinically, alcohol-induced fasting hypoglycaemia is an uncommon problem, but one it is essential to recognise and treat promptly. Patients are characteristically chronically malnourished and habitual drinkers, but exceptionally a single heavy drinking bout may precipitate hypoglycaemia in a normal subject who has missed a meal on two. Habitual intake of a low carbohydrate diet increases susceptibility to hypoglycaemia which may occur after only modest doses of alcohol (McLaughlan, 1973). Children, who are, anyway, more prone to hypoglycaemia, are particularly at risk, and cases have been reported following use of an alcohol-containing mouthwash and even following tepid-sponging with alcohol (Moss, 1970). The mortality in children may be as high as 25 per cent.

The blood alcohol concentration is characteristically not unduly high by the time the diagnosis is made, which is generally many hours after termination of drinking. It is essential to consider the possibility of hypoglycaemia in any unconscious patient known or suspected to have been drinking heavily even though there may be an adequate alternative explanation for the coma such as a head injury or a drug overdose. In children, particularly, treatment should, if necessary, be administered before the result of blood glucose measurement is known. Treatment with glucagon is ineffective and may, in fact, be dangerous since the insulin response to glucagon stimulation is enhanced in the presence of alcohol (Wright et al, 1979). Treatment, therefore, must consist of intravenous glucose, possibly with 100 mg hydrocortisone initially. Recurrent bouts of hypoglycaemia precipitated by alcohol abuse should raise the suspicion of coexisting alcohol-induced ACTH or growth hormone insufficiency (Andreani, 1976), both of which are seemingly reversible with abstinence.

In normally fed subjects in whom starvation has been 'accelerated' by vigorous exercise, modest doses of alcohol (25 g), sufficient to produce a blood alcohol level of no more than about 5 mmol/l, may precipitate hypoglycaemia in some subjects (Haight & Keatinge, 1973), especially when subjected to the cold. In view of the fact that both hypoglycaemia and alcohol inhibit shivering (MacDonald et al 1980), this observation has implications for those involved in activities such as winter sport and mountaineering who should be warned against using alcohol after exercise in the cold.

Alcohol potentiation of drug-induced hypoglycaemia

In normal, healthy subjects, the hypoglycaemic action of insulin is potentiated by simultaneous administration of alcohol either orally or intravenously, resulting not only in a lower blood glucose nadir but also a delayed return to normoglycaemia (Arky et al 1968). Despite the lower blood glucose, the fall in free fatty acid concentration is attenuated by alcohol and this is associated with a diminished growth hormone response.

In a large literature series (Madison, 1968), insulin was by far the commonest drug causing hypoglycaemia in combination with alcohol. There have been a number of deaths reported in insulin-treated diabetics following heavy drinking (Arky et al, 1968) and there are obviously many more which are either unreported or in which severe hypoglycaemia results in permanent brain damage but falling short of death itself.

Alcohol abuse should always be remembered as a possible factor in the development of nocturnal hypoglycaemia, which is being recognised with increased frequency in insulin-treated diabetics. Though frequently asymptomatic, many patients complain of headache and malaise the following morning. 'Morning after' blood glucose concentrations are statistically lower in both alcoholics and irregular drinkers than in non-drinkers, but there is no conclusive evidence that the symptoms of hangover, which are similar in many respects, are attributable to hypoglycaemia.

The combination of alcohol and oral hypoglycaemic agents is less hazardous (Madison, 1968), possibly because many patients treated with these drugs are obese, which protects against the hypoglycaemic effects of alcohol, and because it is younger, usually insulin-dependent, patients who tend to drink more heavily.

'Essential' reactive hypoglycaemia in alcoholics

As already mentioned there is considerable variation in the reported results of standard tests of glucose tolerance in alcoholics. In at least one series, however (Marks & Wright, 1977), there was a high incidence of reactive hypoglycaemia (with otherwise normal carbohydrate tolerance) which was not preceded by an excessive rise in plasma insulin in response to the glucose ingestion. However, the observed reactive hypoglycaemia failed to provoke a rise in plasma cortisol. This failure of hypoglycaemia to provoke a normal plasma cortisol response may be a predisposing factor in the development of alcohol-induced hypoglycaemia in a proportion of alcoholics.

Alcohol-induced reactive hypoglycaemia

It is now clear that the capacity of alcohol to enhance the insulin response to carbohydrate occasionally results in the development of frank reactive hypoglycaemia. Contrary to initial reports (Kühl & Andersen, 1974), priming of the islets is not required and the effect is observed when alcohol and carbohydrate are administered simultaneously. In a group of ten healthy volunteers the insulin response to 60 g of sucrose and 50 g of alcohol was consistently greater than that seen following sucrose alone, despite similar peak blood glucose levels, and the subsequent blood glucose nadir was lower in all except one subject in the presence of alcohol (O'Keefe & Marks, 1977). The tendency to develop true hypoglycaemia, accompanied by typical symptoms of neuroglycopoenia, is subject to considerable individual variation, but in susceptible subjects, it may be precipitated by very modest amounts of alcohol (25 g) when taken with a mainly carbohydrate meal (Marks & Wright, 1979). Although hypoglycaemia usually develops between two and three hours after drinking, by which time blood alcohol may have fallen to a socially acceptable level, the cumulative effects of mild intoxication and hypoglycaemia may produce a dangerous reduction in critical faculties. The importance of repeated metabolic insults of this nature, occurring particularly at night after an evening's drinking, in the development of brain damage in chronic alcoholics has yet to be established.

Sucrose is an important carbohydrate source in most alcohol beverages and 'mixers' (tonic water, ginger ale, etc). Sucrose is a potent stimulus to insulin release in its own right, and substitution of an alternative carbohydrate with less insulin-stimulating properties, such as fructose or starch, for sucrose in drinks results in marked attenuation not only of the plasma insulin response but also of the tendency to hypoglycaemia (Wright & Marks, 1979; Joffe et al, 1981).

ALCOHOL AND DIABETES

Insulin is not required for the oxidation of alcohol which can, therefore, be metabolised normally by diabetics. There is no reason why, in principle, alcohol should be excluded from the diet of diabetic subjects, provided its

Table 7.2 Average carbohydrate, alcohol and energy content of selected alcoholic beverages

Beverage	Alcohol content (v/v)	Contents of a typical 'measure' or drink			
		Volume (ml)	Alcohol (g)	Sugar (g)	Energy (Kcals)
Beer and lager	3.5–5.5%	280	7.5–12.3	8–15	80–120
'Diet' lager	4.0–6.0%	280	9.0–13.4	2–10	90–130
Wine	10–13%	120	9.5	1–3	70–80
Dry sherry	18%	60	8.5	1.5	65
Port	21%	45	7.0	5.0	70
Spirits	40%	24	7.5	Nil	50
Mixers					
regular	Nil	120	0	10	40
sugar-free	Nil	120	0	0	0

The 'strengths' of the beers vary enormously from type to type but the figures given include most of the popular brands in Britain caloric contribution (and that of anything taken with it) is taken into consideration (Table 7.2). Current dietary guidelines encourage liberalisation of the amount of unrefined carbohydrate in the diet of patients with diabetes, but still usually impose strict limitations on refined carbohydrate, particularly sucrose. In view of this, the amount and type of alcoholic beverage permitted to diabetics should be even more carefully controlled than for the population as a whole.

Both diabetes and alcohol abuse predispose to hyperlipoproteinaemia and, in particular, hypertriglyceridaemia. The role of this particular metabolic anomaly in the pathogenesis of vascular disease is uncertain, but it is generally considered desirable to avoid any factors which exacerbate alterations in lipid metabolism. The reported ability of alcohol to raise high-density lipoprotein (HDL)-cholesterol levels has not been shown to reduce the risk of ischaemic heart disease and does not provide grounds for recommending it as a form of treatment in diabetic patients in whom the risk of atherosclerosis is increased.

The ability of alcohol to produce dangerous hypoglycaemia in patients treated with insulin has already been discussed. It is much less of a problem with oral hypoglycaemic agents, but a variable proportion of patients treated with sulphonylureas (particularly, but not exclusively, chlorpropamide) do develop an unpleasant vasoactive reaction (chlorpropamide-alcohol flushing) after ingestion of only small amounts of alcohol. The mechanism of this idiosyncratic phenomenon is unknown but substitution of an alternative sulphonylurea preparation frequently resolves the problem.

Both alcohol and the biguanide drugs (particularly Phenformin) elevate blood lactate levels. Alcohol consumption should be strictly limited in patients receiving treatment with these drugs in view of the danger of precipitating lactic acidosis.

The ability of alcohol to enhance the insulin response to oral carbohydrates may possibly be useful in the treatment of non-insulin dependent diabetes, for whilst excessive drinking may precipitate diabetes (Philips & Safritt, 1977), there is absolutely no evidence that moderate amounts of alcohol, within dietary recommendations, upset diabetic control (Walsh & O'Sullivan, 1974). No studies have, to our knowledge, been performed on the effect of pre- or per-prandial alcohol on the levels of glucose and other metabolites in the blood following a meal, or on the insulin response to feeding in patients with Type II diabetes or those with Type I diabetes and measurable plasma C-peptide levels. In view of the high prevalence of diabetes and the widespread consumption of alcohol, these are major gaps in our knowledge.

REFERENCES

Andreani D, Tamburrano G, Javicola M 1976 Alcohol hypoglycemia: hormonal changes. In: Andreani D, Lefebvre P, Marks V (eds) Hypoglycemia: proceedings of the European symposium, Rome 1974. Hormone and metabolic research supplement series. Georg Thieme, Stuttgart, p 99–105

Arky R A, Veverbrants E, Abramson E A 1968 Irreversible hypoglycemia: a complication of alcohol and insulin. Journal of the American Medical Association 206: 575–578

Dornhorst A, Ouyang A 1971 Effect of alcohol on glucose tolerance. Lancet 2: 957–959

Dymock I W, Cassar J, Pyke D A, Oakley W G, Williams R 1972 Observations on the pathogenesis, complications and treatment of diabetes in 115 cases of haemochromatosis. American Journal of Medicine 52: 203–210

Fink R, Rosalki S B 1978 Clinical biochemistry of alcoholism. Clinics in Endocrinology and Metabolism 7: 297–320

Friedenberg R, Metz R, Mako M, Surmaczynska B 1971 Differential plasma insulin response to glucose and glucagon stimulation following ethanol priming. Diabetes 20: 397–403

Forsander O, Vartia O K, Krusius F E, 1975 Exerimentelle studien über die biologische wirkung von alkohol. Annales Medicinae Experimentalis et Biologiae Fenniae 36: 416–423

Haight J S J, Keatinge W R 1973 Failure of thermoregulation in the cold during hypoglycaemia induced by exercise and alcohol. Journal of Physiology 229: 87

Joffe B I, Shines R, Seftel H C, Heding L G 1977 Plasma insulin C-peptide and glucagon levels in acute phase of ethanol-induced hypoglycaemia. British Medical Journal 3: 678

Joffe B I, Roache L, Baker S, Shires R, Sandler M, Seftel H C 1981 Failure to induce reactive hypoglycaemia by drinking a starch-based alcohol beverage (sorghum beer). Annals of Clinical Biochemistry 18: 22–24

Johnston D G, Alberti K G M M 1976 Carbohydrate metabolism in liver disease. Clinics in Endocrinology and Metabolism 5: 675–702

Klingman G I, Bane R, Haag H B 1959 Studies on severe alcohol intoxication in dogs. III. Effect of adrenalectomy. Quarterly Journal of Studies on Alcohol 20: 13–23

Klingman G I, Goodall M 1975 Urinary epinephrine and levarterenol excretion during acute sublethal intoxication in dogs. Journal of Pharmacology and Experimental Therapeutics 121: 313–318

Krebs H A 1968 The effects of ethanol on the metabolic activities of the liver. Advances in Enzyme Regulation 6: 467–480

Kühl C, Andersen O 1974 Glucose- and tolbutamide-mediated insulin response after preinfusion with alcohol. Diabetes 23: 821–826

MacDonald I A, Bennett T, Gale E A M, Green J H, Walford S 1980 The influence of hypoglycaemia on the regulation of body temperature. Diabetologia 19: 296

Madison L L 1968 Ethanol-induced hypoglycaemia. In: Levine R, Luft R (eds) Advances in metabolic disorders, vol. 3. Academic Press, New York, p. 85–109

Marks V, Wright J W 1977 Endocrinological and metabolic effects of alcohol. Proceedings of the Royal Society of Medicine 70: 337–344

Marks V, Wright J W 1979 Alcohol-provoked reactive hypoglycaemia. In: Andreani D, Lefebvre P J, (eds) Hypoglycaemia: second European symposium. Academic Press, London

McLaughlan J M, Joel F J, Moodie C A 1973 Hypoglycaemia in humans induced by alcohol and a low carbohydrate diet. Nutritional Reports International 5: 331–336

McMonagle J, Felig P 1975 Effects of ethanol ingestion on glucose tolerance and insulin secretion in normal and diabetic subjects. Metabolism 24: 625–632

Mendelson J H, Ogata M, Mello N K 1971 Adrenal function and alcoholism, l. Serum cortisol. Psychosomatic Medicine 33: 145–157

Moss M H 1970 Alcohol-induced hypoglycaemia and coma caused by alcohol sponging. Pediatrics 46: 445–447

Myrsten A L, Hollstedt C, Holmberg L 1975 Alcohol-induced changes in mood and activation in males and females as related to catecholamine excretion and blood alcohol level. Scandinavian Journal of Psychology 16: 303–310

Nikkilä E A, Taskinen M R 1975 Ethanol-induced alterations of glucose tolerance, postglucose hypoglycaemia, and insulin secretion in normal, obese and diabetic subjects. Diabetes 24: 933–943

O'Keefe S J D, Marks V 1977 Lunchtime gin and tonic a cause of reactive hypoglycaemia. Lancet 1: 1286–1288

Palmer J P, Ensinck J W 1975 Stimulation of glucagon secretion by ethanol-induced hypoglycaemia in man. Diabetes 24: 295–300

Philips G B, Safrit M F 1971 Alcoholic diabetes: induction of glucose intolerance with alcohol. Journal of the American Medical Association 217: 1513–1519
Rees L H, Besser G M, Jeffcoate W J, Goldie D J, Marks V 1977 Alcohol-induced pseudo-Cushing's syndrome. Lancet 1: 726–728
Searle G L, Shames D, Cavalieri R R, Bagdade J D, Porte D 1974 Evaluation of ethanol hypoglycemia in man: turnover studies with C-6 ^{14}C glucose. Metabolism 23: 1023–1035
Serenyi G, Endrenyi L 1978 Mechanism and significance of carbohydrate intolerance in chronic alcholism. Metabolism 27: 1041–1046
Shah J H, Wongsurawat N, Aran P O 1977 Effect of ethanol on stimulus-induced insulin secretion and glucose tolerance. Diabetes 26: 271–277
Shanley B C, Robertson E J, Joubert S M, North-Coombes J D 1972 Effect of alcohol on glucose tolerance. Lancet 1: 1232
Singh S P, Patel D G 1976 Effects of ethanol on carbohydrate metabolism. 1. Influence on oral glucose tolerance test. Metabolism 25: 239–243
Smals A, Kloppenborg P, Njo K T, Knoben J M, Ruland C M 1976 Alcohol-induced Cushingoid syndrome. British Medical Journal 2: 1298
Stokes P E 1973 Adrenocortical activity in alcoholics during chronic drinking. Annals of New York Academy of Sciences 215: 77–83
Straus E, Urbach H J, Yalow R S 1975 Alcohol-stimulated secretion of immunoreactive secretin. New England Journal of Medicine 293: 1031–1032
Thomson A D 1978 Alcohol and nutrition. Clinics in Endocrinology and Metabolism 7: 405–428
Walsh C H, O'Sullivan D J 1974 Effect of moderate alcohol intake on control of diabetes. Diabetes 23: 440–444
Wapnick S, Jones J J 1972 Alcohol and glucose tolerance. Lancet 2: 180
Wilson N M, Blown P M, Juul S M, Prestwich S A, Sönksen P H 1981 Glucose turnover and metabolic and hormonal changes in ethanol-induced hypoglycaemia. British Medical Journal 282: 849–853
Wright J W 1978 Endocrine effects of alcohol. Clinics in Endocrinology and Metabolism 7: 351–368
Wright J, Wood P, Marks V 1979 The effect of alcohol on plasma and urinary cyclic AMP and on the cyclic AMP response to glucagon in man. In: Marks V, Williams D (eds) Proceedings of the third European congress on clinical chemistry. British Medical Association, London.

Lipid abnormalities in alcoholism

INTRODUCTION

The liver has an obligatory role in the metabolism of alcohol, the consistent abuse of which leads to marked liver injury and dysfunction. Three types of alcohol-induced liver disease are recognised.

Alcoholic fatty liver

Fat accumulates in the liver (steatosis) in amounts varying from minimal, detectable only by biopsy, to severe accumulation with hepatocellular dysfunction in addition to the abnormal histology. The steatosis is commonly also accompanied by a hyperlipidaemia, usually a hypertriglyceridaemia.

Alcoholic hepatitis

Steatosis is often a feature of alcoholic hepatitis, but most marked are the morphological changes, with centrilobular necrosis, ballooning of hepatocytes and polymorph infiltration. Interesting artefacts are the paranuclear inclusion bodies, or Mallory hyaline bodies, which are thought to be degenerate mitochondria and endoplasmic reticulum.

Cirrhosis

This implies end-stage liver disease of which alcoholic hepatitis is the invariable precursor, and which is characterised by hepatic fibrosis and parenchymal cell regeneration nodules. Progressive fibrosis and hepatocellular destruction leads to the clinical picture of cirrhosis, portal hypertension and hepatic insufficiency (Harinasuta & Zimmerman, 1971)

What is not commonly recognised is that this spectrum of liver disease caused by alcohol-induced toxic injury is accompanied by changes in hepatic lipid metabolism which are in turn reflected by abnormalities of plasma lipids and lipoproteins.

This chapter briefly reviews normal plasma lipoprotein metabolism, including the central role played by the liver, and then describes how alcohol-induced liver injury produces secondary changes in plasma lipoproteins. Further consideration is given to how these changes may cause alterations in peripheral cell metabolism. Finally, the extent to which the changes might serve as markers for monitoring the progress of alcoholic liver disease is discussed.

PLASMA LIPOPROTEIN METABOLISM

Four main classes of plasma lipoprotein are recognised that have a role in transport and metabolism of lipids in the plasma. These macromolecular complexes are defined according to their ability to float in the ultracentrifuge: chylomicrons; triglyceride (TG) rich particles arising in the gut wall from absorbed neutral fat; very low density lipoprotein (VLDL) formed to a lesser extent from dietary lipid, but mainly synthesised in the liver to transport endogenously produced TG; low density lipoprotein (LDL), the final product of VLDL catabolism; high density lipoprotein (HDL) synthesised in the liver and intimately involved in chylomicron and VLDL metabolism and cholesterol transport.

These particles represent a spectrum with regard to size and lipid and apoprotein composition but appear to have a similar general structure. Each is spherical with a hydrophobic cholesterol ester and TG core contained by a phospholipid, unesterified cholesterol and apoprotein monolayer membrane.

The apoproteins

The apoproteins, of which about 10 have been identified, are commonly described by the ABC classification (Alaupovic, 1971). The major ones being: apoA-I and apoA-II in HDL; apoB the sole apoprotein of LDL, but which is also found in VLDL and chylomicrons. The two latter particles also contain polypeptides from the apoC family and apoE which in their turn exchange on to HDL. Apart from their structural role two of the apoproteins have an enzyme cofactor function, apoA-I as an activator of lecithin:cholesterol acyltransferase (LCAT), and apoC-II performing a similar role for lipoprotein lipase (LPL).

In the following sections those aspects of lipoprotein synthesis and metabolism will be discussed that are particularly dependent on the integrity of hepatocellular function. Reference should be made to authoritative reviews (Jackson et al, 1976; Schaefer et al, 1978; Eisenberg, 1979) for detailed information.

Hepatic synthesis and secretion of VLDL

Hepatic TG is the immediate precursor of TG in VLDL; TG which has been formed by esterification of fatty acid derived from one or more of three sources:

1. synthesis in the liver from acetyl-CoA;
2. uptake of non-esterified or free fatty acid from the circulation;
3. free fatty acid liberated by hydrolysis of TG, cholesterol ester or phospholipid contained within chylomicron- or VLDL-remnants taken up by the liver.

The first situation will be dominant in the well fed state when fatty acid synthesis from 2-C precursors, for example, carbohydrate, is high and circulating free fatty acid concentrations are low.

The rate of uptake of free fatty acids by the liver is proportional to their circulating concentration and will be increased when that is increased. This normally only occurs when adipose tissue lipolysis is increased, and to a lesser extent as a result of the action of LPL during uptake of plasma TG into peripheral tissues. Free fatty acids are bound to albumin by a salt linkage to the positively charged lysyl group. Their plasma concentration may range from 100–2000 μmol/l and they represent the fatty acids found in the adipose tissue, i.e. palmitate, stearate, oleate, palmitoleate, linoleate and other polyunsaturated fatty acids in small amounts. Low levels of fatty acid are found in the fully fed state, rather higher concentrations in the post-absorptive state and markedly higher concentrations in the fasting state. These concentrations will determine the rate of hepatic TG synthesis, though it must be borne in mind up to 50 per cent of the body energy requirements are met from fatty acids and the amount of TG synthesised will be determined by the fatty acid availability.

VLDL assembly

Lipid and apoprotein synthesis occur in the smooth and rough endoplasmic reticulum respectively. The enzymes for TG, cholesterol and phospholipid synthesis are situated in the smooth endoplasmic reticulum, while the apoproteins are synthesised with other proteins on polyribosomes in the rough endoplasmic reticulum. The new synthesised products are translocated to the Golgi apparatus where the particles are packaged into secretory vesicles prior to secretion into the perisinusoidal space of Disse. The actual site of lipoprotein assembly is not certain, but is probably within the cisternal channels of the endoplasmic reticulum which provide avenues for intracellular transport of secretory proteins. Final assembly, concentration and glycosylation of the lipoproteins probably occurs within the Golgi apparatus.

VLDL secretion

Electron microscope evidence shows that VLDL translocation from the endoplasmic reticulum to the Golgi apparatus is by vesicles that deliver the particles to the Golgi cisternae, where possibly final assembly occurs before secretion. The new formed VLDL containing vesicles bud off, move through the cytoplasm to bind with the hepatocyte membrane. The VLDL is then released into the space of Disse by reverse pinocytosis.

Nascent VLDL

The nascent VLDL thus released has a similar lipid composition to that found in the plasma, but the apoprotein composition is markedly different. Nascent VLDL contains exclusively apoB, but in the circulation further apoprotein is acquired by exchange, to yield a particle whose main apoprotein is apoC (50 per cent of total protein), apoB is now 40 per cent, and apoE 10–15 per cent.

HDL secretion and the LCAT reaction

HDL is synthesised and secreted by the liver and intestinal wall in a nascent form presumably by processes similar to those outlined for VLDL. Nascent HDL from the intestine does not contain apoC only apoA-I. Nascent HDL from the liver contains apoprotein, large amounts of phospholipid and unesterified cholesterol and traces of cholesterol ester, and consists of chains of discoidal bilayers rather like stacked coins. These particles are similar to those that accumulate in the plasma of patients with LCAT deficiency and obstructive jaundice (McIntyre et al, 1975). LCAT and probably apoA-I from intestinal HDL bind to these discs, and catalyse the formation of cholesterol ester by transferring a polyunsaturated fatty acyl group from the 2 position of lecithin to unesterified cholesterol. The non-polar cholesteryl ester moves into the hydrophobic interior of the bilayer and the lysolecithin transferred to plasma albumin. The continuing reaction generates an expanding non-polar core that pushes the bilayer apart to form a spherical core contained within a surface coat of polar lipid and apoprotein.

In LCAT deficiency plasma lipoproteins accumulate that contain abnormally low cholesteryl ester and increased free cholesterol and lecithin concentrations. Normally esterified cholesterol is transferred from HDL non-enzymatically by a sterol carrier protein to lower density lipoproteins, e.g. VLDL. The LCAT system appears to be primarily involved in the removal of excess unesterified cholesterol from lipoproteins. In LCAT deficiency a large LDL particle accumulates which is rich in unesterified cholesterol (Glomset, 1980).

Cholesteryl ester rich HDL is degraded in Küpffer cells of the liver. This catabolism of HDL involves a sequence of binding, uptake, proteolytic degradation and cholesteryl ester hydrolysis. Binding to the hepatocyte HDL receptor is dependent on recognition of apoE.

Delipidation of TG rich particles

Chylomicrons and VLDL are cleared from the circulation by LPL which progressively hydrolyses the core TG. The liver has a role in this process as the activator of LPL apoC-II is secreted on nascent HDL and acquired by chylomicrons and VLDL in the plasma. LPL is bound to the luminal endothelial surface of capillaries in peripheral tissues and TG hydrolysis occurs while the lipoproteins are adherant to the enzyme on the vessel wall and leads to a loss of about 90 per cent of the TG core. These partially metabolised particles can be isolated from plasma at densities between those of VLDL and LDL; and are similar to those yielded by chylomicron hydrolysis. During this process some surface components are transferred to HDL_3 producing a higher density HDL, HDL_2.

Remnant lipoproteins are removed by the liver, and the remaining TG hydrolysed by hepatic triglyceride lipase (H-TGL). Little is known as yet about this process but there is evidence that the H-TGL and a lipoprotein receptor are in close proximity. Deficiency of H-TGL has been reported in liver disease when TG particles of LDL density accumulate.

LDL is the product of VLDL catabolism, and is degraded in peripheral tissues following binding to specific cell receptors for apoB. After internalisation, the cholesteryl esters of LDL are hydrolysed by a lysosomal cholesterol esterase yielding free cholesterol which regulates cellular cholesterol metabolism (Goldstein & Brown, 1977).

THE ROLE OF THE LIVER IN LIPOPROTEIN METABOLISM

It will be realised from the preceding sections, which have described lipoprotein metabolism in some depth, that the liver has a very important role in lipoprotein metabolism. It secretes nascent VLDL and nascent HDL, and synthesises LCAT and the apoprotein cofactors necessary for intravascular lipoproprotein metabolism. Finally, it takes up the remnant lipoproteins and disposes of their lipids. Alcohol-induced liver injury will inevitably produce lipoprotein abnormalities similar to those discussed in the following sections. Some of these topics have been further reviewed in the volume edited by Avogaro et al (1979).

Prevalence and natural history of development of the lipid disorders in alcoholic liver disease

The frequent occurrence of severe hyperlipidaemia in subjects with alcoholic liver disease is very well documented and beyond question. It is most commonly recognised when a chylous sample is observed following venepuncture or if pancreatitis develops, and occurs in both the well and the ill nourished. The liver is often enlarged and fatty with mild cirrhotic changes present. The fatty liver regresses gradually when drinking is stopped, though the plasma lipids normalise usually within one week. The relationship between the hyperlipidaemia and acute pancreatitis is not clear, though the hyperlipidaemia is usually severe and mixed (Cameron et al, 1973). Any patient with such a severe, mixed hyperlipidaemia should be suspected of alcohol abuse in the absence of any other severe metabolic disorder.

However, it should be borne in mind that severe alcohol-induced hyperlipidaemias invariably develop only in the presence of a pre-existing mild primary hypertriglyceridaemia, and that plasma TG rarely returns to within normal reference ranges.

Fat accumulation

The acute or chronic ingestion of alcohol will produce an accumulation of fat in the liver. Over the years many workers, especially Lieber and co-workers, have studied this field extensively, and there is a very extensive literature, much of it controversial and difficult to relate to the clinical situation. It has been comprehensively reviewed recently by Baraona & Lieber (1979). The general consensus of opinion would now appear to be that alcohol per se can produce steatosis, but that protein and lipotropic factor deficiency may be important in some patients (Lieber & De Carli, 1977).

Alcohol and hepatic TG

Alcohol ingestion increases fasting plasma TG concentrations moderately in otherwise normolipaemic individuals (Schapiro et al, 1965; Belfrage et al, 1977), the magnitude of the increase being proportional to the caloric intake (Ginsberg et al, 1974). Ostrander and co-workers (1974) have shown in an epidemiological study that the mean plasma TG concentration was double that of abstainers in an alcohol consuming group.

This hypertriglyceridaemia reflects altered hepatic TG metabolism and increased hepatic TG storage. The esterified fatty acids that accumulate are primarily endogenous in origin and the raised hepatic TG concentration returns to normality rapidly after the alcohol challenge is discontinued (Scheig & Isselbacher, 1965).

The important mechanisms that can contribute to the alcohol-induced fatty liver are:

1. increased mobilisation of fatty acids from adipose tissue;
2. decreased fatty acid oxidation in the liver;
3. increased hepatic fatty acid esterification;
4. decreased secretion of VLDL by the liver.

All may contribute in some degree; the relative contribution depending on the size and duration of the alcohol challenge, sex and nutritional status.

Enhanced mobilisation of adipose tissue fatty acids, mediated by catecholamines, appears to be an important factor only when large stressful doses of alcohol are administered (Kalant et al, 1975). On the other hand, alcohol is oxidised in preference to all other oxidative substrates. Hepatic oxygen consumption is not increased following alcohol ingestion, so fatty acid, ketone body, and glucose oxidation decreases by about 50 per cent (Wolfe et al, 1976). Thus, in the post-absorptive state when fatty acids are being oxidised almost exclusively, alcohol ingestion will depress their oxidation.

It appears that production of a fatty liver is almost certainly the result of preferential oxidation of alcohol by the liver, thus displacing or sparing the fatty acids that are the normal energy substrate for the hepatic mitochondria. As a result, fatty acids accumulate (Reboucas & Isselbacher, 1961). As alcohol oxidation also depresses citric acid cycle activity and increases the $NADH/NAD^+$, the micro-environment is right for diversion of fatty acids into the esterification pathway. If the rate of TG synthesis is such that lipoprotein assembly is unable to keep pace, TG accumulation will ensue, even though secretion of VLDL is such as to produce a hypertriglyceridaemia. Little is known about the composition of these particles, but there is some evidence that the number of VLDL particles *per se* is not increased, but those that are tend to be TG rich.

The effects described above may be markedly exacerbated by starvation. Alcohol ingestion, in an individual whose hepatic glycogen stores are depleted following a two to three day fast, leads to a marked increase in free fatty acid release from adipose tissue and the liver becomes rapidly fatty, primarily because the rate of secretion of VLDL-TG, though increased, cannot keep pace with incoming free fatty acids.

Paradoxically, a rather similar picture is observed in subjects whose nutritional status is adequate. Under these circumstances, chylomicron derived fatty acids are oxidised at a slower rate when alcohol is being metabolised and are available for esterification. In fact, TG formation from such fatty acids and their subsequent secretion in VLDL is the primary reason for the prolongation of alimentary lipaemia by alcohol (Wilson et al, 1970).

However, plasma TG is not invariably raised in regular drinkers, possibly due to adaptive changes in the rates of TG metabolism. Belfrage et al (1977), in their study of lipid metabolism in healthy young volunteers who were only occasional drinkers, showed that the addition of 75 g alcohol (500 kcal) to their daily diet led to an increase of some 50 per cent in their plasma TG concentration for about two weeks. The concentrations then began to fall, returning to basal values at about five weeks in spite of continuing ingestion of alcohol. Hepatic biopsy showed a tripling of hepatic TG concentration up to about three weeks, then that fell by five weeks. LPL activity in adipose tissue increased progressively until at five weeks it was 30 per cent above the initial rate. It would appear that increased hepatic VLDL secretion is compensated for by an increased capacity for peripheral tissue TG catabolism, thus preventing long-term elevation of plasma VLDL. There must be also a concomitant increase in secretory capacity of nascent VLDL as hepatic TG is normalised.

A similar adaptive increase in LPL was described by Nilsson-Ehle (1979) in chronic alcoholics. The LPL activity fell to the normal range in one to two weeks after stopping alcohol consumption.

Alimentary lipaemia

The alimentary lipaemia that occurs following a standard fat load is exaggerated and prolonged if the meal is taken with alcohol. The hypertriglyceridaemia under these conditions is due to a rise in VLDL with the fatty acid composition of the TG resembling that of the dietary fat. The mechanism involved must be that TG taken up by the liver in chylomicron remnants increases the concentration of intrahepatic fatty acids and they are diverted into VLDL.

It has, however, been noted that in alcoholics the rate of removal of an intravenously injected bolus of TG emulsion is reduced in subjects with alcoholic hyperlipaemia who had a residual hyperlipidaemia after resolution of the severe lipidaemia (Chait et al, 1972). This study emphasises that subjects with a pre-existing mild primary hypertriglyceridaemia, whose capacity to metabolise VLDL is diminished, may be particularly susceptible to alcoholic hypertriglyceridaemia. However, individual susceptibility varies considerably (Kudzma & Schonfeld, 1971; Mendelson & Mello, 1973; Fry et al, 1973). In regular drinkers the rate of alcohol metabolism is markedly increased; this leads to a rapid increase in hepatic VLDL synthesis and secretion, and hence of plasma concentration, which may be exacerbated by a decreased removal rate. The extent to which genetic variation determines this susceptibility is unknown.

The ability of the liver to stabilise steatosis by increasing VLDL secretion will depend on the extent of the assault on the liver and the rate of progression of hepatocellular dysfunction.

LIPOPROTEINS AND PROGRESSIVE LIVER INJURY

With the progression of alcoholic fatty liver to more advanced stages of liver damage changes occur in the plasma lipoproteins that are different to those described above, which can be regarded as the changes in patients without overt liver disease. A marked hypertriglyceridaemia, severe hypercholesterolaemia, low cholesteryl ester concentrations together with a marked HDL deficiency are characteristic of alcoholic hepatitis. This is a plasma picture very reminiscent of LCAT deficiency and indeed evidence of LCAT deficiency in such patients has been demonstrated (Sabesin et al, 1977; Ragland et al, 1978). As a result of this LCAT deficiency, probably due to diminished hepatic secretion, nascent HDL rich in apoE and unesterified cholesterol accumulate in the plasma. In turn, the low plasma cholesteryl ester concentration prevents apoC and apoE transfer to VLDL particles causing accumulation of both nascent VLDL and TG rich LDL particles, hence the hypertriglyceridaemia. Confirmation of such a sequence of events is provided by lipoprotein electrophoresis, which shows a reduced or absent α-globulin band and a broad band with mobility between β and pre-β. The pre-β band may be absent altogether. As shown by Sabesin et al (1977) the

HDL in such cases has an abnormal composition and morphology, and migrates as a component of the broad β band. A slow-migrating HDL was demonstrated by Watanabe (1979) in patients with hepatocellular damage or with cholestasis and was attributed to an abnormal apoprotein composition. Both apoA-I and apoA-II concentrations fall in liver disease (Fujii et al, 1981) and this is thought to reflect the inability of the damaged liver to secrete apoA-I and apoA-II. However, Nestel et al (1980) reported that the diminished apoA-I concentration in alcoholic hepatitis is due not to a diminished synthesis rate, which is normal, but to an increased rate of degradation. The abnormal HDL structure associated with LCAT deficiency could well produce a particle that is particularly susceptible to degradation. However, the evidence suggests that most likely the abnormal HDL is, in fact, nascent HDL, rich in apoE and poor in apoA-I, that cannot be converted to mature HDL as a result of LCAT deficiency. The presence of the broad band must reflect the accumulation of remnant particles due to impaired H-TGL activity (Freeman et al, 1977).

On withdrawal of alcohol and subsequent resolution of the disease, the hypertriglyceridaemia disappears and plasma lipoprotein patterns become normal as hepatic function is regained and LCAT activity increases. It would appear that LCAT deficiency plays a key role in the development of the dyslipoproteinaemia associated with hepatitis. The diagnostic and prognostic value of measuring LCAT activity in the plasma has not been assessed, so it is impossible as yet to suggest its use along with other tests of hepatocellular function. A recent review by Sabesin (1981) considers these aspects in greater detail.

It has been suggested that the transition to more advanced hepatic lesions is accompanied by an early decrease in plasma VLDL and that this could be a useful diagnostic marker (Borowsky et al, 1976) for identification of alcoholics likely to progress to severe hepatic lesions unless drinking is discontinued.

An initial decrease in VLDL is followed by marked changes in plasma lipoprotein and lipid patterns similar to those seen in patients with non-alcoholic liver disease, and directly reflect the degree of hepatic functional impairment. The changes seen in alcoholic hepatitis, and described earlier, are markedly exacerbated (McIntyre, 1978; Sabesin et al, 1980). It can only be concluded that the changes in plasma lipoproteins and lipids seen in chronic alcoholics must be considered along with the more conventional tests of hepatic function. As suggested above, it is too early to state whether measurement of plasma lipoproteins or their metabolising enzymes will be of value in patient management, nor whether the dyslipoproteinaemia has a deleterious effect upon other body systems. There is evidence that the acquired LCAT deficiency associated with liver disease causes not only changes in plasma lipids but also in the lipid composition of erythrocyte and platelet membranes, leading to abnormal cellular function (Owen et al, 1979; 1981). This must inevitably be a fruitful avenue for development.

ALCOHOL AND HDL

There is considerable evidence from epidemiological and clinical studies consistent with the inference that alcohol ingestion is a determinant of plasma HDL concentrations (Hulley & Gordon, 1981). Conversely, epidemiological evidence shows that decreased concentrations of HDL are highly predictive of coronary heart disease and provide a more sensitive indicator than increased concentrations of LDL (Miller & Miller, 1975). This suggests that accumulation of cholesterol in the vessel wall due to impaired removal is a major factor in the aetiology of this disease. It is thus tempting to speculate on the protective role of HDL and the extent to which alcohol-induced elevations of HDL concentration might contribute to this process. However, the relationship between alcohol and HDL is complex (Devenyi et al, 1980). The evidence points to moderate alcohol ingestion increasing plasma HDL concentrations. However, chronic alcoholism associated with supervening progressive liver disease, LCAT deficiency and low HDL concentrations must inevitably negate the HDL-related protection against coronary heart disease. This may explain the association between heavy drinking and ischaemic heart disease (Tibblin et al, 1975; Dyer et al, 1977).

REFERENCES

Alaupovic P 1971 Apolipoproteins and lipoproteins. Atherosclerosis 13: 141–146

Avogaro P, Sirtori C R, Tremoli E (eds) 1979 Metabolic effects of alcohol. Elsevier, New York

Baraona E, Lieber C S 1979 Effects of ethanol on lipid metabolism. Journal of Lipid Research 20: 289–315

Belfrage P, Berg B, Hägestrand I, Nilsson-Ehle P, Tornquist H, Wiebe T 1977 Alterations of lipid metabolism in healthy volunteers during long-term ethanol intake. European Journal of Clinical Investigation 7: 127–131

Borowsky S A, Perlow W, Baraona E, Lieber C S 1976 Disappearance of alcoholic hyperlipemia as a sign of advancing liver damage. Gastroenterology 70: 978 (abstract)

Cameron J L, Capuzzi D M, Zuidema G D, Margolis S 1973 Acute pancreatitis with hyperlipemia. American Journal of Medicine 56: 482–487

Chait A, Mancini M, February A W, Lewis B 1972 Clinical and metabolic study of alcoholic hyperlipidaemia. Lancet 2: 62–64

Devenyi P, Robinson G M, Roncari D A K 1980 Alcohol and high-density lipoproteins. Canadian Medical Association Journal 123: 981–984

Dyer A et al. 1977 Alcohol consumption, cardiovascular risk factors, and mortality in two Chicago epidemiologic studies. Circulation 56: 1067–1074

Eisenberg S (ed) 1979 Progress in biochemical pharmacology: lipoprotein metabolism. Karger, Basel

Freeman M, Kuiken L, Ragland J B, Sabesin S M 1977 Hepatic triglyceride lipase deficiency in liver disease. Lipids 12: 443–445

Fry M M, Spector A A, Conner S L, Connor W E 1973 Intensification of hypertriglyceridemia by either alcohol or carbohydrate. American Journal of Clinical Nutrition 26: 798–802

Fujii S, Koga S, Shono T 1981 Serum apoprotein AI and AII levels in liver disease and cholestasis. Clinica Chimica Acta 115: 321–331

Ginsberg H, Olefsky J, Farquhar J W, Reaven G M 1974 Moderate ethanol ingestion and plasma triglyceride level. Annals of Internal Medicine 80: 143–149

Glomset J 1980 High-density lipoproteins in human health and disease. Advances in Internal Medicine 25: 91–116
Goldstein J L, Brown M S 1977 The low density lipoprotein pathway and its relation to atherosclerosis. Annual Review of Biochemistry 46: 897–930
Harinasuta U, Zimmerman H J 1971 Alcoholic steatonecrosis. Relationship between severity of hepatic disease and presence of Mallory bodies in the liver. Gastroenterology 60: 1036–1046
Hulley S B, Gordon S 1981 Alcohol and high-density lipoprotein cholesterol. Circulation 64 (supplement III): III57–63
Jackson R L, Morrisett J D, Gotto A M Jr 1976 Lipoprotein structure and metabolism. Physiological Reviews 56: 259–316
Kalant H, Khanna J M, Seymour F, Loth J 1975 Acute alcoholic fatty liver — metabolism or stress. Biochemical Pharmacology 24: 431–434
Kudzma D J, Schonfeld G 1971 Alcoholic hyperlipidemia: induction by alcohol but not by carbohydrate. Journal of Laboratory and Clinical Medicine 77: 384–395
Lieber C S, De Carli L M 1977 Metabolic effects of alcohol on the liver. In: Lieber C S (ed) Metabolic aspects of alcoholism. MTP Press, Lancaster, p 31–79
McIntyre N 1978 Plasma lipids and lipoproteins in liver disease. Gut 19: 526–530
McIntyre N, Harry D S, Pearson A G 1975 The hypercholesterolaemia of obstructive jaundice. Gut 16: 379–391
Mendelson J H, Mello N K 1973 Alcohol-induced hyperlipidemia and beta lipoproteins. Science 180: 1372–1374
Miller G J, Miller N E 1975 Plasma high-density lipoprotein concentration and development of ischaemic heart-disease. Lancet 1: 16–19
Nestel P J, Tada N, Fidge N H 1980 Increased catabolism of high density lipoprotein in alcoholic hepatitis. Metabolism 29: 101–104
Nilsson-Ehle P 1979 Alcohol-induced alterations in lipoprotein lipase activity and plasma lipoproteins. In: Avogaro P, Sirtori C R, Tremoli E (eds) Metabolic effects of alcohol. Elsevier, New York, p 175–186
Ostrander L D, Lamphiear D E, Block W D, Johnson B C, Ravenscroft C, Epstein F H 1974 Relationship of serum lipid concentrations to alcohol consumption. Archives of Internal Medicine 134: 451–456
Owen J S, Bruckdorfer K R, McIntyre N 1979 Decreased membrane fluidity in erythrocytes from patients with liver disease. Biochemical Society Transactions 7: 1272–1274
Owen J S, Hutton R A, Day R C, Bruckdorfer K R, McIntyre N 1981 Platelet lipid composition and platelet aggregation in human liver disease. Journal of Lipid Research 22: 423–430
Ragland J B, Heppner C, Sabesin S M 1978 The role of lecithin: cholesterol acyltransferase deficiency in the apoprotein metabolism of alcoholic hepatitis. Scandinavian Journal of Clinical Laboratory Investigation 38 (supplement 150): 208–213
Reboucas G, Isselbacher K J 1961 Studies on the pathogenesis of ethanol induced fatty liver. I. Synthesis and oxidation of fatty acids in the liver. Journal of Clinical Investigation 40: 1355–1362
Sabesin S M 1981 Lipid and lipoprotein abnormalities in alcoholic liver disease. Circulation 64 (supplement III): III72–84
Sabesin S M, Bertram P D, Freeman M R 1980 Lipoprotein metabolism in liver disease. Advances in Internal Medicine 25: 117–146
Sabesin S M, Hawkins H L, Kuiken L, Ragland J B 1977 Abnormal plasma lipoproteins and lecithin: cholesterol acyltransferase deficiency in alcoholic liver disease. Gastroenterology 72: 510–518
Schaefer E J, Eisenberg S, Levy R I 1978 Lipoprotein apoprotein metabolism. Journal of Lipid Research 19: 667–687
Schapiro R H, Scheig R L, Drummey G D, Mendelson J H, Isselbacher K J 1965 Effect of prolonged ethanol ingestion on the transport and metabolism of lipids in man. New England Journal of Medicine 272: 610–615
Scheig R, Isselbacher K J 1965 Pathogenesis of ethanol-induced fatty liver. 3. In vivo and in vitro effects of ethanol on hepatic fatty acid metabolism in rats. Journal of Lipid Research 6: 269–277

Tibblin G, Wilhelmsen R, Werkö L 1975 Risk factors for myocardial infarction and death due to IHD and other causes. American Journal of Cardiology 35: 514–522
Watanabe M 1979 Lipoprotein abnormalities in cholestasis. II Isolation, characterisation and clinical evaluation of additional cholestatic lipoprotein (slow-migrating HDL). Acta Medica Okayama 33: 327–341
Wilson D E, Schreibman P H, Brewster A C, Arky R A 1970 The enhancement of alimentary lipemia by ethanol in man. Journal of Laboratory and Clinical Medicine 75: 264–274
Wolfe B M, Havel R J, Marliss E B, Kane J P, Seymour J, Ahuja S P 1976 Effects of a 3-day fast and of ethanol on splanchnic metabolism of FFA, amino acids and carbohydrates in healthy young men. Journal of Clinical Investigation 57: 329–340

9 *M.R.Moore K.E.L.McColl A.Goldberg*

The effects of alcohol on porphyrin biosynthesis and metabolism

INTRODUCTION

The porphyrin ring is a unique and intriguing biological structure. Porphyrins are found ubiquitously in nature and have been used for very many different biological functions. Their principal role revolves around control of biological oxidation and oxygen transport, but they are used additionally in many other ways, such as in the colouring of the feathers and shells of birds. Because of their importance in biological oxidation reactions, it is of interest to study the influence of ethanol on porphyrin synthesis since ethanol has such profound effects on biological oxidation-reduction potentials. Additionally, ethanol can be metabolised in a small part by oxidative systems which utilise monooxygenases containing haem (Rubin et al, 1970). By virtue of their complex ring structure, porphyrins are capable of binding many metals. The commonest metals bound are iron and magnesium and in these forms, the porphyrins or metalloporphyrins reach their true apotheosis. The iron-containing complex haem is central to all biological oxidations. Since chlorophylls are magnesium-porphyrin compounds, which are central in solar energy utilisation in the biosphere, all known photosynthetic organisms show porphyrin-dependent photosynthesis.

The association between ethanol ingestion and alterations in human haem biosynthesis was first noted by Franke & Fikentschir (1935), who found that after drinking one litre of beer or 90 ml cognac a subject generally doubled his urinary coproporphyrin excretion. This was considered to be the result of ethanol-related increased hepatic production of coproporphyrin. Shanley et al (1968) demonstrated that acute ethanol dosage resulted in increased activity of the rate-controlling enzyme of haem biosynthesis, delta-aminolaevulinic acid (ALA) synthase, in rat hepatic tissue. Patients with any of the hepatic porphyrias, which are due to hereditary abnormalities in the pathway of haem biosynthesis, are particularly sensitive to ethanol. Those with one of the inducible hereditary hepatic porphyrias (acute intermittent porphyria, hereditary coproporphyria or variegate porphyria) may have an acute attack of the disease following the consumption of moderate quantities of ethanol (Eales, 1971; Goldberg, McColl & Moore, 1981). Ethanol is also an important aetiological factor in the development of cutaneous hepatic porphyria. A high percentage of patients presenting with this disorder have a history of excess ethanol consumption (Goldberg & Rimington, 1962; Goldberg & Moore, 1980).

HAEM BIOSYNTHESIS AND BIODEGRADATION

Porphyrin and haem biosynthesis

The basic porphyrin nucleus consists of 4 pyrrole rings linked by 4 methine bridges to form the macrocycle. This represents a rigid planar structure on to which eight side chains can be attached at positions one to eight. The type of side chain determines the physical characteristics of the porphyrin. The four pyrrole rings are designated A, B, C and D and the four methine bridges α, β, γ, and δ (Fig. 9.1). The normal biological intermediate is not this highly conjugated porphyrin, but the hexa-hydro porphyrin, the porphyrinogen, in which each of the methine bridges is reduced. Porphyrinogens are colourless and unconjugated as compared with the highly conjugated and highly coloured porphyrins. More specific details of porphyrin chemistry are given by Smith (1975). The initial biosynthetic sequence for synthesis of the haems, chlorophylls and corrins is the same

Position		1,3,5	2,4	6	7	8
Uroporphyrin	1	Acetyl	Propionyl	Propionyl	Acetyl	Propionyl
"	3	Acetyl	Propionyl	Propionyl	Propionyl	Acetyl
Coproporphyrin	1	Methyl	Propionyl	Propionyl	Methyl	Propionyl
"	3	Methyl	Propionyl	Propionyl	Propionyl	Methyl
Protoporphyrin	9	Methyl	Vinyl	Propionyl	Propionyl	Methyl

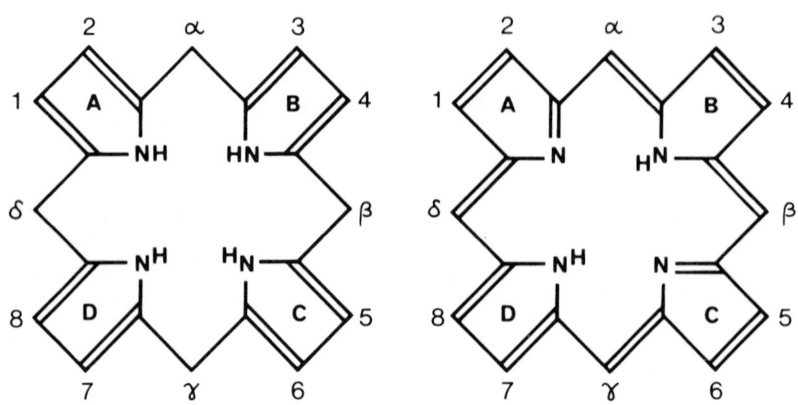

PORPHYRINOGEN PORPHYRIN

Fig. 9.1 The structure of porphyrins and porphyrinogens of biological interest.

and each utilises these porphyrinogens as direct intermediates of the final product. The haem biosynthetic pathway starts with the very basic precursors, succinyl CoA from the tricarboxylic acid cycle and glycine and proceeds through from the compound delta-aminolaevulinic acid to the formation of the monopyrrole porphobilinogen four of which link and cyclise to form the porphyrinogens. The last stage of the sequence is the insertion of iron into the porphyrin ring structure to form haem (Fig. 9.2).

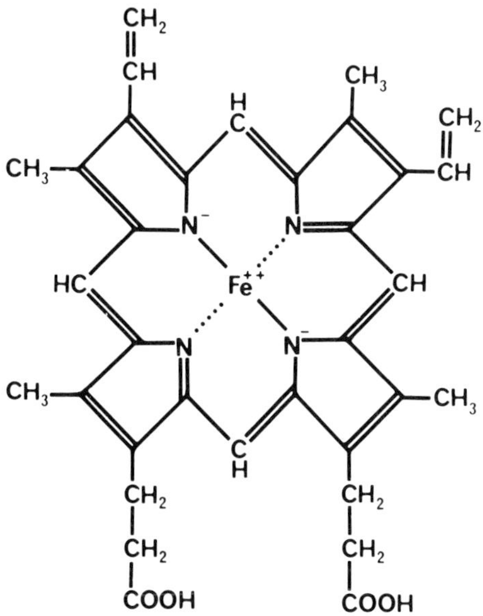

Fig. 9.2 The structure of haem showing ferrous iron at the centre of the protoporphyrin moiety.

Delta-aminolaevulinic acid (ALA) synthase (EC2.3.1.37)

The first and rate-controlling step of haem biosynthesis is the condensation of succinate and glycine to form delta-aminolaevulinic acid. The normal enzyme catalyst for this reaction, ALA synthase, requires pyridoxal phosphate as a cofactor and it is of note that ethanol will impair pyridoxine metabolism. Blood concentrations of pyridoxal phosphate are frequently diminished in alcoholic patients (Hines, 1975; Lumeng & Li, 1974). The reason for this may be related either to impaired phosphorylation in vivo of pyridoxine or alternatively by the accelerated degradation of pyridoxal phosphate by an aldehyde stimulated erythrocyte phosphorylase. An additional co-factor for ALA synthase is iron, which has the capacity to stabilise the pyrodoxal-phosphate α amino β keto apidic acid complex. The basic process of the reaction is that succinate as activated succinyl CoA has an electrophilic carbonyl group which can react with glycine bound to pyridoxal phosphate as a stable carbanion on the enzyme surface. This will produce α amino β keto adipic acid which is then decarboxylated to delta-aminolaevulinic acid (Granick & Sassa, 1971; Jordan & Shemin, 1972). This last stage takes place on the enzyme surface prior to the release of ALA into solution. The ALA produced in this reaction may then by binding to the enzyme surface inhibit the activity of the enzyme (Fanica-Gaignier & Clement-Metral, 1973). Sulphydryl compounds have been found to inhibit the activity of the enzyme, and this may be reversed by pyridoxal phosphate, which forms a Schiff base with the enzyme (Tait, 1978).

Properties and location

The molecular properties of ALA synthase are now becoming clearer following development of techniques for its purification and characterisation. It is a relatively unstable enzyme with a short half life in vivo of about one hour in mammalian species (Granick & Sassa, 1971) and a low basal activity. In mammalian systems, active ALA synthase is found exclusively in the mitochondrion. Low activities in other subcellular fractions are probably due to release of the enzyme from the mitochondrion or alternatively to the activity of precursors of the enzyme synthesised in the cytoplasm in passage to the mitochondrion. Studies on the subcellular location of the enzyme shown that ALA synthase is loosely bound to the inner mitochondrial membrane although it may also be found free within the mitochondrial matrix. The molecular weight of the cytoplasmic enzyme is generally found to be higher than that of the mitochondrial enzyme, which would be consistent with enzyme modification following incorporation into the mitochondrion (Moore, 1980). The activity of ALA synthase may be markedly increased following treatment with various compounds amongst which ethanol is numbered and it is on the basis of the changes of activity of this enzyme by these compounds that one may define the role of this enzyme as a control point for the biochemical pathway (Granick & Sassa, 1971).

An alternative synthesis

In non-mammalian systems, an alternative pathway utilising a C5 pathway from glutamate or glutamate-1 phosphate has attracted some interest. Early work in Shemin's department had suggested that this succinate-glycinecycle could play some part in the synthesis of ALA. Its importance, however, has never been clarified. It could perform two roles, either disposal of synthesised ALA or, by acting in the opposite direction, contributing to general ALA synthesis. The enzyme required for the reaction glutamate dioxovalerate amino-transferase has been characterised (Varticovski et al, 1980) and suggested as part of the system producing ALA from glutamate in plants but which because of competition with pyruvate for binding is non-reversible. No effect of ethanol upon this system has yet been demonstrated.

Delta-aminolaevulinic acid dehydratase (EC4.2.1.24)

Of all the enzymes in the biochemical pathway, this is the one which has been most studied other than ALA synthase, principally because of the profound effect that lead poisoning may have upon its activity (Moore, Meredith & Goldberg, 1980) but also because of the effects of ethanol upon it. The catalytic process has been well covered by the work of Shemin (1976) who has shown that the combination of two molecules of ALA to form porphobilinogen (PBG) takes place in a series of stages. It is an unusual reaction in that two identical substrate molecules are involved. This enzyme is particularly sensitive to the presence or absence of sulphydryl groups and optimum activity in vitro is only obtained after preincubation with sulphydryl containing compounds such as glutathione, cysteine or dithiothreitol. Not only is this enzyme particularly sensitive to the inhibitory effects because of this, but it has also been shown to require zinc for full activation, requiring in the region of 5–6 gram atoms of zinc/mol enzyme (Cheh & Neilands, 1973). The activity of ALA dehydratase in tissues is very much higher than that of ALA synthase and it is thought to play little part in regulating the overall rate of haem biosynthesis. In vitro work has suggested that the redox state within cells will determine the rate at which this reaction may proceed, and, therefore, that this reaction may become rate-limiting in some circumstances (Moore, 1975). This point is of particular importance in consideration of the effects of ethanol.

Since alcohol ingestion may diminish the activity of this enzyme in vivo and in vitro (Moore et al, 1971; Krasner et al, 1975a; Abdulla et al, 1976), it has been suggested that these changes are mediated through a relative increase in reduced glutathione metabolism (Moore, 1975). However, the situation here is complex and the role of zinc must not be forgotten since this has been shown to be essential for ALA dehydratase activity (Abdulla et al, 1976; Meredith & Moore, 1980) and to be depleted in alcoholism through excessive renal excretion (Sullivan, 1974).

Porphobilinogen deaminase (EC4.3.1.8) and uroporphyrinogen 3 cosynthase

Of all the reactions that have interested research workers in porphyrin metabolism. this combined reaction has stretched their ingenuity to the limit and beyond. In normal systems, these two enzymes act concertedly to condense four molecules of porphobilinogen and cyclyse them to form the first of the porphyrins, uroporphyrinogen 3. The importance of the combined reaction is that the tetrapyrrole produced in normal biological sequences is not the symmetrical uroporphyrinogen 1, but the asymmetrical uroporphyrinogen 3, and it is only this that may proceed past the stage of coproporphyrinogen in the biosynthetic sequence that will form haem.

Both of these enzymes are cytoplasmic enzymes, and the activity of the first is the rate-limiting one in normal circumstances. In the paired reaction, porphobilinogen deaminase can only form the symmetrical uroporphyrinogen 1, and it is easy to visualise that the reaction of this enzyme is the sequential head to tail condensation of four units of porphobilinogen to give rise to the cyclic tetramer, during which process, four moles of ammonia will be released. The role of the second enzyme present in higher activities than the first, is to allow an inversion of the D ring of the porphyrin molecule to produce the asymmetrical uroporphyrinogen 3. The currently accepted viewpoint is that, following the initial condensation process, one of the pyrrole groups joins to another in a head-to-head reaction. This implies that the two reactions would have a common basis in the initial stages, and that the porphobilinogen unit incorporated into ring D undergoes intramolecular rearrangement. This is not, however, the complete story ongoing NMR studies have shown that the formation of uroporphyrinogen 3 is by the sequential action of uroporphyrinogen 1 synthase, which produces an hydroxy methyl bilane and uroporphyrinogen co-synthase utilises this as substrate (Battersby et al, 1980). An interesting feature that must also be considered here is that changes in porphyrin isomer ratios occur during alcoholic coproporphyrinuria. Whereas the normal percentage of series 3 isomer is around 70 per cent (Doss & Schermuly, 1976), various conditions of alcohol abuse linked with hepatic cholestasis commonly give percentages of less than 50 per cent (Doss, 1978). This implies that some change has occurred in the pathway at the stage of porphyrinogen deaminase — uroporphyrinogen cosynthase, which has allowed excess synthesis of the series 1 isomer.

Uroporphyrinogen decarboxylase (EC4.1.1.37)

At this stage in the reaction sequence, the basic structure of the porphyrins has been produced and all that remains before iron is inserted to form haem is that a series of decarboxylations and oxidations has to take place to form protoporphyrin. The first of these decarboxylation sequences is catalysed by uroporphyrinogen decarboxylase. In this, four moles of carboxyl are lost from every mole of porphyrin, taking the porphyrin from the octacarboxylic uroporphyrinogen to the tetracarboxylic coproporphyrinogen. This sequence will be followed by both the series 3 and the series 1 isomers of the porphyrins, but because of substrate requirements, the series 3 isomer is decarboxylated more rapidly than the series 1 isomer (Smith & Francis, 1979). This difference in reaction rate might be traced to the asymmetry of the D ring which could effectively give a reaction focus for the processes catalysed by uroporphyrinogen decarboxylase. Thus the decarboxylation of the first acetic acid side chain is the most rapid (Garcia et al, 1973; Smith & Francis, 1979). The rationale for this argument is that studies have shown that the process of decarboxylation of these porphyrins commences on ring D and proceeds through rings A, B and C to give heptacarboxylic, hexacarboxylic and pentacarboxylic intermediates prior to the formation of coproporphyrinogen 3 (Jackson et al, 1976). It is then obvious that if greater quantities of series 1 isomer are synthesised in alcoholism, the rate of this reaction will inevitably be adversely affected. As part of this reaction sequence, it is possible that at the pentacarboxylic porphyrin stage, one of the propionate side chains on ring A is decarboxylated and oxidised to a vinyl grouping, probably by the enzyme coproporphyrinogen oxidase (Elder, 1976). This side-branching results in the isocoproporphyrinogen series of porphyrins, and is of importance in cutaneous hepatic porphyria. This first one is dehydroisocoproporphyrinogen 3. A problem associated with this is that the next enzyme in the pathway is a mitochondrial one, whilst uroporphyrinogen decarboxylase is a soluble cytoplasmic enzyme. The only likely explanation is that in liver damage situations the pentacarboxylic porphyrinogen has become accessible to the mitochondrial enzyme, but this also implies that an unlikely double membrane transfer, cytoplasm to mitochondrion to cytoplasm, would have to occur to allow decarboxylation of the last acetyl grouping.

The activity of this enzyme is inhibited when sulphydryl groups are bound by compounds such as mercury and iodoacetamide. This type of inhibition can be reversed by the addition of glutathione. Oxygen will also inhibit activity of the enzyme by substrate oxidation. In general, little change can be found in the activity of this enzyme but it has been shown that following treatment with hexachlorobenzene, the activity was undetectable (Elder, 1976). It has, in addition, been shown to be relatively stable, with little alteration in activity of a system to which cycloheximide had been added (Smith & Francis, 1979).

Coproporphyrinogen oxidase (EC1.3.3.3)

At this stage of the reaction sequence, the pathway once again re-enters the mitochondrion. The reaction catalysed by a coproporphyrinogen oxidase is a combined oxidation and decarboxylation of two proprionyl residues on rings A and B of the porphyrin nucleus to vinyl groups. This enzyme requires molecular oxygen for activity and will not use any other form of oxygen acceptor (Sano & Granick, 1961). The end product of the reaction is protoporphyrinogen and the enzyme will only act on the 3 isomer of coproporphyrinogen and not on the series 1 isomer. This implies that excess series 1 isomer produced in alcoholism will be excreted either as the porphyrinogen or after auto-oxidation as the porphyrin. An intermediate is the monovinyl porphyrinogen harderoporphyrinogen which was first isolated in the harderian gland of the rat. Studies have shown that this is the 2-vinyl porphyrinogen rather than the 4-vinyl porphyrinogen (isoharderoporphyrinogen) (Jackson, Elder & Smith, 1978). Of these two, it has been shown that isoharderoporphyrinogen is a much less effective substrate for coproporphyrinogen oxidase and has only about 10 per cent of the availability of harderoporphyrinogen.

Protoporphyrinogen oxidase

The penultimate stage of the biosynthetic sequence is the oxidation or dehydrogenation of protoporphyrinogen to protoporphyrin. The existence of this step as specifically enzyme catalysed has only recently been established. In retrospect, however, it was unreasonable to suppose that spontaneous oxidation of protoprophyrinogen would take place in the anaerobic reducing environment of the mitochondrion and equally improbable that the enzyme coproporphyrinogen oxidase would be able to carry out this dehydrogenation in addition to its other duties. Studies have now shown that the reaction is a stereo-specific one taking place from only one side of the porphyrin ring (Jackson et al, 1974), which would not have occurred had it been a purely chemical oxidation. The studies of Poulson & Polglaze (1975) and Poulson (1976) provided evidence that it was an oxygen-dependent enzyme found in mitochondrial extracts. It has a high substrate specificity and does not react with uroporphyrinogens or coproporphyrinogens although it will react with the monovinyl harderoporphyrinogen and isoharderoporphyrinogen, although all are less efficiently metabolised than protoporphyrinogen 9. From these same studies, it has also been shown that substrates with a lipophyllic grouping on the A and B rings of the porphyrinogen are more readily metabolised by this enzyme (Jackson et al, 1978).

Ferrochelatase (EC4.99.1.1)

The last biosynthetic step of this pathway, catalysed by ferrochelatase or haem synthetase, inserts ferrous iron into protoporphyrin to form haem or protohaem. Ferrochelatase is again a mitochondrial enzyme attached firmly to the inner mitochondrial membrane (McKay et al, 1969) and it is probable that reduction of ferric iron to ferrous iron is taking place at this site as well (Barnes et al, 1972). As an enzyme, ferrochelatase is not substrate specific but will catalyse the chelation of a number of different bivalent metals into various dicarboxylic porphyrins such as cobalt into mesoporphyrin. In assay conditions, the natural substrates are not the most convenient for the measurement of activity of this enzyme, and many assays have been described using ferrous iron and mesoporphyrin 9. The soluble form of the enzyme has not yet been isolated, but its activity has been increased by the addition of organic solvents to liver mitochondrial assays. This is consistent with the hypothesis that the presence of lipids is essential for activity of the enzyme (Yoneyama et al, 1969). The exact role of this lipid is not clear, but it may activate the enzyme by alteration of conformation by binding with a metal ion to transfer it from the aqueous environment to a non-aqueous environment or, by increasing the solubility of the relatively water-insoluble protoporphyrin 9, by transfer to a lipophilic medium. Haem biosynthesis is shown in entirety in Figure 9.3.

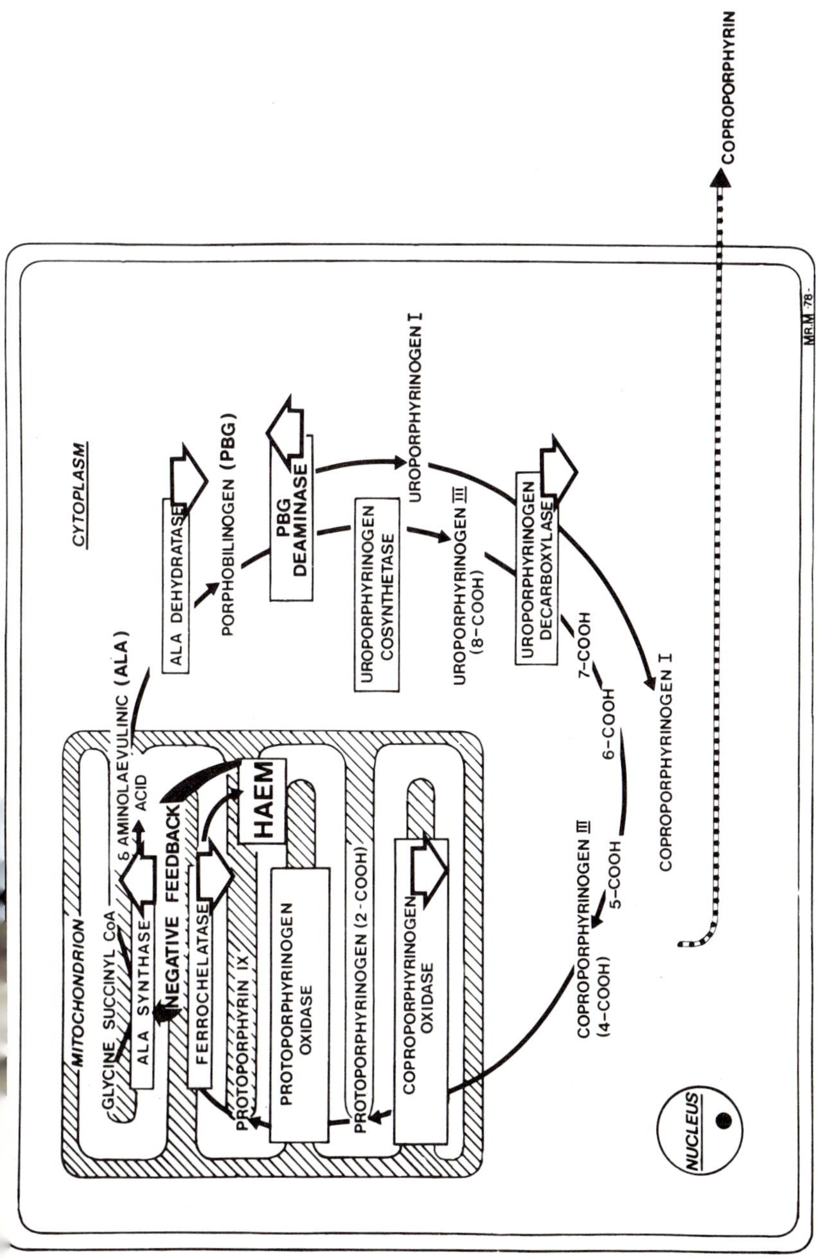

Fig. 9.3 The pathway of haem biosynthesis. This starts within the mitochondrion with the enzyme delta-aminolaevulinic acid synthase which forms delta-aminolaevulinic acid. The pathway then passes out of the mitochondrion and does not re-enter it again until level of coproporphyrinogen oxidase. Control points of the pathway lie at the level of ALA synthase and porphobilinogen deaminase. Where series I-somers of the porphyrins are produced, these cannot proceed beyond the level of coproporphyrinogen and are obligatorily excreted usually in the urine as coproporphyrin I. The effects of acute ethanol ingestion upon the pathway is shown diagrammatically by the arrows. Those enzymes with diminished activity being delta-aminolaevulinic acid dehydratase, uroporphyrinogen decarboxylase, coproporphyrinogen oxidase and ferrochelatase, compensatory rises are observed in delta-aminolaevulinic acid synthase and porphobilinogen deaminase.

Haem oxygenase (EC1.14.99.3)

The catabolic sequence of haem degradation starts with this first step in the reductive breakdown of the haem macrocycle. The position at which this cycle is most open to oxidative attack is at the carbon bridges linking the pyrrole rings, resulting in the formation of the linear tetrapyrroles which are referred to collectively as the bile pigments. Since there are four different ring positions, α, β, γ and δ at which the haem ring may be cleaved, haem oxygenase can potentially produce four different biliverdins (O'Carra, 1975; Tenhunen, 1976). The reaction is normally specific, for cleavage between rings A and B, to produce biliverdin 9 α. It is of interest to note that cobalt and other metal ions are potent inducers of activity of this enzyme (Maines & Kappas, 1974; Maines & Kappas, 1976). These studies suggest that there is an SH-active regulatory component controlling the activity of haem oxygenase which is blocked by combination with such metal ions. Little direct evidence for the effect of ethanol upon haem oxygenase are available. There is however, sufficient indirect evidence to suggest that ethanol will probably diminish activity of this enzyme. Firstly, because of interactions with the SH-active regulatory component and secondly because of the requirements for NADPH cytochrome C reductase in this reaction (Yoshida & Kikuchi, 1978a & b), which enzyme will certainly be influenced by the availability of reducing equivalents produced during ethanol oxidation. Another feature which will influence the activity of this enzyme will be ascorbic acid availability, which is diminished during ethanol oxidation (Krasner et al, 1975).

BIOLOGICAL CONTROL OF HAEM BIOSYNTHESIS

The principal control of haem biosynthesis resides in the low activity and ready inducibility of the first enzyme of the pathway, ALA synthase, coupled with a negative feedback system. The end product of the pathway, haem, acts by repression of synthesis and inhibition of activity of ALA synthase. Thus any compound that depletes hepatic haem by increasing haem catabolism or decreases haem formation will cause an increase in the activity of ALA synthase which can usually be prevented by inhibitors of protein synthesis or haemin (Granick & Sassa, 1971). The potential for ALA synthase to control this pathway can be more readily understood by consideration of the activities of each of the enzymes of the pathway in sequence. Of all enzymes of the pathway, ALA synthase clearly has the lowest activity in vivo although other factors may also act on the rate of progress of the pathway. The rate of haem synthesis mat be altered by impairing the supply of substrate to ALA synthase. There is little evidence to suggest that lack of either glycine or succinyl CoA can limit its activity under any circumstances. One should, however, bear in mind that the Km of ALA synthase for glycine lies between 4–19 mmol/l and that the intracellular glycine concentration, though variable is generally around 1 mmol/l. One should also remember that during ethanol metabolism the citric acid cycle ceases to function. This implies that the availability of substrate for the pathway will be severely compromised and will potentially inhibit overall function of the haem biosynthetic pathway in the limited period of high circulating ethanol concentrations. Alternatively, there is some evidence to suppose that diminution of pyridoxal phosphate availability will decrease enzyme activity and thus produce a pyridoxine deficiency anaemia. The only other enzyme in the sequence which has markedly lower activity than any of the other enzymes of the pathway is porphobilinogen deaminase. This enzyme can be considered to be the secondary control point for this pathway. The reasons for this can be found in consideration of the activities of the enzymes of the pathway in normal subjects and in some of the diseases in which porphyrin metabolism is deranged (Moore et al, 1980).

If one then considers the patterns of activities in each of the porphyrias, in lead poisoning and in alcoholism, one feature becomes immediately clear. Porphobilinogen deaminase activity either normal or depressed in the acute porphyrias is raised in alcoholism, in the non-acute porphyrias and in lead poisoning. The importance of this finding is that in these diseases where the activity of the initial enzyme is raised, thus feeding greater quantities of substrate to the pathway, it is essential that some of this excess substrate

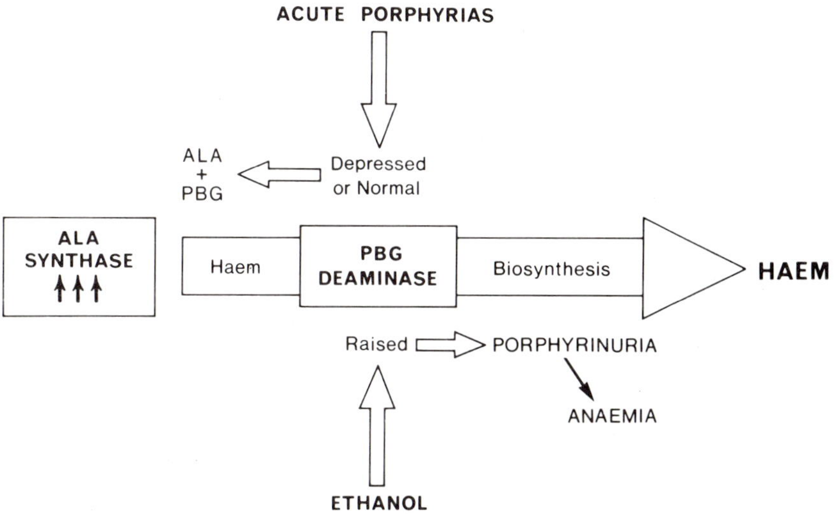

Fig. 9.4 Control of haem biosynthesis. During ethanol exposure the activity of the enzyme porphobilinogen deaminase is raised whilst at the same time, negative feedback has raised the activity of ALA synthase. The obligatory increase in precursor synthesis results in a porphyrinuria and with associated anaemia due to inability of the system to utilise copious stores of protoporphyrin and of iron. In the acute porphyrias, porphobilinogen deaminase activity is lower than normal and there is an accumulation of the porphyrin precursor delta-aminolaevulinic acid and porphobilinogen.

be excreted either as porphyrin precursor or as formed porphyrin, since the quantities of substrate entering into the pathway are in excess of the biological requirement for haem. Since in the acute porphyrias the activity of porphobilinogen deaminase is low (acute intermittent porphyria) or normal (hereditary copropophyria and variegate porphyria). the excessive production of ALA and subsequently PBG accumulates in the body. In hereditary coproporphyria and variegate porphyria, sufficient of the free porphyrin will then be formed and accumulate, as a function of depressed activity of either coproporphyrinogen oxidase or protoporphyrinogen oxidase, to allow photosensitisation lesions to occur. In each of the non-acute porphyrias, lead poisoning ard alcoholism porphobilinogen deaminase activity is raised and there is no accumulation of porphyrin precursors (Brodie et al, 1977; Doss, 1978). In lead poisoning there is also diminution of the activity of ALA dehydratase resulting in some accumulation of ALA but not of PBG (Moore et al, 1979) (Fig. 9.4).

This view of control of the pathway does not take into consideration other features within the cell that could alter the rate of pathway functioning. Principal amongst these are the changes in cellular compartmentation involved between the different stages of the pathway. ALA synthesised within the mitochondrion has to pass out into the cytoplasm to react with ALA dehydratase, and coproporphyrinogen synthesised in the cytoplasm then has to pass once more into the mitochondrion where the latter stages of the pathway occur. In these circumstances, it is possible that substrates could be lost from the appropriate intracellular compartment. Equally, the transfer from one compartment to another must to some extent limit the progress of the pathway. Generally, in invivo situations, there is a dynamic equilibrium where the synthesis of ALA exactly balances both the production of haem and the excretion of intermediates from the pathway. This is normally a most efficient pathway with little of the intermediate being excreted prior to formation of haem. In alcoholism, however, the pathway becomes inefficient with some of the throughput being excreted principally as coproporphyrin (Brugsch, 1937; Orten et al, 1963; Sutherland & Watson, 1951). An intriguing additional feature is that such changes in the haem biosynthetic pathway may be altered by administration of Vitamin E. Mezey et al (1971) found that the urinary excretion of ALA and PBG was unaltered in ethanol fed rats given Vitamin E although there were large drops in coproporphyrinogen excretion. Cytochrime P450 induction was unaltered.

The pattern of control in all tissues is unlikely to be the same. The general principles will still hold, but there will be quantitative differences, according to the pattern of haem utilisation by the tissue. Thus, in the liver the principal requirement is for haemoproteins with a rapid turnover which are crucial to oxidative metabolism. These will have to change quickly in response to specific environmental change, and therefore require a more finely tuned control system than that for the haemopoietic system, which principally needs haem synthesis to take place to co-ordinate with the rate of α and β globin chain synthesis, or for nervous tissue which will again require only small amounts of haem synthesis for maintenance of its energy production system.

ETHANOL AND PORPHYRIN BIOSYNTHESIS IN NORMAL SUBJECTS

Information on the effect of acute ethanol ingestion on the activity of the enzymes of the haem biosynthetic pathway is limited. Acute ethanol dosage has been shown to depress the activity of ferrochelatase and ALA dehydratase (Moore, 1973; Moore et al, 1971) and increase the activity of ALA synthase (Shanley, Zail & Joubert, 1968) in rat hepatic tissue. We have previously reported the depressant effect of acute ethanol ingestion on ALA dehydratase in human peripheral erythrocytes (Moore et al, 1974; Krasner et al, 1975). The development of methods for the measurement of other enzymes of haem biosynthesis in peripheral blood cells has allowed a more detailed examination of the effects of acute ethanol ingestion on the biochemical pathway. Our results demonstrate that the consumption of a moderate quantity of Vodka (1319 mmol ethanol) results in significant alterations in the activity of the enzymes of haem biosynthesis in the pattern shown in Figures 9.5 and 9.6 (McColl et al, 1980).

Several mechanisms may be responsible for the rise in ALA synthase activity seen following alcohol consumption. ALA synthase is under negative feedback control by haem, and ethanol depletes free haem in at least two ways. Firstly, by reducing haem synthesis due to its inhibitory effect on four of the enzymes of the pathway, and secondly by increasing haem utilization due to its induction of the haemoprotein cytochrome P450 (Rubin, Hutterer & Lieber, 1968). Increased hapatic concentrations of cytochrome P450 have been noted within 2 h of enteral ethanol dosing of rats (Pennington, Smith & Tappscott, 1978). It is probable that ethanol, by either or both of the above mechanisms, could increase the activity of ALA synthase 6 h after ingestion. A third mechanism may be important. ALA synthase activity is affected by the intramitochondrial NADH/NAD ratio (Labbe et al, 1970) and the alteration in the redox state produced by the metabolism of ethanol could result in increased enzyme activity (Shanley et al, 1968). The only other enzyme noted to increase in activity following the ethanol ingestion was PBG deaminase. This was a phenomenon of late onset when no detectable ethanol remained in the blood. This delayed rise indicates that the rise in activity of PBG deaminase is a secondary compensatory phenomenon. PBG deaminase plays a secondary rate-controlling role in the pathway when ALA synthase is derepressed (Moore et al, 1980). It is, therefore, interesting to note that the two enzymes which increased in activity are the two enzymes which are of importance in controlling the rate of the pathway.

The other enzymes studied, the mitochondrial enzymes ferrochelatase and coproporphyrinogen oxidase and the cytosolic enzymes ALA dehydratase and uroporphyrinogen decarboxylase were all depressed following the ethanol consumption. Ferrochelatase showed the most dramatic depression,

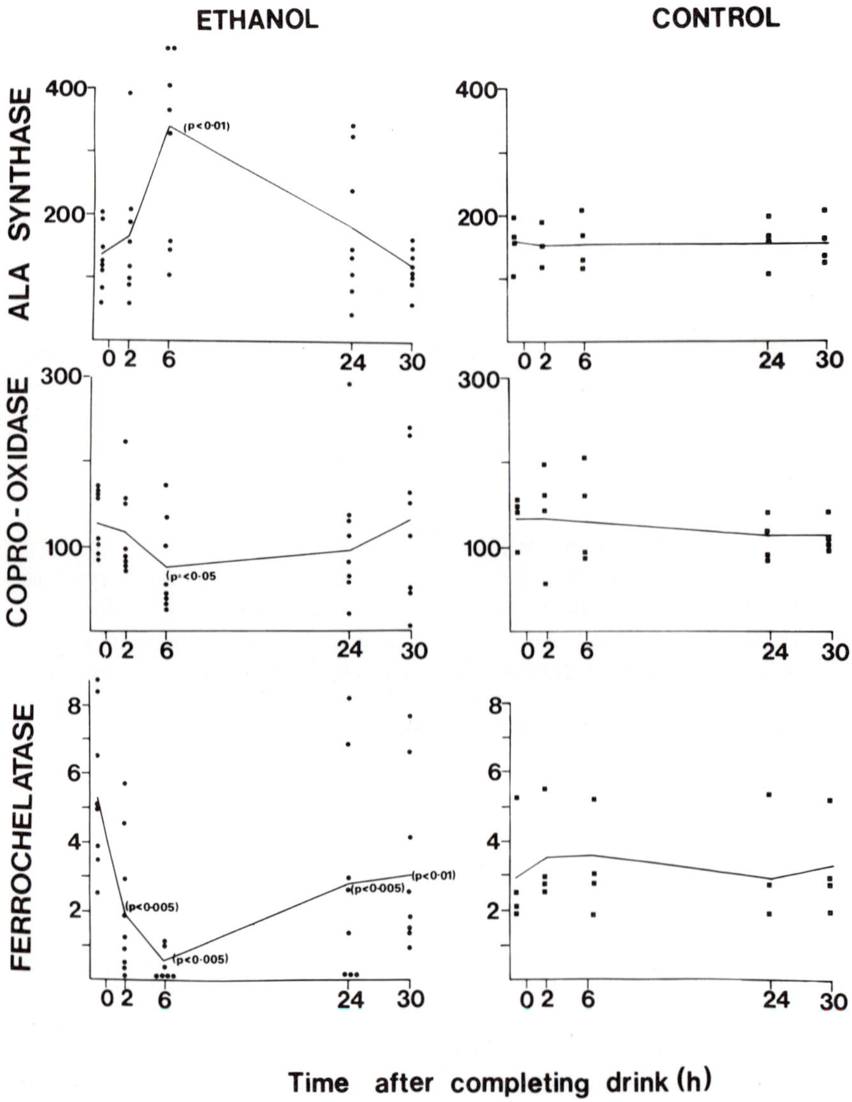

Fig. 9.5 The effect of consumption of 200 ml Vodka on the activity of ALA synthase coproporphyrinogen oxidase and ferrochelatase in peripheral leucocyte. Ethanol was consumed at time O. The values at each time studied had been compared with the pre-ethanol values uring the Wilcoxon paired samples ranking test. Acitivity of these enzymes in four of the subjects over a similar control period is also shown. ALA synthase activity is expressed as nmol of ALA g protein/hour, coproporphyrinogen oxidase as nmol protoporphyrin/g/hour and ferrochelatase as pmol meso haem/g protein/h.

remaining low at 30 h. The mechanism by which ethanol or its metabolites exert this effect on these enzymes is unclear.

Increased urinary excretion of coproporphyrin, a feature common to many porphyrinurias, was observed during the 24 hours following ethanol

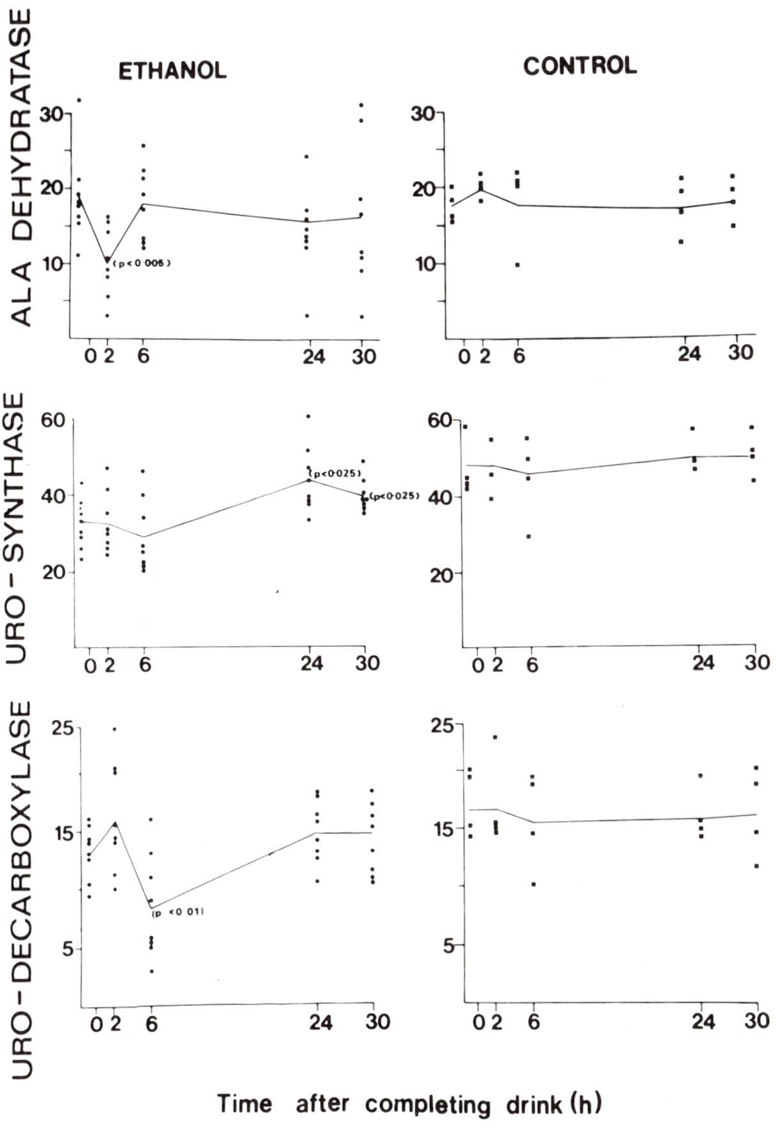

Fig. 9.6 The effect of consumption of 200 ml Vodka on the activity of delta-aminolaevulinic acid dehydratase, prophobilinogen deaminase and uroporphyrinogen decarboxylase in the peripheral erythrocytes of normal subjects. ALA dehydratase activity is expressed as nmol ALA/1 red blood cells/min., porphobilingoen deaminase as nmol URO/1 red blood cells/h and uroporphyrinogen decarboxylase as nmol COPRO/1 red blood cells/h.

consumption. This is due to increased synthesis of this porphyrin, especially the series 1 isomer, and possibly to increased renal excretion. There is no information available on the mechanism of renal handling of coproporphyrin. If tubular reabsorption is important, the ethanol-induced diuresis might temporarily increase renal clearance. However, the relative magnitude of the increase in coproporphyrin excretion compared to the increased urine volume is against a purely renal explanation.

Effects on erythropoiesis

The enzyme changes in blood cells may be relevant to the known haematological effects of ethanol ingestion. Ethanol is known to depress erythropoiesis (Myrhed, Berglund & Bottinger, 1977). Houribane & Weir (1970) observed that well nourished chronic alcoholics had an elevated serum iron concentration which, on cessation of drinking, fell with an associated rise in the reticulocyte count. The depression of erythropoiesis by ethanol is thought to be the result of primary depression of haem biosynthesis with resultant consequent depression of protein synthesis (Ibrahim, Spieler & Freedman, 1979). The very marked depression of ferrochelatase may be of particular importance in the aetiology of ethanol-related sideroblastic anaemia, which has also been found to have increased activity of ALA synthase in bone marrow (Fraser & Schacter, 1977) and accumulation of protoporphyrin and coproporphyrin in erythrocytes (Ali & Sweeney, 1974). All these changes could be explained by depression of ferrochelatase activity.

Comparison with other tissues

It is probable that ethanol ingestion produces similar alterations in the enzymes of haem biosynthesis in hepatic cells. In rats, acute ethanol ingestion is known to produce similar changes in hepatic ALA synthase, ALA dehydratase and ferrochelatase to those which have been observed in human peripheral blood cells. Since ethanol resulted in increased urinary coproporphyrin excretion coproporphyrinogen oxidase activity is probably reduced in hepatic cells. If similar changes are occurring in hepatic as well as in peripheral blood cells, these are relevant to our understanding of the mechanisms of certain ethanol related hepatic disorders, such as its role as an aetiological agent in the development of cutaneous hepatic porphyria. Patients with this condition have a genetic deficiency of hepatic uroporphyrinogen decarboxylase (Kushner, Barbuto & Lee, 1976; Elder, Lee & Tovey, 1978). A further acquired factor such as alcohol excess, certain drugs and chemicals or liver disease, is necessary before patients excrete excess urinary uroporphyrin and develop symptoms of the disease. The finding of ethanol-related depression of uroporphyrinogen decarboxylase activity and increase of ALA synthase activity may explain the mechanism by which alcohol can precipitate this condition in patients possessing the genetic trait.

Hepatic siderosis is also a feature of this disease, and ethanol has been incriminated as a factor in its development. Alcoholism and alcoholic liver disease are associated with increased hepatic iron deposition and alcohol is an important aetiological factor in the development of the so called idiopathic haemochromatosis (McDonald, 1964). The ethanol-related depression of ferrochelatase may play an important role in the accumulation of non-haem in hepatic tissue.

CUTANEOUS HEPATIC PORPHYRIA

Having considered the effects of ethanol upon porphyrin metabolism in normal subjects, it is now appropriate to view the metabolic changes associated with ethanol in disease states. One of the most interesting of these is cutaneous hepatic porphyria. This is a relatively common porphyria associated with liver damage and hepatic siderosis in which the primary aetiological agent is ethanol. Although controversy existed in the past on whether or not this was an acquired or inherited metabolic disease, evidence now exists to prove the presence of both forms. In the inherited condition, uroporphyrinogen decarboxylase activity is found to be around 50 per cent of normal (Kushner, Barbuto & Lee, 1976; DeVerneuil et al, 1978; De Verneuil & Grandchamp, 1981) and in the sporadic or acquired condition such changes can only be detected in the liver with no change being found in the red cells (Elder, Lee & Tovey, 1978). The sporadic form of the disease appears when liver damage is caused by disorders such as alcoholic liver disease, but since not all patients with alcoholic liver disease develope porphyria, it is probable that some latent genetic pre-disposition exists which may be activated by drugs or chemicals.

Szodoray & Sumegi (1944) were the first to associate this disease with alcoholism. Since that time, many other foreign compounds such as hexachlorobenzene and oestrogens have been linked with its exacerbation. Liver disease plays an important part in the association of cutaneous hepatic porphyria with alcoholism. This was emphasised by Brunsting (1954). Liver damage is indicated by raised levels of serum transaminases. This is found in combination with increased hepatic iron storage which plays a central role in the development of the disease. Indeed, current methods of treatment of cutaneous hepatic porphyria depend upon removal of iron, usually by venesection, to deplete liver iron stores (Ramsay et al, 1974) which results in remission of the disease associated with changes in ALA synthase activity (Moore et al, 1972).

The clinical picture in this disease is typical. The features are of increased susceptibility to minor mechanical damage to the skin, hypertrichosis, changes in skin pigmentation, photosensitivity to light of around 400 nm and pseudo-scleroderma. The biochemical picture in this disease is very typical. As a consequence of the diminished activity of uroporphyrinogen decarboxylase, excess concentrations of porphyrins lying between the octacarboxylic uroporphyrin and tetracarboxylic coproporphyrin are found

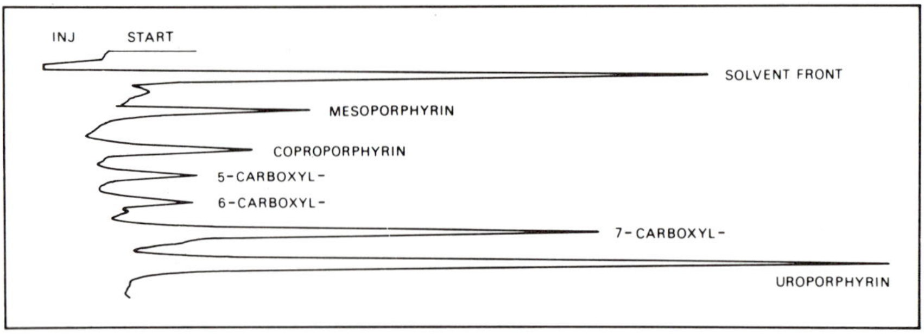

Fig. 9.7 High pressure liquid chromatographic separation of porphyrins in the urine of a patient with cutaneous hepatic porphyria. Note the excessive excretion of high carboxyl number porphyrin, especially uroporphyrin and 7-carboxyl porphyrin. This trace does not show the characteristic peak of the isocoproporphyrins.

(Fig. 9.7). The greatest concentration lies at the upper end of this range, that is of the 8 and 7 carboxyl porphyrins (Fig. 9.3), but in particular the tetracarboxylic isocoproporphyrin series is found in this disease. The reasons for alcohol excess precipitating the sporadic disease, must relate therefore not only to its effects upon uroporphyrinogen decarboxylase, but also upon its ability to diminish ferrochelatase activity and thus allow the accumulation of iron in hepatic tissue. This is all coupled with increased activity of ALA synthase, which supplies the biosynthetic pathway with increased concentrations of substrate for porphyrin synthesis. Since in this disease no excess concentrations of either delta-aminolaevulinic acid or porphobilinogen are produced, one must assume that the diminution in activity of ALA dehydratase has no serious metabolic consequences.

In summary, the disease will develop in susceptible persons in response to an external agent such as hepatotoxic compounds like hexachlorobenzene or ethanol, in combination with excess iron stores. The extent of uroporphyrin accumulation caused by stimulation of delta-aminolaevulinic acid synthase will not cause porphyria in the normal individual but is certainly sufficient to cause exacerbation of the disease in those with the genetic trait. It should also be borne in mind that agents such as ethanol and iron will act synergistically upon the activity of uroporphyrinogen decarboxylase. Whereas iron or ethanol alone will only cause minimal changes in uroporphyrinogen decarboxylase, a combination of these two have a much more pronounced effect upon the biosynthetic pathway. This is equivalent to the effects found with the porphyrinogenic agent hexachlorobenzene, which given alone will only produce a minimal porphyria in animals, but in combination with iron will rapidly produce hepatic porphyria in rats.

ALCOHOL-INDUCED ANAEMIA AND HAEM BIOSYNTHESIS

A variety of mechanisms may be responsible for anaemia in chronic alcoholics, including nutritional deficiencies, gastrointestinal blood loss, haemolysis (Zieve's syndrome) and haemodilution due to liver disease. In addition, alcohol can directly depress haematopoiesis and this is porbably the result of its inhibitory effect on the biosynthesis of haem. Evidence for direct depression of erythropoiesis by alcohol was presented by Houribane & Weir (1970), based on their studies on alcohol withdrawal in chronic alcoholic subjects without haematinic deficiency. Cessation of drinking was associated with disappearance of haemosiderin granules in erythrocyte precursors and a precipitous fall in serum iron, suggesting that the alcohol had been inhibiting the marrow's utilization of iron. These findings were confirmed by Myrhed et al (1977) who noted a reticulocytosis and fall in serum iron on cessation of drinking in well-nourished alcoholics.

Alcohol-induced sideroblastic anaemia

A proportion of alcoholics develop sideroblastic changes in the marrow, which may be associated with anaemia and which quickly reverse with alcohol withdrawal (Chanarin, 1969). The sideroblastic marrow is characterised by the presence of ringed-sideroblasts which are erythroblasts containing a peri-nuclear ring of iron which stains strongly with Prussian Blue (Fig. 9.8). Electron microscopic studies show that these erythroblasts are overloaded with ferritin which is distributed in microvesicles throughout the cytoplasm and within the mitochondria (Grasso & Hines, 1969; Hines & Cowan, 1970).

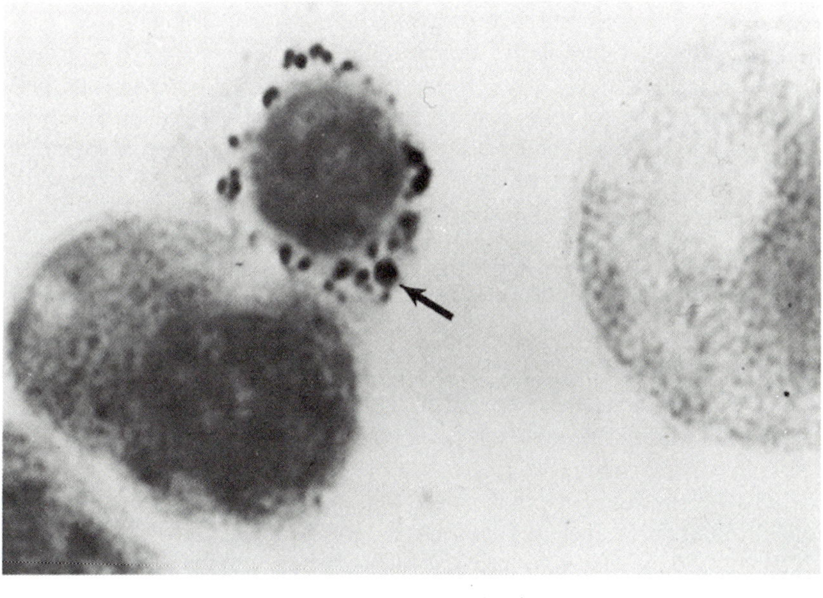

Fig. 9.8 Alcohol induced ring sideroblast.

Hines (1969) found ringed-sideroblasts in the marrow of 24 out of 33 severe chronic alcoholics examined within 36 hours of alcohol withdrawal. These marrow findings were associated with increased saturation of the serum iron-binding capacity. Re-examination of these subjects after 7–20 days of alcohol withdrawal and institution of a normal diet showed no remaining sideroblasts and normal iron saturation. Three of the subjects who received only intravenous glucose and saline solution showed a similar resolution, indicating that the improvement was the result of withdrawing alcohol rather than the improved nutrition. These observations provide strong evidence that chronic alcohol ingestion can block the incorporation of iron within erythrocyte precursors.

Haem biosynthesis in alcohol-related sideroblastic anaemia

There is considerable evidence indicating that the underlying biochemical mechanism of alcohol-related sideroblastic anaemia is inhibition of haem biosynthesis within the erythroblasts. Ali & Sweeney (1974) demonstrated markedly elevated levels of protoporphyrin and coproporphyrin in erythrocytes of subjects with alcoholic sideroblastic anaemia. They postulated that the anaemia and accumulation of iron, protoporphyrin and coproporphyrin could all be explained by depressed activity of the mitochondrial enzyme ferrochelatase which inserts iron into protoporphyrin to form haem. Fraser & Schacter (1977) provided further evidence for a block in haem biosynthesis by noting increased activity of the initial and rate-controlling enzyme of haem biosynthesis delta-aminolaevulinic acid (ALA) synthase in the marrow of 3 alcoholics with sideroblastic anaemia. Alcohol is only one of many causes of sideroblastic anaemia, and it is of interest that several of these other causes also inhibit haem biosynthesis eg, deficiency of pyridoxine which is a cofactor for ALA synthase (Cartwright & Wintrobe, 1948), chloramphenicol which inhibits ferrochelatase (Manyan & Arimura, 1972) and lead poisoning which interferes with several of the enzymes of haem biosynthesis (Moore, Meredith & Goldberg, 1980).

In vitro studies of alcohol and erythropoiesis

Excessive exposure to ethanol has been shown to inhibit human reticulocyte protein (Freedman et al, 1975), and globin chain synthesis (Ali & Brain, 1974) in vitro. This effect is prevented by the addition of haemin, indicating that the inhibition of protein synthesis is secondary to the alcohol inhibiting reticulocyte haem synthesis. Haem is known to regulate reticulocyte protein synthesis by retarding the formation and reversing the action of a translational repressor of protein synthesis (Freedman et al, 1974). Ibrahim et al (1979) studied the effects of ethanol of haem biosynthesis in a rabbit reticulocyte in vitro preparation. They noted that the alcohol inhibited the activity of ALA synthase in intact reticulocytes, and that this was prevented by the addition of dibutyryl cyclic AMP (adenosine monophosphate). They also noted that there was reduced incorporation of ^{14}C ALA into haem, indicating that the alcohol was also inhibiting the pathway more distally. The concentrations of alcohol used in these studies were high and approached the fatal dose in man.

ALCOHOLISM

As haematological complications of alcohol are usually seen in relation to chronic rather than acute alcohol ingestion, we have also studied haem biosynthesis in peripheral blood cells of chronic alcoholics (McColl et al, 1981). This was performed on eleven male alcoholics who were admitted to hospital for alcohol withdrawal. All subjects had been drinking heavily up until 24 h prior to their admission. The haemoglobin concentration was reduced in 3 subjects; in one this was explained by iron deficiency but the other two had no haematinic deficiency and indeed had elevated plasma iron saturation. On admission the activity of ALA synthase was significantly increased and the activities of ALA dehydratase and uroporphyrinogen

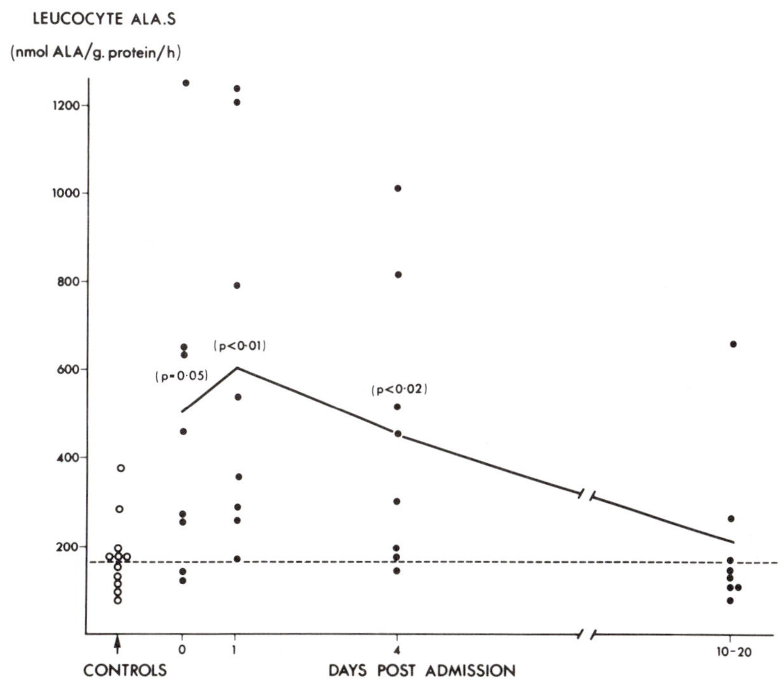

Fig. 9.9 Longitudinal examination of delta-aminolaevulinic acid synthase activity in a group of chronic alcoholics followed for up to 20 days after admission to a psychiatric ward. All were withdrawn from ethanol upon admission. Significances were compared by Mann-Whitney 'U' Test on the control group where the dotted line shows the mean control activity.

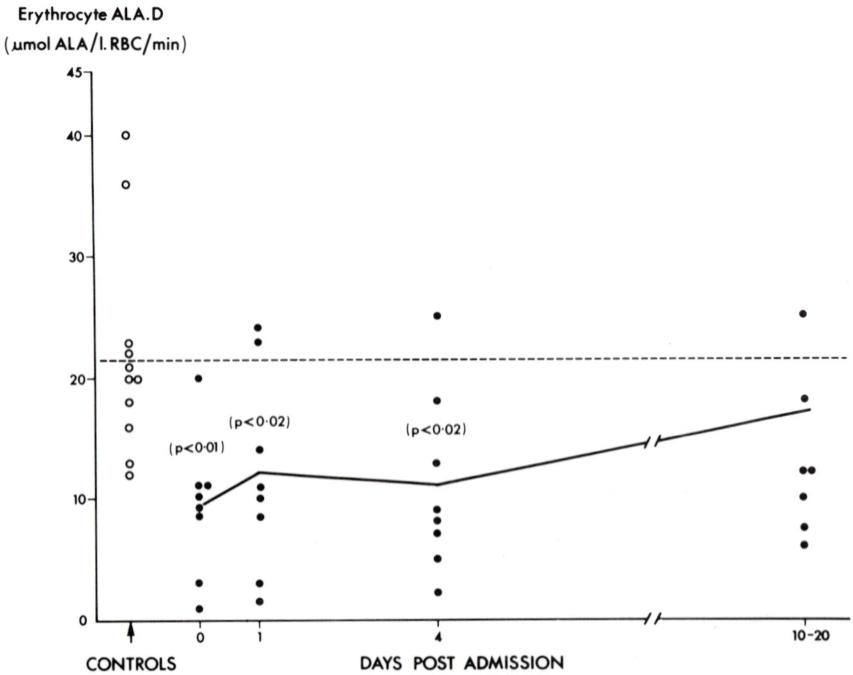

Fig. 9.10 Longitudinal examination of changes in erythrocyte delta-aminolaevulinic acid dehydratase in a group of chronic alcoholics during alcohol withdrawal. Significances were calculated by Mann Whitney 'U' Test, the dotted line shows the mean control activity.

decarboxylase significantly decreased in the alcoholics compared with control subjects (Fig. 9.9, 9.10, 9.11). These enzymatic abnormalities returned to normal between the tenth and twentieth day post admission (McColl et al, 1981).

The changes in porphyrin metabolism and enzymes of haem biosynthesis were different and particularly interesting in the two anaemic alcoholics. Both had a macrocytic anaemia with normal levels of Vitamin B12 and folic acid and markedly increased plasma iron saturation. They also had increased erythrocyte concentrations of protoporphyrin and coproporphyrin. In addition to increased activity of ALA synthase, both these subjects had markedly depressed activity of ferrochelatase and one of them also had markedly depressed coproporphyrinogen oxidase activity. The anaemia and associated biochemical changes all reverted to normal with alcohol withdrawal. It would appear, therefore, that in these 2 patients the chronic alcohol ingestion was depressing the activities of ferrochelatase and coproporphyrinogen oxidase, resulting in accumulation of their substrates (coproporphyrin, protoporphyrin and iron) and anaemia due to deficient haem synthesis. Both of these enzymes have been noted to be inhibited by acute alcohol ingestion in normal subjects (McColl et al, 1980), and it is likely that

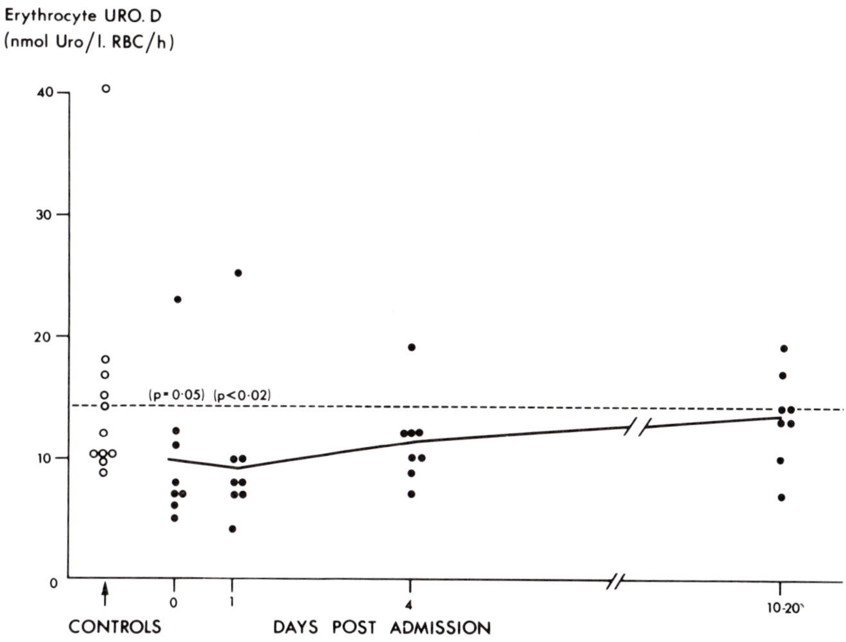

Fig. 9.11 A longitudinal examination of erythrocyte uroporphyrinogen decarboxylase in a group of chronic alcoholics after withdrawal. Significance was calculated by Mann Whitney 'U' Test, the dotted line is the mean control activity.

in certain patients this persists with chronic alcohol ingestion, resulting in alcohol-induced anaemia. The biochemical changes previously noted in patients with alcoholic sideroblastic anaemia, i.e. increased bone marrow ALA synthase activity (Fraser & Schacter, 1977) and accumulation of protoporphyrin and coproporphyrin in erythrocytes, can all be explained by the depression of ferrochelatase and coproporphyrinogen oxidase activities.

CONCLUSIONS

The ability to synthesise haem is an important function of every cell in the body and, as was stated at the beginning of this chapter, any dyshaemopoietic effects must ultimately reflect upon capacity of the body to carry out oxidative reactions in which haem is involved as much as in its requirement for oxygen transport within the body. In this chapter we have brought together the various effects of ethanol upon porphyrin synthesis. We have shown that ethanol enhances the production and excretion of coproporphyrin and the deposition of iron in cells. We have shown that these changes may be directly related to specific alterations in the enzymes of the pathway which synthesise porphyrins and ultimately haem. The chapter has finally linked over-exposure to ethanol with a number of disease states, which include cutaneous hepatic porphyria, sideroblastic anaemia and of course alcoholism.

The overwhelming overall impression that one gets in considering the multiple effects of ethanol upon porphyrin synthesis, is that these are of sufficient magnitude to be of consequence in the maintenance of cellular homeostasis. We have tried to convey to the reader that, as a consequence of certain metabolic effects, ethanol is interfering with the synthesis of one of the basic building blocks of the body, essential in energy metabolism and in gas transport, and without which life could not have evolved or existed on this planet.

REFERENCES

Abdulla M, Haegar-Aronsen B, Svensson S 1976 Effect of ethanol and zinc on ALA-dehydratase activity in red blood cells. Enzyme 21: 248–252

Ali M A M, Brain M C 1974 Ethanol inhibition of haemoglobin synthesis. In vitro evidence for a haem correctable deficit in normal subjects and in alcoholics. British Journal of Haematology 28: 311–316

Ali M A M, Sweeney G 1974 Erythrocyte coproporphyrin and protoporphyrin in ethanol-induced sideroblastic erythropoiesis. Blood 43: 291–295

Barnes R, Connelly J L, Jones O T G 1972 The utilisation of iron and its complexes by mammalian mitochondria. Biochemical Journal 128: 1043–1055

Battersby A R, Fookes C J R, Matcham G W J, McDonald E 1980 Biosynthesis of the pigments of life: formation of the macrocyte. Nature 285: 17–21

Brodie M J, Moore M R, Goldberg A 1977 Enzyme abnormalities in the porphyrias. Lancet 2: 690–701

Brunsting L A 1954 Observations on porphyria cutanea tarda. AMA Archives Dermatologia Syphilogica 70: 551–564

Brugsch J 1937 Toxic porphyrinuria following chronic alcoholism. Procedural Staff Meeting Mayo Clinic Proceedings 12: 609

Carwright G E Wintrobe M M 1948 Studies on free erythrocyte protoporphyrin, plasma copper and plasma iron in normal and in pyridoxine deficient swine. Journal of Biological Chemistry 172: 557–565

Chanarin I 1969 Alcohol and haemopoeisis. British Journal of Haematology 17: 515

Cheh A, Neilands J B 1973 Zinc, an essential metal ion for beef liver delta-aminolaevulinate dehydratase. Biochemical and Biophysical Research Communications 55: 1060–1063

De Verneuil H, Aitken G, Nordmann Y 1978 Familial and sporadic porphyria cutanea tarda. Two different diseases. Human Genetics 44: 145–151

Doss M 1978 Relationships between acute hepatic porphyrias due to genetic variability of primary enzyme defects and limiting function of uroporphyrinogen synthase. International Journal of Biochemistry 9: 911–916

De Verneuil H, Nordmann Y 1981 Porphyrie cutanée symptomatique. Nouvelle Presse Medicale 10: 3541–3544

Doss M 1978 Alkoholbedingte Störungen des Porphyrinstoffwechsals. Leber Magen Darmstadt 8: 278–285

Doss M Schermuly E 1976 Urinary porphyrin excretion pattern and isomer distribution of I and III in human porphyrin disorders. In: Doss M (ed) Porphyrins in human diseases. Proceedings international porphyrin meeting. Karger, Basel, p 189

Eales L 1971 Acute porphyria. The precipitating and aggravating factors. South African Journal Laboratory Clinical Medicine 17: 120–125

Elder G H 1976 Acquired disorders of haem synthesis. Essays in medical biochemistry 2: 75–114

Elder G H, Lee G B, Tovey J A 1978 Decreased activity of hepatic uroporphyrinogen decarboxylase in sporadic cutanea tarda. New England Journal of Medicine 299: 274–278

Fanica-Gaignier M, Clement-Metral J 1973 Delta-aminolaevulinic acid synthetase of rhodopseudomonas spheroides Y. European Journal of Biochemistry 40: 19–24

Franke K, Fikentscher R 1935 Die bedeutung der quantitativen porphyrinbestimmung mit der lumineszensmes-sung für die prüfund der leberfunktion und für ernäh-rungsfragen. Münch en Medizinische Wochenschift 83: 171

Fraser M B, Schacter B A 1977 Increased bone marrow delta-aminolaevulinic acid synthetase activity in the acute reversible sideroblastic anaemia for alcoholics. Blood 50: 92

Freedman M L, Cohen H S, Rossman J, Forte F J 1975 Ethanol inhibition of reticulocyte protein synthesis. The role of haem. British Journal of Haematology 30: 351–362

Garcia R C, San Martin de Viale L C, Tomio J M, Grinstein M 1973 Porphyrin biosynthesis X. Biochimica Biophysica Acta 309: 203–210

Goldberg A, Moore M R (eds) 1980 The porphyrias. Clinics in haematology 9. Saunders, London

Goldgerg A, Rimington C 1962 Diseases of porphyrin metabolism. Springfield, Illinois, p 241

Goldberg A, McColl K E L, Moore M R 1981 Alcohol and porphyria. Lancet 2: 925

Granick S, Sassa S 1971 Delta-aminolaevulinic acid synthetase and the control of heme and chlorophyll synthesis. In: Vogel H J (ed) Metabolic regulation. Academic Press, New York

Grasso J A, Hines J D 1969 A comparative electron microscopic study of refractory and alcoholic sideroblastic anaemia. British Journal of Haematology 17: 35–44 (1969)

Hines J D 1969 Reversible megaloblastic and sideroblastic marrow abnormalities in alcoholic patients. British Journal of Haematology 16: 87–100

Houribane D O, Weir D G 1970 Suppresion of erythropoiesis by alcohol. British Medical Journal 1: 86–89

Ibrahim N G, Spieler P J, Freedman M L 1979 Ethanol inhibition of rabbit reticulocyte haem synthesis at the level of delta-aminolaevulinic acid synthetase. British Journal of Haematology 41: 235–243

Jackson A H, Elder G H, Smith S G 1978 The metabolism of coproporphyrinogen III into protoporphyrin IX International Journal of Biochemistry 9: 988–882

Jackson A H, Games D E, Couch P, Jackson J R, Belcher R B, Smith S G 1974 Conversion of coproporphyrinogen III to protoporphyrin IX. Enzyme 17: 81–87

Jackson A H, Sancovich H A, Ferramola A M, Evans N, Games D E, Matlin S A, Elder G H, Smith S G 1976 Macrocyclic intermediates in the biosynthesis of porphyrins Philosophical Transactions of the Royal Society of London 273: 191–206

Jordan P M, Shemin D 1972 Delta-aminolaevulinic acid synthetase. In: Boyer P D (ed) The enzymes, 3rd edn. Academic Press, New York, vol 7, p 339–356

Krasner N, Moore M R, Thompson G G, Goldberg A 1974 Depression of erythrocyte delta-aminolaevulinic acid dehydratase activity in alcoholics. Clinical Science & Molecular Medicine 46: 415–418

Krasner N, Moore M R, Dow J, Goldberg A 1974 Ascorbic-acid saturation and ethanol metabolism. The Lancet 2: 693–694

Kushner J P, Barbuto A J, Lee G R 1976 An inherited enzymatic defect in porphyria cutanea tarda: decreased uroporphyrinogen decarboxylase activity. Journal of Clinical Investigations: 58: 1089–1097

Labbe R F, Nutter J, Cowger M L, Neilson L D 1970 Control of haem biosynthesis. Effect of nicotinamide adeninc dinucleatide on the induction of delta-aminolaevulinic acid synthetase. Biochemical medicine 3: 465–474

Lumeng L, Li T 1974 Vitamin B_6 metabolism in chronic alcohol abuse. Pyridoxal phosphate levels in plasma and the effects of acetaldehyde on pyrodixal phosphate synthesis and degradation in human erythrocytes. Journal of Clinical Investigations 53: 693–704

Maines M D, Kappas A 1974 Cobalt induction of hepatic heme oxygenase; with evidence that cytochrome P-450 is not essential for this enzyme activity. Proceedings of the National Academy of Sciences 71: 4293–4297

Maines M D, Kappas A 1976 The induction of heme oxidation in various tissues by trace metals: Evidence for the catabolism of endogenous heme by hepatic heme oxygenase. Annals of Clinical Research 8: 39–46

Manyan D R, Arimura G K 1972 Chloramphenicol-induced erythroid suppression and bone marrow ferrochelatase activity in dogs. Journal of Laboratory and Clinical Medicine 79: 137–144

McColl K E L, Thompson G G, Moore M R, Goldberg A 1980 Acute ethanol ingestion and haem biosynthesis in healthy subjects. European Journal of Clinical Investigation 10: 107–112

McColl K E L, Moore M R, Thompson G G, Goldberg A 1981 Abnormal haem biosynthesis in chronic alcoholics. European Journal of Clinical Investigation 11: 461–468

McDonald R A 1964 Haemochromatosis and haemosiderosis. Thomas, Springfield, p 300–310

McKay R, Druyan R, Getz G S, Rabinowitz M 1969 Intramitochrondrial localisation of ALA synthase, delta-aminolaevulinate synthase and ferrochelatase in the rat liver. Biochemical Journal 114: 455–461

Meredith P A, Moore M R 1980 Effects of zinc on erythrocyte delta-aminolaevulinic acid dehydratase in man. International Archives of Occupational Environmental Health 45: 163–168

Mezey E, Quartner J, Nair P P 1971 Effect of vitamin E on porphyrinuria induced by ethanol in the rat. Biochemical medicine 5: 30

Moore M R 1974 The effects of ethanol on heme biosynthesis. In: Thurman R, Yonetani T, Williamson J R et al (eds) International symposium on alcohol and aldehyde metabolizing systems. Academic Press, New York, p 543

Moore M R 1975 Lead ethanol and delta-aminolaevulinic acid dehydratase. In: Recent advances in the assessment of the health effects of environmental pollution. Commission of the European Communities, Luxembourg, p 1171–1176

Moore M R 1980 The biochemistry of the porphyrins. In: Clinics in haematology, The porphyrias 9: 227–252

Moore M R, Beattie A D, Thompson G G 1971 Depression of delta-aminolaelvulinic acid dehydrase activity by ethanol in man and rat. Clinical Science 40: 81–88

Moore M R, Barnardo D, Magnus I A, Turnbull A L, Beattie A D, Goldberg A 1972 Hepatic delta-aminolaevulinic acid synthetase activity in porphyria cutanea tarda. Lancet 2: 97–100

Moore M R, McColl K E L, Goldberg A 1979 The porphyrias. Diabetes and Metabolism 5: 323–336

Moore M R, McColl K E L, Goldberg A 1980 The activities of the enzymes of haem biosynthesis in the porphyrias and during treatment of acute intermittent porphyria. International Journal of Biochemistry 12: 941–946

Moore M R, Meredith P A, Goldberg A 1980 Lead and heme biosynthesis. In: Singhal R D, Thomas J A (eds) Lead toxicity. Urban & Schwartzenberg, Baltimore, p 79–114

Myrhed M, Berglund L, Bottinger L E 1977 Alcohol consumption and haematology. Acta Medica Scandanavica 202: 11–15

O'Carra P 1975 Heme cleavage: biological systems and chemical analogs. In: Smith K M (ed) Porphyrins and metalloporphyrins. Elsevier, Amsterdam, p 123–153

Orten J M S, Doehr A, Bond C, Johnson H, Pappas A 1963 Urinary excretion of porphyrins and porphyrin intermediates in human alcoholics Quarterly Journal of Studies in Alcohol 24: 598

Pennington S N, Smith C P, Tapscott E B 1978 Effects of an acute dose of ethanol on rat liver microsomal mixed function oxygenase components and membrane lipid composition. Alcoholism: Clin and Exper Res 2: 311–316

Poulson R, Polglaze W J 1975 The enzymic conversion of protopotphyrinogen IX to protopotphyrin IX. Protoporphyrinogen oxidase activity in mitochondrial extracts of saccharomyces cerevisiae. Journal of Biological Chemistry 250: 1269–1274

Poulson R 1976 The enzymic conversion of protoprophyrinogen IX to protoporphyrin IX in mammalian mitochondria. The Journal of Biological Chemistry 251: 3730–3733

Ramsay C A, Magnus I A, Turnbull A, Baker H 1974 The treatment of porphyria cutanea tarda by venesection. Quarterly Journal of Medicine 36: 29–57

Rubin E, Hutterer F, Lieber C S 1968 Ethanol increases hepatic smooth endoplasmic reticulum and drug-metabolizing enzymes. Science 159: 1469

Rubin E, Bacchin P, Gang H 1970 Induction and inhibition of hepatic mircrosomal and mitochondrial enzymes by ethanol. Laboratory Investigations 22: 569–580

Sano S, Granick S 1961 Mitochondrial coproporphyrinogen oxidase and protoporphyrin formation. Journal of Biological Chemistry 236: 1173–1180
Shanley B C, Zail S S, Joubert S M 1968 Effect of ethanol on liver delta-aminolaevulinic synthetase in rats. Lancet 1: 70–71
Shemin D 1976 Delta-aminolaevulinate dehydratase: structure function and mechanism. Philosophical Transactions of the Royal Society of London B 273: 109–115
Smith A G, Francis J E 1979 Decarboxylation of porphyrinogens by rat liver uroporphyrinogen decarboxylase Biochemical Journal 183: 455–458
Smith K M Porphyrins and metalloporphyrins. Elsevier, Amsterdam, p 3–58
Sullivan J F 1974 Zinc deficiency and chronic alcoholism. In: Pories W J, Strain W H, Hsu J M et al (eds) Clinical applications of zinc metabolism. Thomas, Springfield, p 113–118
Sutherland C A, Watson C J 1951 Studies on coproporphyrin VI. The effect of alcohol on the per diem excretion and isoner distribution of the urinary coproporphyrins. Journal of Laboratory and Clinical Medicine 37: 29
Szodoray L, Sumegi S 1944 Uber die Nosologie der chronischen kutanen porphyrie. Dermatologica 90: 224–232
Tait G H 1978 The biosynthesis and biodegradation of heme. In: De Matteis F, Aldridge W N (eds) Heme and hemoproteins. Springer Verlag, Berlin, p 1–48
Tenhunen R 1976 The enzymic conversion of heme to bilirubin in vivo. Annals of Clinical Research 8: 2–9
Varticovski L, Kushner J P, Burnham B F 1980 Biosynthesis of prophyrin precursors. The Journal of Biological Chemistry 255: 3742–3747
Yoneyama Y, Sawada H, Takeshita M, Sugita Y 1969 The role of lipids in heme synthesis. Lipids 4: 321–326
Yoshida T, Kikuchi G 1978 Purification and properties of heme oxygenase from pig spleen microsomes. Journal of Biological Chemistry 253: 4224–4229

10

Peter R. Ryle Allan D. Thomson

Nutrition and vitamins in alcoholism

INTRODUCTION

Clinical and biochemical evidence of malnutrition is frequently found in chronic alcoholics, and alcoholism is the major cause of nutritional deficiency in countries with an adequate food supply. The mechanisms underlying such deficiency are multifactoral, involving decreased intake, poor absorption, decreased conversion of vitamins to their metabolically active forms, increased requirements, decreased storage, increased breakdown and increased excretion of vitamins. The ultimate consequence of these effects is impairment of normal physiological and biochemical function at the cellular level, so that cells are less able to carry out their normal functional role, and are less able to relicate or repair the damage caused by chronic alcohol abuse (Fig. 10.1).

Various organisations have defined normal daily requirements for each of the vitamins in terms of mg/1000 kcal consumed or simply as mg/person/day. In the alcoholic, however, the assessment of requirement is complicated by the various factors mentioned above that in fact mean that the alcoholic has an increased requirement for vitamins when compared with a non-alcoholic consuming equivalent calories. Ethanol metabolism requires a number of vitamins (Fig. 10.2). Although ethanol has a calorific value of 7.1 kcal/g, it is not equivalent nutritionally to an isocaloric amount of fat, protein or carbohydrate, as ethanol interferes with energy production by uncoupling oxidative phosphorylation in the mitochondria. Also, a proportion of the calorific content of ethanol is dissipated as heat due to induction of the Cytochrome-P450 mediated microsomal ethanol oxidising system (MEOS) in alcoholics. The MEOS pathway involves utilisation of reducing equivalents (NADPH) for drug metabolism and heat production rather than for ATP synthesis as in oxidative phosphorylation.

Thus, the alcoholic has an increased requirement for vitamins and nutrients, yet he often derives 50 per cent or more of his calorie intake from ethanol. Alcoholic beverages are very poor sources of vitamins and minerals. To obtain one's daily recommended requirement of the B vitamins, for example, one would have to ingest about 40 litres of beer or 200 litres of

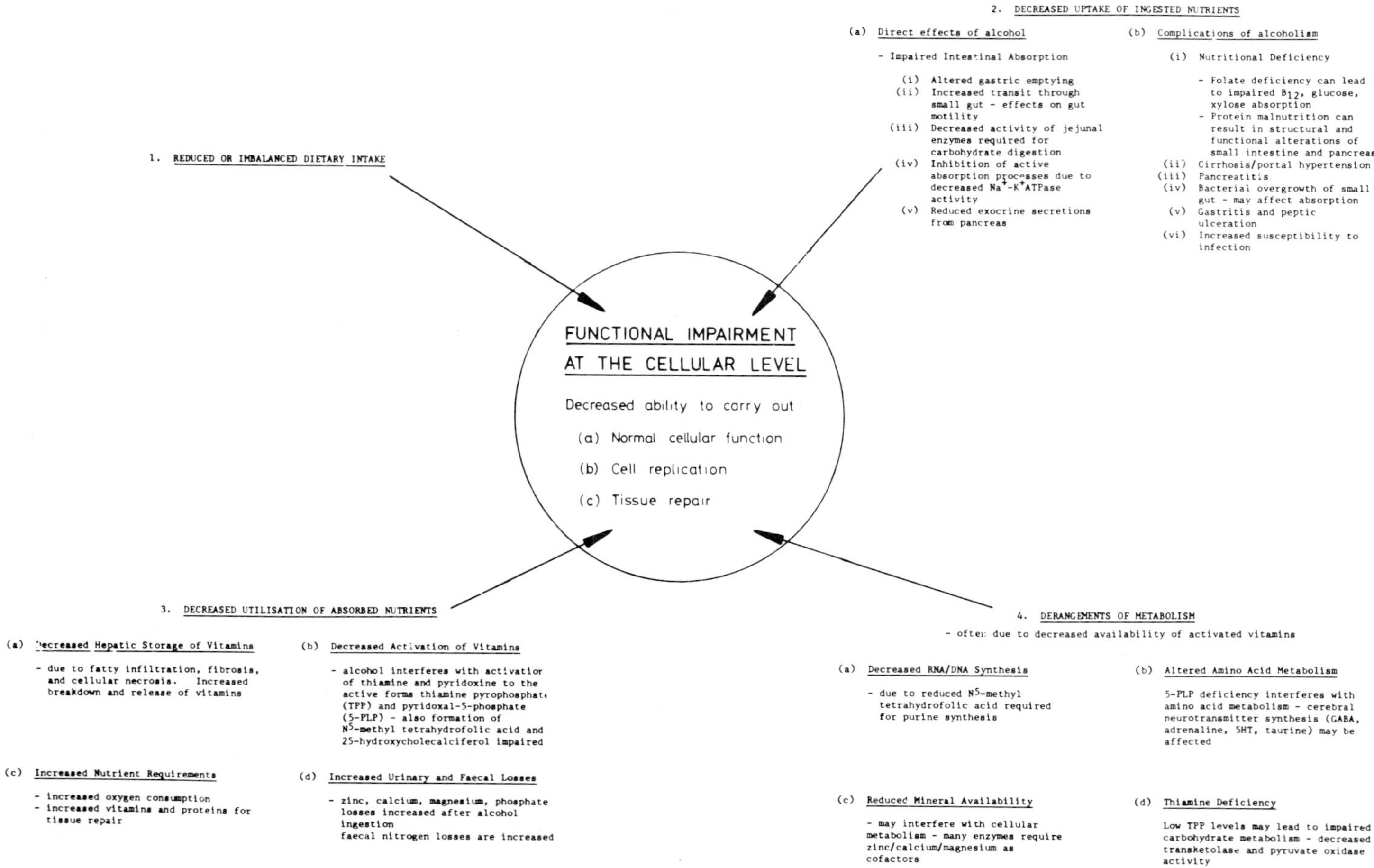
1. REDUCED OR IMBALANCED DIETARY INTAKE
2. DECREASED UPTAKE OF INGESTED NUTRIENTS
(a) Direct effects of alcohol
- Impaired Intestinal Absorption
(i) Altered gastric emptying
(ii) Increased transit through small gut - effects on gut motility
(iii) Decreased activity of jejunal enzymes required for carbohydrate digestion
(iv) Inhibition of active absorption processes due to decreased Na+-K+ATPase activity
(v) Reduced exocrine secretions from pancreas
(b) Complications of alcoholism
(i) Nutritional Deficiency
- Folate deficiency can lead to impaired B12, glucose, xylose absorption
- Protein malnutrition can result in structural and functional alterations of small intestine and pancreas
(ii) Cirrhosis/portal hypertension
(iii) Pancreatitis
(iv) Bacterial overgrowth of small gut - may affect absorption
(v) Gastritis and peptic ulceration
(vi) Increased susceptibility to infection
FUNCTIONAL IMPAIRMENT AT THE CELLULAR LEVEL
Decreased ability to carry out
(a) Normal cellular function
(b) Cell replication
(c) Tissue repair
3. DECREASED UTILISATION OF ABSORBED NUTRIENTS
(a) Decreased Hepatic Storage of Vitamins
- due to fatty infiltration, fibrosis, and cellular necrosis. Increased breakdown and release of vitamins
(b) Decreased Activation of Vitamins
- alcohol interferes with activation of thiamine and pyridoxine to the active forms thiamine pyrophosphate (TPP) and pyridoxal-5-phosphate (5-PLP) - also formation of N5-methyl tetrahydrofolic acid and 25-hydroxycholecalciferol impaired
(c) Increased Nutrient Requirements
- increased oxygen consumption
- increased vitamins and proteins for tissue repair
(d) Increased Urinary and Faecal Losses
- zinc, calcium, magnesium, phosphate losses increased after alcohol ingestion
faecal nitrogen losses are increased
4. DERANGEMENTS OF METABOLISM
- often due to decreased availability of activated vitamins
(a) Decreased RNA/DNA Synthesis
- due to reduced N5-methyl tetrahydrofolic acid required for purine synthesis
(b) Altered Amino Acid Metabolism
5-PLP deficiency interferes with amino acid metabolism - cerebral neurotransmitter synthesis (GABA, adrenaline, 5HT, taurine) may be affected
(c) Reduced Mineral Availability
- may interfere with cellular metabolism - many enzymes require zinc/calcium/magnesium as cofactors
(d) Thiamine Deficiency
Low TPP levels may lead to impaired carbohydrate metabolism - decreased transketolase and pyruvate oxidase activity

Fig. 10.1 Mechanisms contributing to vitamin deficiency and malutilisation in chronic alcoholism.

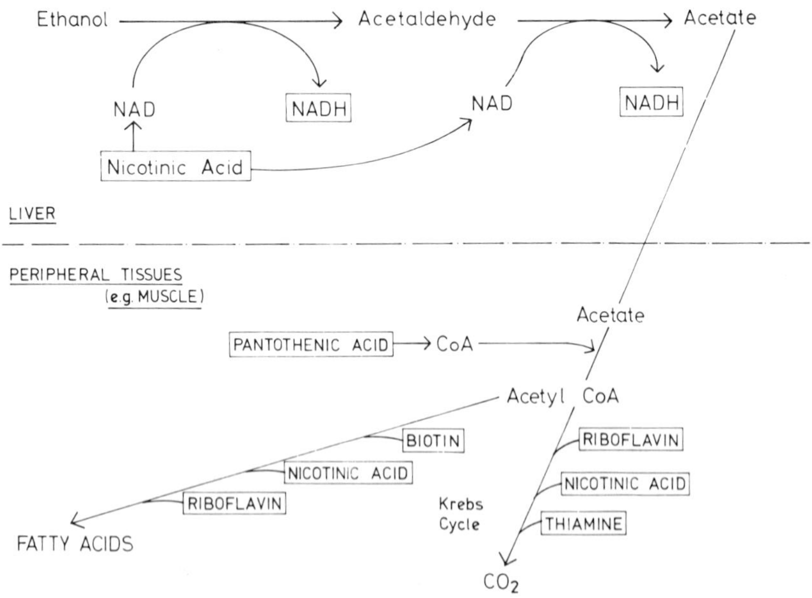

Fig. 10.2 Vitamin requirements in ethanol oxidation.

wine. Spirits contain virtually no vitamins at all (Thomson, 1978). So the problem the alcoholic has is that he is ingesting a smaller amount of vitamins than a normal person yet actually needs more. The problem facing the clinician or chemical pathologist is how to recognise when a chronic alcoholic is at risk from the consequences of nutrient depletion. Various clinical signs can be attributed to specific or generalised vitamin deficiencies, but very often by the time these are evident, irreversable neurological damage has occurred. Measurement of blood vitamin levels can be useful, a deficiency state often showing up as a low circulating level long before clinical evidence of the deficit shows itself. However, this approach to the problem can be fraught with misleading anomalies and problems of interpretation. Ultimately, what is important is whether enough of a vitamin or nutrient is available in a utilisable form at a subcellular level, and blood levels can be misleading in this respect.

An alternative approach is to attempt to diagnose deficiency or define nutrient requirements by assessing function. It is evident that ethanol can lead to gross changes in brain structure and function as well as affecting the liver, and these brain changes may be taking place at the same time or even earlier (Thomson et al, 1980; Thomson, 1982). Detailed psychometric testing may be able to pick up these disturbances long before a full-blown vitamin deficiency syndrome, such as the Wernicke-Korsakoff psychosis develops, and thus allow the clinician to take appropriate action, in the form of vitamin supplementation, to prevent permanent neurological damage.

MECHANISMS UNDERLYING NUTRIENT DEFICIENCY IN THE ALCOHOLIC

The major cause of nutritional deficiency in many alcoholics is reduced dietary intake, although alcoholics consuming a normal diet may also show evidence of malnutrition. Ethanol consumption itself places large metabolic demands on the liver and other tissues, yet the calorie intake derived from ethanol is rarely accompanied by adequate amounts of vitamins and other essential nutrients to cope with these demands. This, in conjunction with other factors that will be discussed below, means that the alcoholic has increased nutrient requirements (Mezey, 1980)

Decreased uptake of ingested nutrients

Ethanol has a number of direct effects on the gastrointestinal tract which lead to impaired absorption of ingested nutrients (see also Chs 11 and 12). Loss of ingested food frequently can occur due to vomiting secondary to gastric irritation. In addition, ethanol affects gastric emptying, and increases small gut motility, so that transit time is reduced. Acute ethanol administration interferes with normal pancreatic and biliary secretion so that fat absorption is impaired and steatorrhoea may occur.

Nutrients are absorbed from the gut lumen either by simple passive diffusion or by an energy-requiring carrier mediated process. Ethanol is not thought to have any direct effect on passive diffusion although in the long term, absorption of nutrients by this mechanism may be reduced in the alcoholic due to ethanol's effects on intestinal morphology. Work in man and animals has shown that chronic ethanol administration causes multiple mucosal erosions in the upper gastrointestinal tract. Furthermore, shortening of the villi in the jejunum has been observed in animal experiments, the consequence being a reduced surface area over which passive diffusion can occur (Halsted et al, 1975). Ethanol inhibits uptake by carrier-mediated processes as it impairs adenosine triphosphate (ATP) hydrolysis by the $Na^{+}K^{+}$ ATPase complex that provides the energy required for uptake of nutrients by this mechanism. Uptake of glucose, amino acids and low concentrations of thiamine involve carrier-mediated processes and inhibition of intestinal transport of these nutrients by ethanol has been shown (Schultz, 1977; Kuo & Shanbour, 1978; Hoyumpa et al, 1975). The ethanol molecule contains both hydrophilic and hydrophobic groups. The hydrophobic end of the molecule can embed itself in the lipid bilayer of cell membranes, and, depending on the concentration of ethanol in the gut lumen, an increase in membrane fluidity in the mucosal cells results. It has not been established whether this effect has any influence on nutrient absorption by passive diffusion, although it may play a part in altering absorption where a specific carrier or membrane-bound enzyme is involved, as membrane fluidity is crucial in maintaining normal function of these mucosal cell surface constituents. Impaired carrier-mediated absorption due to ethanol has already been mentioned, although a different mechanism is implicated, whilst on the other hand, lactose malabsorption in rats has been reported due to reduced jejunal lactase activity following acute ethanol administration (Rubin et al, 1972).

In addition to these direct effects of ethanol, impaired absorption can result from the complications of long term alcohol abuse. Biliary and pancreatic disease can lead to fat malabsorption. Alcoholic gastritis and peptic ulceration, changes in the gut microflora, cirrhosis and portal hypertension, can all contribute to malabsorption of ingested nutrients (Fig. 10.1). In addition, a continuing state of malnutrition becomes significant in reducing absorption due to poor tissue repair and may operate in conjunction with any of the above factors. For a more detailed discussion of the effect of ethanol on intestinal absorption and utilisation of nutrients, the reader is referred to the recent review by Thomson & Majumdar (1981).

Decreased utilisation of absorbed nutrients

Apart from the problems of decreased intake and uptake of nutrients, the alcoholic also faces the problems of ethanol interfering with normal storage, activation and excretion of nutrients, especially vitamins. The liver is a major storage site for many water and fat-soluble vitamins, and in alcoholic liver disease a large proportion of the body vitamin stores may be lost into the circulation and excreted, due to hepatocellular necrosis which accompanies steatonecrosis, alcoholic hepatitis and cirrhosis.

Many vitamins are not active in the form in which they are ingested or absorbed. The liver is a major site for the activation of thiamine, pyridoxine and folic acid. Many of these processes involve phosphorylation by ATP. Hepatic levels of ATP fall during ethanol oxidation due to uncoupling of oxidative phosphorylation, and, in addition, activation of some vitamins, for example pyridoxine, depends on enzymes which require other vitamins (e.g. riboflavin), as cofactors so that in multiple vitamin deficiency, activation will be further impaired. A combination of these specific effects allied to a poor hepatic metabolic function, that is commonly associated with chronic alcoholism, means that availability of activated vitamins is reduced. In addition, in the case of pyridoxine, it seems that ethanol, or its metabolite acetaldehyde may actually increase the degradation of the activated form of the vitamin once it has been formed. Ethanol may also increase renal clearance of vitamins due to the osmotic diuresis that it induces.

In the ensuing discussion, we will consider the biochemical and physiological role of vitamins and the way in which ethanol interferes with their role. The hospitalised alcoholic will nearly always receive an adequate intake of fat, protein, carbohydrate and trace elements following admission. The potentially dangerous clinical situations, such as acute Wernicke-Korsakoff syndrome, may arise because this large calorie intake is not balanced with sufficient utilisable vitamins at the cellular level. The alcoholic may have complications such as liver disease or pancreatitis so that he is unable to utilise vitamins given in the diet or as medication and there may be failure to identify that the patient's vitamin requirements may be much greater than those available. It should be appreciated that whilst the alcoholic is drinking heavily, and deriving possibly 70–80 per cent of his calorie intake from ethanol, his vitamin intake may be sufficient to support metabolism of calories from other sources, yet once hospitalised, a large intake of calories from carbohydrate, fat and protein may precipitate an acute vitamin deficiency state due simply to imbalance and inadequate vitamin reserves. For example, it is possible to precipitate Wernicke's encephalopathy in an alcoholic by administering a glucose load without giving any thiamine at the same time. When we consider the role of vitamins in intermediary metabolism, it will be seen that the crucial factor is that metabolic demands have to be balanced by an adequate supply of vitamins in a utilisable form. If there is an imbalance, derangements of metabolism will occur, followed by cellular dysfunction and cell damage; ultimately a clinical syndrome may develop.

THE BIOCHEMICAL AND PHYSIOLOGICAL ROLE OF VITAMINS: THEIR INTERACTIONS WITH ETHANOL

Vitamin A (retinol)

Vitamin A originates in the diet as retinol or as a carotenoid precursor, β-carotene. β-carotene is absorbed and hydrolysed in the small intestine epithelial cell to retinaldehyde and reduced to the alcohol form, retinol. Approximately 75 per cent of the retinol is then esterified with palmitic acid or other long-chain fatty acids in the mucosal cell and transported through the lymph system to the liver. The liver efficiently removes retinol esters from the circulation and stores them, bound to a specific intracellular protein, in vesicles within the hepatocyte. Virtually the whole of the body pool of vitamin A is located in the liver. Retinol ester hydrolases release retinol from these storage complexes, the vitamin then binds to the specific transport protein, retinol binding protein (RBP). The retinol-RBP complex is then secreted into the blood where it forms a 1:1 molar complex with prealbumin, thus preventing filtration and loss of retinol at the glomerulus.

The pigment epithelial cells have a specific receptor for retinol-RBP complex on their surface, the cells taking up retinol and leaving RBP at the cell surface. To be photochemically active in the rods and cones of the retina, retinol has to be converted to its aldehyde, retinal, which requires the zinc-dependent enzyme, alcohol dehydrogenase. Zinc may also be involved in vitamin A metabolism at the hepatic mobilisation stage (Russell, 1980). Normal vitamin E status may also be required for normal retinol function, so as to prevent peroxidation of vitamin A in the retina which receives a plentiful supply of oxygen (Robison et al, 1980).

Vitamin A, as retinal, also plays an important role in spermatogenesis, in vitro work showing that it acts synergistically in collaboration with insulin, follicle-stimulating hormone and testosterone, to stimulate production of androgen binding protein by the Sertoli cells (Karl & Griswald, 1980). The vitamin also appears to have a systemic role, concerned with maintenance of life, growth and general health. The vitamin seems to have a number of protective actions, for example preventing hypercholesterolemia, and inducing the Glutathione-S-transferase enzymes in the liver that help protect the body against chemical carcinogens (Elliott & Lachanse, 1980; Siddik et al, 1980). Deficiency of the vitamin may present in the form of poor dark adaptation, although this may be due to other causes. In adults, a skin lesion, follicular hyperkeratosis, is found, and in children, xerophthalmia.

Hypogonadism and poor dark adaptation are often found as complications of chronic alcoholism, and are probably associated with poor vitamin A status. Ethanol may interfere with absorption of this fat-soluble vitamin due to hepatic and pancreatic insufficiency. Hepatocellular damage produces large losses of the vitamin, particularly as prealbumin synthesis by the liver may well be impaired in the alcoholic, so that increased urinary losses of the retinol-RBP complex occur. The alcohol dehydrogenase enzyme that converts retinol to retinal, has an affinity for ethanol 50 times that for retinol, so ethanol in the circulation acts as a competitive inhibitor of the enzyme. Ethanol inhibition of retinal formation has been shown to occur in vitro at concentrations of ethanol far below those found in the plasma of chronic alcoholics (Leathen, 1970). Ethanol consumption also causes increased urinary losses of zinc, furthering impairing vitamin A function.

Vitamin A status in alcoholics, as assessed by plasma or serum concentrations, reveals only slightly low or normal values (Russell, 1980; Devgun, 1981). However, these values may not be a true reflection of vitamin status, for reasons that will be discussed in the methodology section.

Vitamin B_1 (thiamine)

An adequate supply of thiamine is probably of more importance to the alcoholic than any other vitamin, because of the association of the Wernicke-Korsakoff syndrome with chronic thiamine depletion. The clinical features of Wernicke's encephalopathy incluse a confusional state, variable degrees of ophthalmoplegia, ataxia and polyneuropathy. The central feature of the Korsakoff psychosis is a memory defect specifically involving short term memory. It is now considered that the Korsakoff psychosis is usually a sequel to Wernicke's encephalopathy, hence the term Wernicke-Korsakoff syndrome is commonly used. The disease usually evolves over a period of a few days or weeks in chronic alcoholic patients who have been drinking steadily, sometimes for years, in the face of nutritional depletion. If recognised early, many of the clinical features can be reversed by rapid and effective repletion of thiamine. However, the syndrome is fairly rare, only a small percentage of alcoholics being affected, so it may well not be diagnosed until irreversible neurological damage has occurred. Chronic alcoholism is the commonest cause of the Wernicke-Korsakoff syndrome, although cases have been reported in patients who have become thiamine depleted due to other reasons, such as lesions of the stomach, duodenum and jejunum or suffering from prolonged intractable vomiting. At autopsy, the picture is one of haemorrhages in the mamillary bodies and in the walls of the third and floor of the fourth ventricles of the brain. In chronic cases, there may be gross atrophy of the mamillary bodies, which are considered to be the anatomical site of lesion as far as the Korsakoff memorising defect is concerned (Victor & Adams, 1971).

Thiamine must be supplied in the diet and is absorbed in the small intestine, chiefly the jejunum, by a saturable, carrier-mediated process requiring energy derived from ATP hydrolysis by the Na^+-K^+-ATPase system. This mechanism is the main one for uptake of thiamine at low or physiological concentrations, but at higher or pharmacological concentrations, transport across the intestine is thought to be by a nonsaturable passive diffusion process. However, work in malnourished alcoholic patients has shown ineffective absorption of water-soluble thiamine derivatives given in large doses, whereas lipid-soluble derivatives were effectively absorbed by simple diffusion (Thomson et al, 1971a). This suggests that for water soluble derivatives, passive diffusion is not the major mechanism of uptake in such patients and this contrasts with findings in the rat (Hoyumpa, 1980). Some phosphorylation of thiamine to tri-, di- (thiamine pyrophosphate: TPP) and monophosphate forms takes place in the enterocyte, although dephosphorylation may occur before free thiamine passes out of the serosal side of the cell. About half the thiamine in the portal blood appears to be phosphorylated. Subsequently, further phosphorylation of thiamine to TPP or to the triphosphate form, thiamine triphosphate (TTP) occurs in the liver and other tissues. The liver is the principal storage depot for thiamine. Thiamine, in the form of TPP, serves as a cofactor for a number of important enzymes. The three major enzymes involved are transketolase, in the hexosemonophosphate shunt, pyruvate dehydrogenase, important in the conversion of pyruvate to Acetyl CoA, and α-ketoglutarate dehydrogenase in the Kreb's cycle. TPP is also thought to be a necessary cofactor for the oxidative decarboxylation of branched chain α-ketoacids such as leucine, isoleucine and valine (Connelly & Johnson, 1975; Hoyumpa, 1980). Thiamine also has a functional role in nervous tissue, TTP playing a part in nerve conduction (Cooper & Pincus, 1979).

The clinical features of thiamine deficiency range from the classical Wernicke-Korsakoff syndrome to less well-defined brain changes, peripheral neuropathy and beri-beri heart disease. Biochemically, one sees a fall in tissue and red blood cell transketolase activities, an increased 'TPP effect' (see methodology section), low circulating thiamine levels and there may be increased blood levels of pyruvate, particularly after a carbohydrate load, although this is not a reliable marker for thiamine depletion. There are a number of ways in which alcoholism can lead to a thiamine deficiency state (Hoyumpa, 1980). Again, insufficient dietary intake and increased metabolic demands due to alcohol consumption (which provides only 'empty' calories) are contributory factors. Ethanol is known to inhibit the Na^{+}-Ka^{+}-ATPase system in the gut, thereby preventing efficient uptake of thiamine by the carrier-mediated process. A similar mechanism is thought to operate in the transfer of thiamine across the blood-brain barrier, so ethanol may inhibit thiamine uptake by the brain which could be of great importance in terms of explaining the lesions seen in the Wernicke-Korsakoff syndrome (Sharms & Quastel, 1965; Greenwood et al, 1981). In addition, decreased hepatic ATP availability may inhibit conversion of thiamine to its active form, TPP, and hepatocellular damage can cause loss of thiamine reserves. There also appears to be a correlation between nutritional deficiency and thiamine uptake. Normal folate status appears to be necessary for efficient thiamine absorption (Thomson et al, 1971b). Thus, a state of general nutritional deficiency, as is commonly found in the chronic alcoholic, may affect thiamine transport secondarily.

The exact mechanism linking thiamine deficiency with the functional and histological changes seen in the Wernicke-Korsakoff syndrome remains unknown. Various hypotheses have been proposed. Thiamine deficiency may lead to decreased activity of the cerebral enzymes that require TPP as a cofactor. The activity of pyruvate dehydrogenase and transketolase have been shown to fall in the brain in thiamine deficiency, yet high energy phosphate (ATP) levels seem unaffected. Recent animal work has shown that cerebral glucose utilisation is impaired in thiamine deficiency, the regions of the brain which show lesions in the Wernicke-Korsakoff syndrome being most affected (Hakim & Pappius, 1981). It may be that reduced transketolase activity impairs generation of NADPH by the hexosemonophosphate shunt, so that lipid synthesis for myelination is impaired. However, the hexosemonophosphate shunt seems unimpaired in thiamine deficiency, and the neurological signs can often be reversed rapidly with thiamine treatment, this neurological recovery being much more rapid than the turnover of myelin constituents. Decreased pyruvate dehyrogenase activity may limit acetyl CoA availability for acetylcholine synthesis, but work still has to be done to prove or otherwise this hypothesis.

The syndrome may arise as a result of deficient TTP levels in the brain which interferes with thiamine's proposed role in nerve conduction. In subacute necrotizing encephalomyelopathy (Leigh's disease), subjects have an inherited inability to form TTP from TPP. This is due to secretion of a lipoprotein that specifically inhibits the enzyme TPP-ATP phosphoryl transferase in the brain and post mortem examination reveals a lowered level of TTP in the brain compared to controls. The brain lesions in Leigh's disease are similar to those seen in Wernicke-Korsakoff syndrome. However, animal work has shown that in thiamine deficiency, brain levels of TTP seem to be maintained as total thiamine declines, so the hypothesis that the Wernicke-Korsakoff syndrome is attributable to insufficient TTP is not fully convincing (Pincus, 1972).

Recent work has shown that genetic factors may be involved. Blass & Gibson (1977) showed that cultured fibroblasts from four patients with Wernicke-Korsakoff syndrome contained transketolase apoenzyme that had a greatly reduced affinity for its cofactor, TPP, when compared with fibroblasts from control subjects. Thus, it appears that certain people may be genetically predisposed to the effects of thiamine depletion, and this may explain why only some alcoholics develop Wernicke-Korsakoff syndrome and not others. However, to date, only Blass & Gibson's four original patients have been studied, and further work is required before this hypothesis receives widespread acceptance (Schenker et al, 1980).

Whatever the physiological implications of thiamine deficiency are, there is widespread clinical and biochemical evidence of thiamine depletion in alcoholics. Biochemically, there is often a low red blood cell transketolase activity, an increased 'TPP effect' (see later), and circulatory levels of thiamine may be low. Patients with the Wernicke-Korsakoff syndrome may show very low transketolase activities, yet a normal or only slightly elevated TPP effect, thus giving some support to Blass & Gibson's hypothesis (Wood et al, 1977). On the other hand, a more recent study has shown that Wernicke-Korsakoff subjects may have an increased TPP effect compared with non-Korsakoff alcoholics (Leigh et al, 1981). When we come to discuss thiamine methodology, we will see that there are many anomalies surrounding tests of thiamine status. It will be important to attempt to resolve these difficulties in assessing thiamine status over the next few years, as the risks associated with thiamine deficiency in alcoholics are starting to become realised more universally, yet one study has shown that a large proportion of cases of Wernicke-Korsakoff syndrome are not diagnosed until after death (Harper, 1979).

Vitamin B_2 (riboflavin)

Vitamin B_2 or riboflavin is derived from the diet, milk, eggs and vegetables being good sources of the vitamin. Absorption takes place chiefly in the ileum by passive diffusion. The vitamin is converted in the liver to one of its active forms, flavin mononucleotide (FMN), a phosphorylation being involved. FMN serves as a cofactor for a number of enzymes, for example NADH dehydrogenase, important in the electron transport chain of the mitochondria, NADPH-dependent cytochrome-P450 reductase, important in microsomal drug de-toxification, and dihydroorotate oxidase in the pathway leading to the pyrimidines, important for DNA and RNA synthesis. However, a large proportion of the FMN formed by the liver is esterified with ATP to form flavin adenine dinucleotide (FAD), which serves as a cofactor for a large number of key enzymes in intermediary metabolism.

Among the large number of FAD-dependent enzymes are succinate dehydrogenase in the Kreb's cycle, dihydrolipoyl dehydrogenase involved in the conversion of pyruvate to acetyl CoA, acyl-CoA dehydrogenase, the first enzyme in the oxidation of fatty acids, and amino acid oxidase in the interconversion of amino acids to their corresponding ketoacids which can then be fed into Kreb's cycle. It is also of importance to notice that FAD serves as cofactor for one enzyme that converts pyridoxine to its active form pyridoxal-5-phosphate (5-PLP), pyridoxol phosphate oxidase. Storage of riboflavin in the body takes place in many tissues, the liver, kidney, heart and muscle being principle sites. Most of the stored vitamin is in the form of FAD or FMN bound to their respective apoenzymes, although small amounts of riboflavin itself are found in most tissues. Retention of riboflavin seems to depend, amongst other things, on a good dietary intake of good quality protein. If there is breakdown of protein, as in malnutrition, negative nitrogen balance occurs and this seems to be associated with increased urinary excretion of the vitamin (Goldsmith, 1975; McCormick, 1975).

Riboflavin deficiency has been studied in many animals and, bearing in mind the many coenzyme functions the vitamin has to perform, depletion always results in failure to grow. In man, intake of the vitamin must be low for many months for clinical symptoms to appear. The clinical signs are not very specific to riboflavin deficiency, concurrent deficiencies of other vitamins probably being implicated as well. Riboflavin deficiency is frequently seen in association with pellagra, and other symptoms include angular stomatitis, glossitis and dermatitis progressing to anaemia and possibly peripheral neuropathy. Personality disturbances, depression, hysteria, psychopathic deviation, hypomania and reduced hand grip strength have also been reported in experimental riboflavin deficiency in humans (Lane et al, 1964). Anaemia in riboflavin deficiency may be related to disturbances in folic acid metabolism, due to reduced activity of flavoprotein enzymes that are required for utilisation of folic acid. On the other hand, FAD is a cofactor for the red cell enzyme glutathione reductase that forms reduced glutathione, which is important for maintaining integrity of the red cell membrane. Reduced in vivo survival time of red blood cells in riboflavin deficiency has been reported (Powers & Thurnham, 1980).

Clinical evidence of riboflavin deficiency in alcoholics is often lacking directly, because of confusion of the symptoms with those of other associated nutritional deficiencies and alcohol-related disease. Ethanol may interfere with absorption and utilisation of riboflavin in similar ways that it does that of other vitamins. The same factors of decreased uptake and storage, decreased activation and increased requirement are probably involved. Data from our own patients shows some biochemical evidence of a deficiency in terms of a low erythrocyte glutathione reductase activity and increased response of the enzyme activity to the in vitro addition of FAD to the assay system.

Vitamin B_6 (pyridoxine)

Pyridoxine is absorbed chiefly in the jejunum and ileum by simple passive diffusion. The vitamin is then converted to its active form, pyridoxal-5-phosphate (5-PLP), in the tissues, the liver being the main site. The red blood cell is able to form pyridoxal-5-phosphate from pyridoxine (Anderson, 1980), and it has been suggested that there is wide individual variation in the ability of red cells to convert pyridoxine, and also riboflavin, to their respective active forms, so that genetic factors may predispose certain individuals to the effects of deficient vitamin intake (Nutrition Reviews, 1981). The conversion of pyridoxine to 5-PLP is shown in Figure 10.3. 5-PLP serves as cofactor for a large number of enzymes (Table 10.1), and is

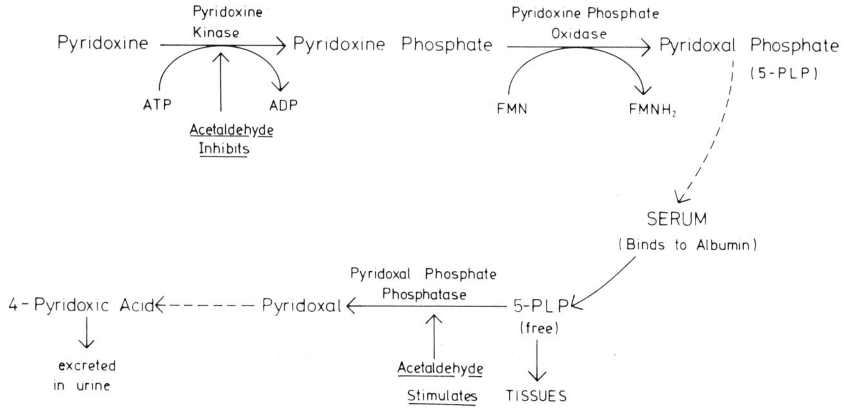

Fig. 10.3 The activation and breakdown of pyridoxine.

the main circulating form of the vitamin. Like riboflavin, pyridoxine is of great importance in maintaining normal cellular metabolism, and is required for normal growth and development, particularly of the brain and central nervous system (Loo, 1980; Chang et al, 1981). Pyridoxine may also have other functions in addition to its role as a cofactor. 5-PLP appears able to modulate tbe binding of cytosolic steroid-receptor complexes to DNA, and in deficiency more rapid binding of glucocorticoid-receptor complexes to cell nuclei is found (Cake et al, 1978). Reduced cellular transfer of amino acids, important for normal growth, is found in deficiency, and this has been shown to be due to inadequate growth hormone secretion from the pituitary. This effect may be due to decreased dopamine synthesis arising from B6

Table 10.1 Some enzymes requiring pyridoxal-5-phosphate (5-PLP) as a cofactor

Enzyme	Function
△-aminolevulinic acid synthetase	Heme biosynthesis
Alanine transaminase	Transamination of amino acids
Aspartate transaminase	
Leucine transaminase	
Tyrosine transaminase	
Kynureninase	Tryptophan metabolism: involved in nictotinamide synthesis
Threonine synthetase	Synthesis of threonine from aspartate
Serine hydroxymethyl-transferase	Synthesis of threonine from glycine and acetaldehyde
Cysteic acid decarboxylase	Taurine synthesis
Glutamate decarboxylase	Gamma amino butyric Acid (GABA) synthesis
Dihydroxyphenylalanine (DOPA) decarboxylase	Dopamine/noradrenaline/adrenaline synthesis
5-Hydroxytryptophan decarboxylase	5-Hydroxytryptamine (5-HT, serotonin) synthesis

deficiency, as dopamine stimulates growth hormone secretion. It has also been postulated that B6 is necessary for normal insulin secretion, impaired glucose tolerance being found in pyridoxine-deficient rats, although the mechanism is not understood (Heindel & Riggs, 1978; Tezuka & Makino, 1959). Pyridoxine deficiency is also associated with alterations in functions of the immune system (Robson & Schwarz, 1980). Pyridoxine may also act as an antithrombotic agent.

Clinical symptoms of pyridoxine deficiency include neuromuscular irritability, peripheral neuropathy, dermatitis, cheilosis and stomatitis, depression of immune response and anaemia. As with riboflavin, specific signs of pyridoxine deficiency may not be recognised in alcoholics to other complications. Depression is a common feature of chronic alcoholism and this could be due to pyridoxine deficiency. As will be seen from Table 10.1, 5-PLP is required for synthesis of various brain neurotransmitters including taurine, GABA, noradrenaline and serotonin (5HT). Biochemically, depression has been subdivided into noradrenergic, due to a functional deficiency of noradrenaline, serotonergic, due to lack of serotonin, or of a mixed type. It is interesting that 5-PLP deficient alcoholics have been reported to have hyperprolactinaemia. It is now known that the so-called prolactin inhibitory factor (PIF) is in fact dopamine, the precursor of noradrenaline (Williams, 1976). Lack of dopamine might explain the increased prolactin secretion, and may be the basis of a noradrenergic type of depression in alcoholics. Serotonergic depression may also occur. Oral contraception can induce depression as oestrogen and progesterone induce the hepatic microsomal enzymes that favour metabolism of tryptophan down the pathway leading to nicotinamide rather than along the pathway leading to serotonin. In this situation, there is increased substrate load on the 5-PLP-requiring enzymes in the nicotinamide pathway, and redistribution of 5-PLP from enzymes in the serotonin pathway to those in the nicotinamide pathway may occur. Administration of pyridoxine to oral contraceptive users reverses depression, presumably by restoring the activity of 5-hydroxytryptophan decarboxylase to normal, so that serotonin synthesis is increased.

From the above discussion, it will be appreciated that biochemical implications of pyridoxine deficiency are wide ranging, and include decreased haemoglobin synthesis, decreased neurotransmitter synthesis and derangements of amino acid metabolism. Chronic ethanol consumption can lead to deficiency by various mechanisms, including the usual effects of decreased intake, uptake, utilisation and storage. However, in the case of pyridoxine, ethanol appears to have specific effects on the activation and breakdown processes involved in utilisation of the vitamin. Lack of hepatic ATP may decrease pyridoxine kinase activity in the liver, and associated riboflavin deficiency may decrease pyridoxine phosphate oxidase activity (Fig. 10.3). Acetaldehyde, the oxidation product of ethanol, inhibits pyridoxine kinase, and stimulates pyridoxal phosphate phosphatase, thereby decreasing activation and stimulating breakdown of the active vitamin. Lowered serum albumin, common in alcoholic liver disease, may decrease serum binding of 5-PLP, so that losses can occur. In addition, alcohol consumption appears to cause an inability to liberate the bound form of the vitamin from food in the gastrointestinal tract so that reduced uptake occurs. Chronic alcoholics often show laboratory evidence of pyridoxine deficiency in terms of low circulating level of 5-PLP, although interestingly, red cell activity of the 5-PLP dependent enzyme, aspartate aminotranferase (AST) is often normal or even increased. Also, in vitro stimulation of red cell AST in alcoholics by adding 5-PLP to the assay system seems to result in a lower response than in normal subjects. These anomalies will be discussed more fully in the methodology section.

Nicotinamide

The pyridine coenzymes, nicotinamide adenine dinucleotide (NAD) and nicotinamide adenine dinucleotide phosphate (NADP) are necessary cofactors in virtually every metabolic pathway in the cell and contain the vitamin nicotinamide. Nicotinamide can be synthesised endogenously from tryptophan, and feeding a tryptophan rich diet can prevent deficiency occurring when nicotinamide is removed from the diet. However, if protein intake is low, deficiency soon develops, and most people require some dietary intake of the vitamin.

There is evidence of nicotinamide deficiency in alcoholics due to decreased uptake, decreased conversion to active coenzyme form (ATP is required), decreased storage and increased requirement. Ethanol metabolism involves many NAD dependent reactions (Fig. 10.2). Deficiencies of other vitamins, principally pyridoxine, in alcoholism may also reduce endogenous synthesis of nicotinamide. Classically, pellagra has been associated with nicotinamide deficiency in man, although other vitamin deficiencies are probably involved in this condition. The mental changes include memory impairment, hallucinations, and melancholia. Cerebral atrophy may be involved, ophthalmoplegia can develop in severe cases, and patients may be left with memory defects, including encephalopathy which resembles acute Wernicke-Korsakoff psychosis. However, these changes can be successfully treated with nicotinic acid (Jolliffe, 1941). Clinical studies have shown that improvement in mortality rates can be achieved with nicotinic acid therapy in alcoholics who present with severe impairment of consciousness, delirium, cogwheel rigidity of the limbs and uncontrollable graspings or sucking reflexes.

Biotin

Biotin functions as a prosthetic group in enzymes involved in carboxylation reactions. These enzymes include pyruvate decarboxylase, important in gluconeogenesis and transfer of acetyl CoA across the mitochondrial membranes, and acetyl-CoA carboxylase, the first enzyme in the pathway of fatty acid synthesis.

Biotin is manufactured by intestinal bacteria, and complete removal of biotin from the diet for a long period is often necessary to induce a deficiency state. Large consumption of raw egg whites can, however, produce deficiency as they contain a protein, avidin, which specifically binds biotin very tightly and prevents absorption from the intestine. Deficiency causes reduced activity of the biotin-dependent enzymes, pyruvate carboxylase being the first to be affected, and pyruvate and lactate may accumulate in the blood and tissues as a result. Biotin-deficient animals show reduced growth and reproductive performance. Clinically, a deficiency may produce dermatitis which is exacerbated by pressure or abrasion, so that the soles of the feet are preferentially affected. Other lesions resemble those of deficiency of the other B vitamins, and characteristic clinical signs are only evident when severe depletion has occurred. Experimentally induced biotin deficiency in humans produces a range of symptoms including mild depression, lassitude, hallucinations, muscle pain, hyperesthesia and eventually severe anorexia ensues.

There is little evidence of biotin deficiency in alcoholics. Most reported cases are in subjects who have consumed an excessive amount of raw egg whites or who have received inadequate parenteral nutrition regimes (Tanaka, 1981; Whitehead, 1981).

Pantothenic acid

Pantothenic acid is formed by many plants and bacteria, but is required in the diet of vertebrates. The vitamin combines with β-mercaptoethylamine and ATP to form coenzyme A which acts as a carrier for two carbon fragments in a large number of metabolic processes. The enzyme acetyl-CoA synthetase links acetate to coenzyme A to form acetyl CoA. Acetyl CoA is a key molecule in intermediary metabolism, all foodstuffs, whether carbohydrate, fat or protein, having to be converted to acetyl CoA before further catabolism by the Kreb's cycle can occur. Acetyl CoA has synthetic functions as well, being the precursor for fatty acid, cholesterol and acetylcholine synthesis.

Pantothenic acid deficiency reduces acetylations and leads to various pathological changes, including adrenal cortical insufficiency, lowered cholesterol synthesis, impaired glucose tolerance and anaemia. Most of these changes have been demonstrated in rats, however, and although some clinical studies have shown low circulating levels of the vitamin in hospital in-patients, similar severe symptoms have not been reported in humans. Alcoholics may well be deficient in the vitamin, due once again to decreased uptake and utilisation, and liver biopsies from patients with fatty liver or cirrhosis show decreased tissue levels of the vitamin. The liver is a major storage site for panthothenic acid and hepatocellular damage in alcoholics may actually increase circulating levels of the vitamin (Baker & Frank, 1968).

Vitamin B_{12} and folic acid

Vitamin B_{12} (B_{12}, cyanocobalamin) and folate (pteroylglutamic acid) are required for normal erythrocyte formation. DNA synthesis in the bone marrow, essential for normal hemopoiesis, depends upon the cyclic oxidation-reduction of one-carbon units attached to the active form of folate, tetrahydrofolic acid (THFA). This cyclic process is shown in Figure 10.4.

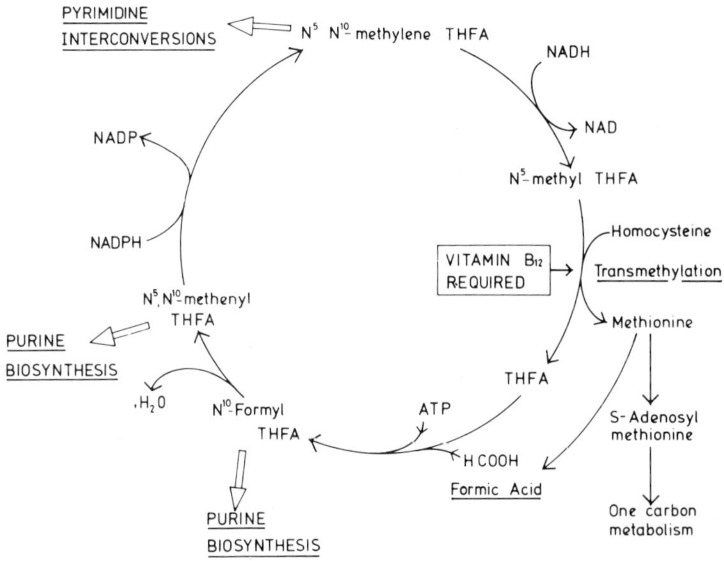

Fig. 10.4 The role of vitamin B_{12} and folic acid in one-carbon metabolism (after Chanarin et al, 1980).

Ethanol oxidation in the liver generates large amounts of NADH which causes pyruvate to be reduced to lactate. Lactate passes out into the tissues, including the bone marrow, so that increased NADH levels will also be found in the periphery. This excess NADH drives the metabolism of THFA to its most reduced form, N^5 methyl THFA, so that one-carbon fragments are trapped at this point in the cycle, as the rate of reduction exceeds the rate of B_{12}-mediated transmethylation (Fig. 10.4). Thus, one-carbon units are diverted away from pyrimidine and purine synthesis, so that DNA formation is impaired. This direct toxic effect of ethanol on folate metabolism is probably a contributory factor to the two major haematological disorders found in the alcoholic, macrocytosis and megaloblastic anaemia. Macrocytosis (mean corpuscular volume, MCV, raised to 95–105 fl) without anaemia or evidence of megaloblastic changes in the bone marrow, is very common amongst drinking alcholics, and is a sensitive index of alcohol intake (see also Ch. 4). The exact mechanisms underlying this macrocylosis are not clear, but effects of ethanol on folate metabolism, ethanol-induced plasma lipoprotein changes, changes in lipid content of the red cell membrane, or persistent toxic effects on erythroid presuprecursors have all been suggested. This mild macrocytosis, without anaemia, takes several weeks to normalise after cessation of alcohol consumption, so direct toxic effects to ethanol probably do not play an important part. In megaloblastic anaemia, however, the MCV is often in excess of 105 fl, and there are visible signs of megaloblastic change in the bone marrow which are reversed rapidly by the withdrawal of alcohol and folate and B_{12} supplementation. Megaloblastic anaemia is thought to be a direct consequence of folate deficiency associated with ethanol's impairment of folate metabolism. Most cases show hypersegmentation of the neutrophils on the blood film, and a small percentage of patients have a marked shift to the left in the leucocyte differential count. The red cells are macroovalocytic in nature. Serum folate levels are usually low, though may be normal due to complicatory factors (see later). Red cell folate is a better guide to vitamin status, low normal to deficient values usually being seen in patients with megaloblastic anaemia, and may be associated with normal or elevated B_{12} serum levels. Severe cases of megaloblastic anaemia (MCV greater than 112 fl) may involve B_{12} deficiency as well as poor folate status, but particularly in the alcoholic this is often not reflected in serum B_{12} levels.

Vitamin B_{12} originates mainly from the diet, although significant amounts are synthesized by the microflora of the small intestine, and vegetarians depend on this source, as well as ingested microorganisms, for their B_{12} nutriture. B_{12} ingested in food has to be released from its bound form by the action of gastric and intestinal enzymes. The free vitamin is bound to intrinsic factor (IF), a glycoprotein produced by the fundal and cardiac glands of the stomach. IF protects the vitamin from utilisation or destruction by the gut bacteria and facilitates uptake of B_{12} in the terminal ileum. Normal pancreatic function is probably important in ensuring effective B_{12}

absorption, as recent work has shown 'R proteins' present in saliva, gastric juice, bile and intestinal juices bind cobalamins more avidly than IF, and pancreatic proteins have been shown to degrade 'R proteins' in vitro, allowing B_{12} to bind to IF (Allen et al, 1978). Normal bile secretion may also be of importance in B_{12} absorption (Teo et al, 1980). True pernicious anaemia is due to lack of IF secretion. The IF-B_{12} complex binds to a receptor on the mucosal cell wall, this being a calcium-mediated process, and a releasing factor than cleaves B_{12} from IF and permits its uptake into the circulation. B_{12} is carried in the plasma by specific α_1 and α_2-globulin-binding proteins, the transcobalamins. The active form of B_{12} or coenzyme B_{12} is 5-deoxyadenosylcobalamin, although various non-active derivatives are also found in the body. 'Coenzyme B_{12}' is required for the transmethylation of homocysteine to methionine, of great importance in the one-carbon metabolism of folate and S-adenosyl-methionine (Fig. 10.4), and is also a cofactor for the enzyme methylmalonyl-CoA mutase in the oxidation of odd-numbered fatty acids. Coenzyme B_{12} is formed in the liver, and is the major storage form of the vitamin, the liver being the principle storage site.

B_{12} deficiency is relatively uncommon in alcoholics when compared with folate deficiency. Various studies have shown that serum B_{12} is normal in 85–100 per cent of chronic alcoholics tested. This may be a reflection of the fact that there is a release of stored B_{12} from necrotic liver cells in alcoholic liver disease which causes a high circulating level of the vitamin, when in whole body terms, there may be a deficiency. It has been suggested that serum B_{12} could be used as a marker for hepatocellular necrosis elevated levels being indicative of damage in a similar way to increased serum activity of the transaminases. In addition, overestimation of serum B_{12} concentration may have occurred in studies where unreliable radio-dilution assays were used. Alcohol abuse can lead to B_{12} deficiency from decreased intake and poor absorption due to intestinal lesions, pancreatic or biliary disease, up to 50 per cent of patients with pancreatic insufficiency showing B_{12} malabsorption in a Schilling test (Lindenbaum, 1980). Ethanol has been shown to interfere with binding of the IF-B_{12} complex to intestinal homogenates, and may reduce in vivo uptake of B_{12} by active transport. Alcoholic liver disease reduces hepatic B_{12} storage and excretion losses are increased, although hepatic stores of the vitamin are sufficient for several years, so hepatic loss is probably only important where severe liver disease is present. The neurological features of B_{12} deficiency are identical to those of folate deficiency but, in addition, subacute degeneration of the cord is found. Folate deficiency, as indicated by low circulating levels, is present in 20–50 per cent of chronic alcoholics. Low serum levels may be present in as many as 87 per cent of alcoholics, and they correlate with reduced hepatic levels. There is a well-defined course of events in folate depletion, serum levels falling first, followed by a progressive decline in tissue levels before bone marrow changes are seen. However, folate intake during the course of this depletion may rapidly correct serum levels, when tissue deficiency is still present. In such a situation, serum folate is not a good indicator of tissue vitamin status (Herbert et al, 1963). Beer drinkers are less liable to folate depletion than wine or spirit drinkers, due to higher content of the vitamin in the beverage. Folate is found as folylpolyglutamates in food and is deconjugated before absorption. Absorption takes place in the jejunum by an energy requiring process, and some activation of the vitamin takes place during absorption. There are several active forms of folate, principle ones being N^5 -methyl THFA, N^5, N^{10} -methylene THFA, N^5, N^{10} -methenyl THFA and N^{10} -formyl THFA. The one-carbon fragments attached to these THFA derivatives originate from various sources, including serine, glycine, histidine, formyglutamate and purines (Baker & Frank, 1968). N^5 forimino THFA is formed from THFA and N-formimino-glutamic acid (FIGLU), and is a precursor for the coenzyme form of THFA. In folate and B_{12} deficiency, FIGLU accumulates and is excreted in the urine. Histidine, the precursor of FIGLU, can be given in a loading test to diagnose folate or B_{12} deficiency. The active THFA derivatives carry out a large number of one-carbon transfer reactions in metabolism, including introduction of C2 and C8 into the purine ring, methylation of uracil ribotides to form thymidylate, interconversion of glycine and serine, methylation of homocysteine to methionine, and methylation of ethanolamine to choline. As already described, folate deficiency leads to reduced replication of rapidly dividing cells and to megaloblastic anaemia and lesions of the intestinal mucosa. The latter can reduce brush border thickness and the area available for absorption, so that uptake of folate itself and other nutrients such as thiamine, glucose and sodium is impaired. The important role folate plays in DNA and RNA synthesis may mean that folate deficiency could limit repair of tissues such as the liver and the brain that are damaged during chronic alcohol abuse.

In alcoholism, folate deficiency arises because of poor dietary intake and decreased body stores due to liver damage, the hepatic stores accounting for much of the total body folate. Intestinal malabsorption is also a major contributing factor due to ethanol's impairment of active transport and the morphological changes induced, and a prolonged state of folate deficiency aggravates this situation even further. Thus, the malabsorption aspect of folate deficiency consists of two components, firstly the effects of ethanol on absorption processes, and secondly there is a vicious circle in which folate malabsorption leads to folate deficiency which in turn aggravates folate absorption. Folate circulates as 5-methyl THFA bound to a variety of proteins including a specific β-globulin. In cirrhosis, serum binding of folate is decreased even though serum levels of the binding protein are unaltered, so increased urinary losses can occur. Hepatic uptake of folate is often reduced after ethanol administration or in cirrhosis, and altered hepatic folate metabolism in alcoholism may result in 'trapping' of folate that has been taken up. There is some evidence also that ethanol reduces the enterohepatic circulation of folate (Halsted, 1980). The toxic effect of ethanol on cyclic metabolism of folate has already been described (Fig. 10.4). Although degeneration of the cord is not usually found in folate deficiency, unlike in B_{12} deficiency, various neurological symptoms are thought to be associated with folate depletion (see Thomson et al, 1980).

Vitamin C (ascorbate)

Ascorbic acid is found in fresh fruit and vegetables and is necessary to prevent scurvy. Most plants and some mammals, but not man, can synthesise the vitamin from endogenous glucose. Ascorbic acid can be reversibly oxidised in vivo to dehydro-ascorbic acid which also has antiscorbutic activity. The vitamin is easily destroyed by heat and oxidation and deficiency is sometimes found in old people living on poor incomes who do not eat fresh fruit and vegetables and who tend to cook in frying pans, where the combination of heat and the large area of food in contact with the air oxidises the vitamin. Ascorbate is thought to act in biological systems as a hydrogen carrier. It has a definite coenzyme function in proline hydroxylase, which forms hydroxyproline for collagen synthesis. Production of defective collagen is thought to underly many of the symptoms seen in scurvy. It may be involved in noradrenaline synthesis, folate metabolism and is thought to be involved in iron metabolism by reducing ferric ion upon its transfer from plasma transferrin to liver transferrin. Ascorbate may also play a role in drug metabolism and steroid synthesis, as it seems to preserve microsomal cytochrome P450 (Omaye & Turnbull, 1980). Other functions appear to be a role in cholesterol biosynthesis, a co-operative action with vitamin E to prevent lipid peroxidation, and finally, roles in cyclic nucleotide metabolism and interferon production have been proposed.

Deficiency of ascorbate leads to scurvy, the main features of which are vascular wall fragility, haemorrhages, swollen and bleeding gums, poor wound healing, osteoporosis and anaemia. There has recently been much controversy over ascorbate requirements in man. An intake of 10 mg or less per day prevents scurvy, although some workers have suggested megadoses of 10–15 g per day to maintain health. Megadoses are thought to protect against acetaldehyde toxicity which is of importance to alcoholics and smokers (Sprince et al, 1975). On the other hand, excessive ascorbate has been shown to lead to increased urinary oxalate excretion, and thus may predispose to kidney stone formation (Schmidt et al, 1981). Excessive ascorbate intake also increases requirments of other vitamins, such as vitamin E (Chen, 1981), and in vitro work has shown high levels of the vitamin in food and serum can cause destruction of vitamin B_{12} (Marcus, 1980; Schorah, 1981; Baker & Frank, 1968).

Low leucocyte levels of ascorbate are found in alcoholics (Devgun et al, 1981). Reduced intake, malabsorption, decreased storage and utilisation all contribute to produce this deficiency state.

Vitamin D (cholecalciferol) (see also Ch. 14)

Cholecalciferol is synthesized endogenously in the Malpighian layer of the epidermis by the photolysis of 7-dehydrocholesterol. The major function of cholecalciferol is hormonal in nature, in that it maintains plasma calcium and phosphate levels so that calcification of bone can proceed. The active form of cholecalciferol acts in combination with parathyroid hormone (PTH) to mobilise calcium from bone, and the vitamin is also necessary for intestinal absorption and renal tubular reabsorption of calcium. The vitamin also has a phosphaturic effect. The active form of the vitamin is 1,25 dihyroxy-cholecalciferol which is formed from 25-hydroxycholecalciferol by mitochondrial cytochrome P450 in the proximal convoluted tubule cells in the kidney. 25-hydroxycholecalciferol is formed from cholecalciferol by microsomal cytochrome P450 in the liver. In the kidney, intestine and cartilage, 25-OH cholecalciferol can also be converted to 24,25 dihydrocholecalciferol which is not as active as 1,25 dihydroxycholecalciferol, and is thought to be an inactivated form of the vitamin which is produced when there are adequate levels of 1,25 dihydroxycholecalciferol. 24-hydroxylation of 25-hydroxycholecalciferol does not take place when there is vitamin D deficiency, so constant levels of 1,25 dihydroxycholecalciferol can be maintained by regulation of the various hydroxylations of 25-OH cholecalciferol. In addition, PTH regulates metabolism of the vitamin by stimulating hydroxylation at the 1α-position in the kidney, thereby increasing levels of the active form, 1,25 dihydroxycholecalciferol.

Most of the total body vitamin D comes from endogenous synthesis by the photolysis of 7-dehydrocholesterol, and it has been questioned whether dietary intake of the vitamin is necessary for normal health. There is a considerable seasonal variation in circulating vitamin D, highest levels being found in August/September and lowest in January/February. In spite of the importance of endogenous synthesis in determining vitamin D status, consumption of animal liver and fish products, rich in the vitamin, can contribute significantly to the body pool. Absorption of dietary vitamin D takes place in the small intestine and requires bile salts. Absorbed vitamin D is transported to the liver bound to a specific α-1-globulin in the blood. The vitamin is stored in unchanged form, cholecalciferol, in the liver and muscles, or else metabolised to one of the hydroxylated forms. Hydroxylated forms of cholecalciferol are not stored but are carried in the plasma bound to the specific carrier protein. 25-hydroxycholecalciferol is the major circulating form, 1,25 dihydroxy-and 24,25 dihydroxycholecalciferol being found at much lower levels in the plasma. For a comprehensive review of cholecalciferol metabolism and action, the reader is referred to the recent articles by Deluca (1980) and Raisz (1980).

Vitamin D deficiency arises because of inadequate exposure to sunlight, poor dietary intake, or poor absorption due to gastrointestinal disorders such as Crohn's disease, coeliac disease, pancreatic insufficiency or biliary obstruction. Low circulating levels of 25-hydroxycalciferol have been reported in alcoholics (Griffiths, 1981; Devgun et al, 1981), and are probably due mainly to poor exposure to sunlight, although impaired absorption and reduced storage may also be involved. It should be remembered that 25-hydroxycholecalciferol is not the most active form of the vitamin, and measurement of 1,25 dihydroxycholecalciferol levels, technically difficult to perform, is necessary in alcoholics to see whether this possible apparent deficiency is of any physiological importance.

Vitamin E (tocopherol)

Vitamin E (α-tocopherol) is principally an antioxidant of natural fats. It inhibits oxidation of unsaturated fatty acids as well as other oxygen sensitive compounds such as vitamin C and vitamin A. Animal work has shown that deficiency produces infertility in male and female rats, although the role of tocopherol deficiency in causing infertility in man has not been established. However, since the vitamin is of importance in preventing lipid peroxidation of membranes, it is of fundamental significance in maintaining the integrity of all cells in the body. Tocopherol exerts its antioxidant effect by interacting with selenium and ascorbate and also has free radical scavenging properties, in its own right.

Deficiencies of vitamin E are found mainly in patients with malabsorption syndromes, or in premature infants as there is poor placental transfer of the vitamin. The symptoms of deficiency are not always specific but may include haemolytic anaemia, increased erythrocyte fragility, creatinuria and deposition of ceroid in smooth muscles. These symptoms can often be reversed by administration of synthetic antioxidants showing that the antioxidant property of tocopherol is not specific. The red cell changes seen may be simply as a result of increased lipid peroxidation in the deficiency state, whilst on the other hand it has been suggested that tocopherol may have a specific role in erythropoiesis (Drake & Fitch, 1980). The vitamin may also have a cardioprotective effect by favouring redistribution of cholesterol into the high-density lipoprotein (HDL) fraction (Hermann et al, 1979).

Vitamin K

Vitamin K, like vitamin E, is a fat soluble isoprenoid compound. At least three forms of the vitamin, designated K_1, K_2 and K_3, are known and differ only in the length of the isoprenoid side-chain on the molecule. Vitamin K deficiency is fairly uncommon as synthesis by intestinal microflora can supply much of the body requirements. The vitamin acts as a cofactor for the hepatic microsomal carboxylase enzyme that converts specific glutamyl residues of precursor prothrombin. As the vitamin contains a quinone ring, it may function as an electron carrier in some specialised electron carrier system, but this has not been proven.

Vitamin K deficiency is accompanied by a bleeding tendency and a prolonged prothrombin time. Fat malabsorption, for whatever reason, can lead to deficiency due to insufficient uptake of the vitamin whether it is of bacterial or dietary origin. Vitamin K deficiency is common in alcoholics as demonstrated by a prolonged prothrombin time on hospital admission which is rapidly corrected by administration of vitamin K supplements. However, in severe cases of alcoholic liver disease, correction of the prothrombin time by vitamin K treatment may not occur due to decreased hepatic synthesis of coagulation factors.

TREATMENT OF VITAMIN DEFICIENCY IN THE ALCOHOLIC

Commercially available vitamin preparations are commonly used to treat hospitalised alcoholics whether they show signs of specific deficiencies or not. These usually take the form of high potency oral, intravenous or intramuscular preparations containing high concentrations of the B vitamins and ascorbic acid. Less potent oral preparations, containing amounts of B vitamins, ascorbate and possibly vitamins A, D and E that are approximately equivalent to the recommended daily intake for a normal person, are often used to treat alcoholics in the community as a prophylactic measure. However, bearing in mind the problems of impaired utilisation and increased requirements that occur in alcoholism, this latter course of action may not be totally effective in preventing vitamin deficiencies occurring. Many of these preparations do not contain folic acid, necessary for normal absorption of many other vitamins. In addition, most of the vitamins in all types of preparation, oral or parenteral, are in the form of salts and will have to be activated before they can be utilised, and impaired hepatic function in the alcoholic may reduce vitamin activation.

In the case of thiamine, rapid and clinically effective repletion of a deficiency state can be achieved by oral administration of allithiamines, that is lipid-soluble thiamine derivatives such as thiamine propyl disulphide or thiamine tetrafurfuryl disulphide. Oral administration of water soluble thiamine (e.g. thiamine hydrochloride) does not restore thiamine activity in blood or cerebrospinal fluid in chronic alcoholics, due probably to impaired uptake by active transport and poor hepatic activation (Baker & Frank, 1976; Thomson et al, 1971a). Rapid repletion of thiamine status is obviously important in the hospitalised alcoholics so as to reduce the risk of Wernicke-Korsakoff syndrome developing.

In patients where there is severe liver disease, poor utilisation of administered vitamins may occur. In such cases the active forms of the vitamin, rather than the parent form, may need to be given (e.g. 5-PLP rather than pyridoxine) parenterally in order to correct the deficiency signs. Unfortunately, preparations of activated vitamins are not easily available at present.

There are occasions when toxicity from vitamin therapy might develop, such as when megadoses of ascorbate are used (see earlier) or when vitamin D is given in its active form, 1,25 dihydroxycholecalciferol.

The general points that should be borne in mind when considering vitamin repletion in the alcoholic are: (1) there may be poor intestinal absorption of orally administered water-soluble vitamins, particularly where active transport is involved; (2) malabsorption of orally administered fat-soluble vitamins may occur, particularly if there is pancreatic or biliary disease; (3) administration of pharmacological doses of one vitamin may increase requirements for other vitamins or minerals (e.g. vitamin E supplementation may increase the requirements for ascorbate and selenium); (4) in alcoholic liver disease, the functional liver mass will be reduced so that decreased activation and storage of administered vitamins occurs; (5) parenteral administration of high potency vitamin preparations is generally better than oral preparations, particularly where long-term malnutrition is indicated; (6) where specific vitamin deficiency syndromes are indicated, parenteral administration of the vitamin in its activated form (e.g. thiamine pyrophosphate or pyridoxal-5-phosphate) may be the most effective course of treatment where available, and could dramatically improve the prognosis in conditions such as the Wernicke-Korsakoff syndrome; (7) earlier work has shown that in certain situations that may be encountered in alcoholics, such as delirium, confusion or coma, intravenous administration of large doses of the B vitamins and ascorbate can give rapid improvement. This may indicate that in such extreme conditions, there may be a greatly increased demand for vitamins (Gould, 1954).

ASSESSMENT OF VITAMIN STATUS: METHODS AND INTERPRETATION

In this section we will outline the methods available for assessment of vitamin status in man. Some general points regarding interpretation of vitamin assay results obtained in alcoholics must be borne in mind when using such methods. Serum levels of vitamins can be misleading in assessing overall vitamin status. Hepatic cell damage in alcoholism causes release of stored vitamins into the circulation, and a normal circulating level of a vitamin can also be due simply to recent intake or therapy when tissue deficiency can still be present. For example, plasma levels of tocopherol rise after therapy, yet penetration into tissues is poor, only 2 per cent of the dose passing into the body pool. Ascorbate shows poor penetration into the red cells after intravenous administration (Baker et al, 1969). Conversely, administered vitamins can be rapidly sequestered by the tissues so that plasma levels revert to below normal soon after therapy, even though tissue status has been improved. Tissue repletion of the vitamin may be necessary before plasma or serum levels are consistently normal.

Thus, for some vitamins red blood cell activity or white cell levels are a better reflection of status. It should also be borne in mind what the method actually measures. Very often, total vitamin derivatives or a form of the vitamin which is not biochemically or physiologically active is measured. This can give misleading information about vitamin status in the alcoholic, where there are often problems with vitamin activation.

Vitamin A

Retinol gives a colour reaction with most strong acids, and many methods for its estimation have been based on this reaction. Currently, methods based on the reaction between the vitamin and trichloroacetic acid or trifluoroacetic acid are accepted as being sensitive and accurate (Bayfield & Cole, 1980; Pitt, 1981). Care is necessary to ensure stability of the reagents in these methods, and measurement of β-carotene is needed to correct for the interference of this substance in the assay. Alternatively, vitamin A and carotene can be measured in serum by removal from proteins with ethanolic potassium hydroxide, followed by extraction with petroleum ether and colorimetric estimation with 1,3 dichloro-2-propanol containing acetyl chloride (Oliver, 1980). Where facilities are available, retinol and α-tocopherol can be determined simultaneously by high pressure liquid chromatography following a total lipid extraction from either plasma or red cells. This latter method is probably the one of choice where large numbers of samples are involved, for example in nutritional surveys (Bieri et al, 1979).

Plasma estimations of vitamin A have their limitations. Mechanisms operate which keep plasma levels fairly constant so as to supply the tissues, even though depletion of hepatic stores may be taking place. Only when hepatic stores are severely depleted do plasma levels fall substantially. Thus, a low plasma retinol concentration is indicative of low liver reserves. Hepatocellular damage in the alcoholic may also give rise to normal or elevated plasma levels when there is in fact tissue depletion. Conversely, low plasma levels may be due to inadequate secretion of prealbumin or retinol binding protein by the liver, so that urinary loss is increased. Low dietary protein is thought to correlate with low RBP synthesis in the liver (Pitt, 1981).

Vitamin B_1 (thiamine)

Blood pyruvate levels were originally used to detect thiamine deficiency, particularly where a glucose load test was used. This test is not very reliable however, and over the last few years, erythrocyte transketolase activity (ETK) measurements have been employed. Addition of TPP to the assay system gives an increase in enzyme activity which is related to the degree of saturation of the enzyme with the cofactor. This increase in activity upon in vitro addition of TPP to the assay system is termed the 'TPP effect' and is expressed as a percentage of the basal activity, ie; the ETK activity in

ETKo = Transketolase activity with no added Thiamine Pyrophosphate (TPP)

ETK+ = Transketolase activity with added Thiamine Pyrophosphate (TPP)

$$\text{'TPP Effect'} = \left(\frac{ETK_{+} - ETK_{o}}{ETK_{o}} - 1\right) \times 100$$

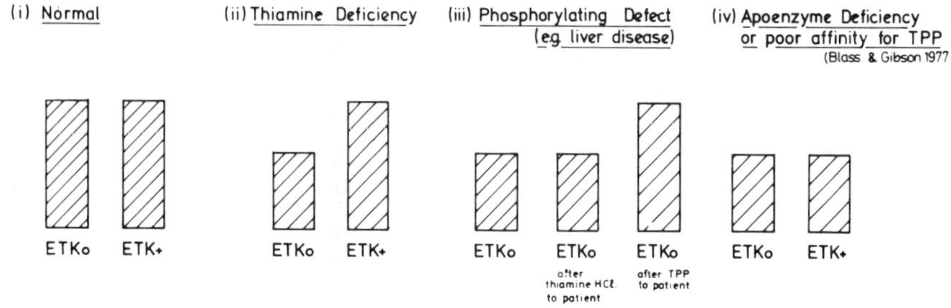

Fig. 10.5 Erythrocyte transketolase activity and 'TPP effect'.

the absence of added TPP (Fig 10.5). A high TPP effect is indicative of thiamine depletion, although it may not always be a reliable marker. Animal work has shown that thiamine depletion results in a fall in basal ETK that is not always accompanied by an increased TPP effect. The study of Wood et al (1977) on thiamine status in alcoholics found a better correlation between ETK and thiamine status evaluated by clinical observations, than if TPP effect was used. Other studies have shown an inverse relationship between ETK and the TPP effect. A lack of correlation of ETK or TPP effect with clinical signs of deficiency could be due to several factors. In liver disease, apoenzyme deficiency or a defective apoenzyme has been suggested, so that a low ETK will be found with a low or normal TPP effect. Genetic factors may determine binding of TPP to the apoenzyme (Blass & Gibson, 1977), so that false indications could arise where TPP effect is used to diagnose deficiency. Comparison of ETK and TPP effect values between various studies shows that there is wide variation in quoted normal ranges. The normal range obviously depends on the method employed and the subjects used to determine it. Hospital staff tend to be used for this purpose, whom it is assumed are not thiamine depleted. In view of this wide variation found in normal values, it is of great importance that any laboratory setting up a transketolase method should carefully screen individuals used for determining the normal range in terms of normal dietary thiamine intake and drinking habits. Methods used for assessing dietary thiamine are not always reliable, owing to the use of outdated methodology for determining the thiamine content of food, and losses in cooking are not always taken into account. Age, body weight and concomitant disease should be given due consideration when assessing what might be 'normal' in terms of vitamin status. Careful thought should be given as to at which level of either ETK or TPP effect, a deficiency state is indicated. From our own experiences a TPP effect of greater than 10 per cent indicates deficiency, although some laboratories maintain that a TPP effect of as much as 40 per cent is still 'normal'.

Transketolase activity can be determined in red cell hemolysates by either colorimetric or enzymatic methods. The former (Shouten et al, 1964) employs incubation with ribose-5-phosphate, and the sedoheptulose 7-phosphate formed is complexed with 87 per cent (v/v) sulphuric acid, this complex then being reduced with cysteine to produce a pink colour. Extreme care is necessary to produce reliable results by this method. The heating stage after the addition of sulphuric acid has to be timed accurately, and the final colour production can be variable. Generally, the colormetric method has the advantage of being cheap and the reagents are stable for long periods once made up. Enzymatic methods tend to produce more consistent and reproducible results however. Incubation with ribose-5-phosphate and xylulose-5-phosphate is used and the glyceraldehyde-3-phosphate formed by the transketolase reaction is measured by a linking enzyme system, triose phosphate isomerase: glycerol phosphate dehydrogenase, the dehydrogenation step being followed by the change in absorbance at 340 nm. This procedure is described by Smeets et al (1971) and modified methods for clinical use have been comprehensively described by Bayoumi & Rosalki (1976) and by Williams (1976). These modified procedures do not include xylulose-5-phosphate in the reaction mixture, this incurring a considerable cost-saving in reagents compared with the original procedure. The presence of haemoglobin in the assay mixture may effect the molar extinction coefficient for NADH, and this should be borne in mind when calculating ETK values using these methods (Buttery et al, 1980). Generally, ETK measurements determined by enzymatic methods are reliable and are useful indicators of thiamine depletion, providing care is taken in ensuring stability of reagents and the assay is carried out as soon as possible after collection of the specimen, as the transketolase apoenzyme is not stable for long periods in vitro. Also, ETK decreases as the red cell ages, and increased ETK is found in iron deficiency, which could be of relevance in the alcoholic (Thurnham, 1981).

Measurement of ETK and TPP effect is an indirect way of looking at utilisable thiamine (i.e. TPP) status. More recently, plasma measurement of TPP itself has been employed to assess thiamine status, and avoids many of the shortcomings of the transketolase assay in the clinical situation. TPP can be measured either by an enzymatic method employing yeast pyruvate decarboxylase, or by high pressure liquid chromatography (McLaren et al, 1981). Plasma TPP still awaits full evaluation as a marker of thiamine status, but may supercede ETK and TPP effect in coming years.

Other methods of thiamine analysis include a fluorimetric method employing the reaction of the vitamin with thiochrome, and a microbiological assay using Ochromonas Danica. Both these methods measure total thiamine, the thiochrome method not being very specific and prone to interference from other constituents of biological samples. A semiautomated modification of the thiochrome method, employing high pressure liquid chromatography to overcome interference problems, has recently been reported, and may be of great value clinically (Schrijver et al, 1982). The O. Danica method is difficult to perform, but is very sensitive and has been used for research purposes, including clinical nutrition surveys (Baker & Frank, 1968). Properly carried out, this protozoalogical method offers the advantages of reliability, low cost, specificity and reproducibility.

Riboflavin and pyridoxine

Riboflavin and pyridoxine status can be assessed in a similar way to that of thiamine by measuring the red cell activity of the vitamin dependent enzymes glutathione reductase (EGR) and aspartate aminotransferase (EAST) in both the absence and presence of FAD and 5-PLP respectively. The enzyme activity in the presence of the added vitamin cofactor can be divided by the basal activity when no cofactor is added to give activation coefficients (expressed as α-EGR and α-EAST) of the enzymes. This is analogous to TPP effect in the case of ETK, a high activation coefficient being indicative of a deficiency state. These methods for assessing riboflavin and pyridoxine status are described in detail by Bayoumi & Rosalki (1976) and also by Williams (1976). In addition, pyridoxine status can be assessed by measurement of red cell 5-PLP levels. The latter can be achieved by incubating a protein-free red cell extract with 1-^{14}C-tyrosine in the presence of tyrosine decarboxylase apoenzyme and collecting the $^{14}CO_2$ released in the reaction, which will be proportional to the amount of 5-PLP in the extract. This method gives a direct measure of a tissue level of the utilisable vitamin, but has the disadvantage of being time consuming to perform and expensive in terms of reagents. EAST methods can be set up on an autoanalyser, but very often EAST and α-EAST are normal in alcoholics, whereas 5-PLP levels are low. For reasons that are not understood, EAST in chronic alcoholics is often high, and α-EAST low, and following vitamin therapy, EAST increases and α-EAST decreases even further, suggesting that in spite of high activities in the first place, there is still some degree of deficiency in this situation. Thus, in the alcoholic, 5-PLP is a better indicator of tissue status. Alternatively, urinary levels of kynurenine can be determined after tryptophan load, raised values indicating pyridoxine deficiency. This test has various limitations though, the administration of tryptophan load causing an imbalance in amino acid metabolism and excess kyrurenine excretion may be seen when there is no clinical evidence of deficiency (Baker & Frank, 1968). Recently, a fluorimetric assay for the B6 vitamins has been reported which may prove more convenient and economical to carry out than enzymatic methods (Chanhan & Dakskinamarti, 1981).

As far as riboflavin is concerned, α-EGR is a good measure of vitamin status, frequently being elevated in alcoholics, and returning to normal following vitamin supplementation. Riboflavin can be determined microbiologically using tetrahymena pyriformis, and the same organism can be used to determine pyridoxine in biological samples (Baker & Frank, 1968).

Folate and B_{12}

Measurement of circulating levels of folate and B_{12} can be achieved by microbiological methods, using Lactobacillus casei for folate, and either Lactobacillus leichmannii, Ochromonas malhamensis or Euglena gracilis for B_{12}. More recently radioassay methods, in the form of commercially available kits have been used. The latter are generally more convenient to use, require less technical expertise than the microbiological methods, do not suffer the problems of interference by cytotoxic drugs or antibiotics, but tend to be expensive and particularly in the case of B_{12}, can give erroneous results. There have recently been many reports of serum B_{12} levels being normal in patients with evidence of megaloblastic anaemia where radioassay procedures have been used (England & Linnell, 1980; Rose, 1981). This has been thought to be due to overestimation of cobalamin due to contamination of the intrinsic factor, used as the competitive protein binder in many radioassays, with 'R proteins' that bind non-active forms of the cobalamins. This problem has largely been overcome by introduction of assay kits containing purified intrinsic factor or 'blocked R binders'. Whether these modifications will overcome the problems of lack of correlation between biochemical and clinical data remains to be seen in the long term, and it should be remembered that some radioassay methods employ chicken serum R-protein as the binder yet give satisfactory results. Many of the problems of interpretation may have stemmed from measurement of total serum B_{12} after release from the binding proteins, usually by heating, when there is transcobalamin II deficiency. Serum B_{12} is distributed between the two binding proteins, transcobalamin I (about 70–80 per cent cobalamins being bound to this carrier protein), and transcobalamin II (10–30 per cent of B_{12} bound). The B_{12} fraction bound to transcobalamin II is the metabolically important fraction, having a higher turnover than the transcobalamin I bound fraction. In transcobalamin II deficiency, megaloblastic anaemia develops. Radioassay and microbiological techniques do not distinguish between these bound proteins, as the assay usually measures total B_{12} after release from the transcobalamins by heating, and in transcobalamin II deficiency, serum B_{12} may be normal. Patients with transcobalamin II deficiency show abnormal absorption in a Schilling test. Transcobalamin I is produced by the leucocytes, and, in chronic myeloid leukaemia, serum B_{12} is raised when there is in fact tissue deficiency of the vitamin (England & Linnell, 1980).

As far as alcoholics are concerned, B_{12} deficiency may have been under-diagnosed due to inaccuracy in the serum assay. Most deficiency in alcoholics, when present, is due to dietary insufficiency which can be ascertained from a dietary survey, or malabsorption which can be diagnosed with the Schilling test. Determination of the serum B_{12} level can be useful where a reliable radioassay or a sensitive microbiological assay is used. Many modified radioassay procedures for B_{12} have recently been reported including assays using oyster toadfish serum as binder (Ithakissio et al, 1980), assays requiring no pretreatment of serum (Houts & Carney, 1981) or assays based on transcobalamin II (Paltridge et al, 1980). As far as microbiological methods are concerned, the protozoan Ochromonas malhamensis is probably the organism of choice, being easier to maintain than Euglena, extremely sensitive, 1 pg being detectable, and this sensitivity means that transcobalamin bound B_{12} can be determined directly if unheated serum is assayed (i.e. free B_{12}) as well as heated (i.e. total B_{12}), the difference being transcobalamin bound B_{12}. The method is described in detail (Baker & Frank, 1968) and these authors have recently reaffirmed their confidence in the method, and claim that it is not technically difficult to perform, and it does have a cost advantage over the radioassay method (Baker et al, 1981).

A valine loading test can be of value in detecting cobalamin deficiency. Increased urinary excretion of methyl malonic acid is found in B_{12} deficiency and is easily detected by a simple thin layer chromatographic method (Gutteridge & Wright, 1970; Balfour & Lane, 1980).

As far as folate is concerned, measurement of red cell levels are usually a better indicator of vitamin status than serum levels. Microbiological and radioassay procedures have been reported (for reviews see Shane et al, 1980; Dawson et al, 1980), the latter often being performed using commercial kits. As for B_{12}, the values obtained on biological samples using radioassay depend on the binder used and which vitamin derivative is used as a standard, so it is vital when these procedures are used that each laboratory determines its own reference range. Microbiological methods give an identical response to all folate monoglutamates, but a poor response to polyglutamates. This can be overcome by treatment of sampes with folate conjugase prior to assay so that total folate is determined. A suitable modification of the microbiological method for routine use is reported by Chen et al (1978). As far as alcoholics are concerned, folate deficiency will probably be easily detectable by either radioassay or microbiological estimation of red cell levels, providing the normal range has been accurately determined in the first place. Microbiological methods tend to give slightly higher values for serum and red cell folate than radioassay techniques. Care should always be taken to avoid loss of folate from samples before analysis takes place. Minimal loss occurs if the blood sample is stored whole in the case of red cell folate, or if ascorbate is added to the separated specimen when serum folate is being measured. For red cell folate, most accurate values are achieved with a freshly prepared haemolysate, or a haemolysate that has been frozen immediately after preparation (Kubasik et al, 1979).

Assays for other vitamins

Serum levels of ascorbate generally reflect recent intake, and determination of leucocyte levels is normally used to assess overall status of the vitamin. Leucocytes are commonly prepared by sedimentation of the cells with dextran, which results in a platelet contaminated preparation, so possibly one should refer to 'buffy-coat ascorbate' rather than 'leucocyte ascorbate'. Ascorbate can be estimated by using the reducing potential of the vitamin with an indicator such as a 2,6 dichlorophenol indophenol, or the formation of an osazone between dehydroascorbate and 2,4, dinitrophenyl hydrazine. Both procedures have drawbacks in terms of lack of specificity. More recently, a specific enzymatic method employing ascorbate oxidase has been reported which should prove accurate, specific and suitable for automation (Avigliano et al, 1978). It should be remembered that low reserves of ascorbate may often be found in late winter and early spring in some populations, due to the expense of fresh fruit and vegetables at this time of year. Leucocyte ascorbate is a good measure of ascorbate status in alcoholics, and deficient levels are frequently found which improve after therapy (Majumdar et al, 1981).

Vitamin D is usually estimated in plasma or serum as 25-hydroxycholecalciferol, the major circulating form which is not as metabolically active as 1,25 dihydroxycholecalciferol. Most methods entail a competitive protein binding radioassay following extraction of the vitamin from the sample using organic solvents (Fairney et al, 1979). Radioimmunoassay has been reported, but antiserum is difficult to obtain. Considerable seasonal variation in plasma 25-hydroxycholecalciferol levels are seen in alcoholics, but may not be of any physiological significance, due to mechanisms which regulate production of the active vitamin, 1,25 hydroxycholecalciferol. The latter is present in plasma at only about one thousandth the concentration of 25-hydroxycholecalciferol, thus is much more difficult to measure. Procedures for measurement of 1,25 dihydroxycholecalciferol have been described based on high pressure liquid chromatography followed by quantitation, either by ultraviolet spectrophotmetry (Avioli & Haddad, 1977), or radioassay. Such techniques are possibly too sophisticated for routine clinical use at present.

α-tocopherol can be determined simultaneously with retinol by high pressure liquid chromatography (Bieri et al, 1979). Other methods are based on separation of the various tocopherols following extraction by thin-layer chromatography, the spots then being eluted from the chromatography plate and quantitated by either colorimetric or fluorimetric methods (Combs,

1981). Again, these techniques are probably too technically present for routine clinical use.

Vitamin K and its derivatives can be quantitated by sp methods. (Hassan, 1980), but, for clinical use, an exten time is as good an indicator of deficiency as any estimat vitamin levels, and is, of course, a far easier test to carry out.

SUMMARY AND CONCLUSIONS

Chronic alcoholics frequently have evidence of nutritional deficiency due to decreased intake, reduced uptake and impaired utilisation of nutrients. The alcoholic has increased nutrient requirements due to greater metabolic demands and the need for tissue repair. Chronic alcohol-related brain damage can often be a direct result of nutrient depletion, particularly of the vitamins thiamine, B_{12}, nicotinamide and pyridoxine. Lesser degrees of brain damage are frequently unrecognised, and by the time a vitamin deficiency syndrome has developed and been diagnosed, irreversible damage has often occurred. The development of suitable computerised psychometric tests may allow earlier detection of brain malfunction associated with malnutrition, which can be reversed by nutrient repletion before permanent damage occurs.

Circulating levels of vitamins can be a valuable guide to nutritional status, although care is needed when interpreting the results of such tests in the alcoholic. Sensitive microbiological and biochemical tests for assessing vitamin status in man have been available for some years, and in addition, new biochemical methods are constantly being developed. It is important that such methods are evaluated, and possibly adapted for clinical use where appropriate. Newer methods may have significant advantages over older, more established techniques. For thiamine and pyridoxine, for example, methods now exist to determine accurately circulating levels of the active forms of these vitamins, which could give more direct assessment of vitamin status than earlier methodology that uses indirect measurements, such as red cell enzyme activities.

On the other hand, in the case of folate and B_{12}, there has been a tendency to opt for the easy-to-perform radioassay techniques, when in fact the earlier microbiological methods offer greater sensitivity and probably also better accuracy. Technically difficult assays should not be disregarded if they can give information which is of greater clinical use than a simpler assay technique. Clinical laboratories should always bear in mind what their vitamin methods are actually measuring, particular consideration being given to whether metabolically inactive forms or analogues are determined in the assay. This can be of importance to the interpretation of vitamin data in the alcoholic, who often has problems forming active vitamins from their precursors.

hemoglobin on NADH absorbance in the transketolase assay. Clinica Chimica Acta 102, 221–225
Cake M H, Disorbo D M, Litwack G 1978 Effect of pyridoxal phosphate on the DNA binding site of activated hepatic glucocorticoid receptor. Journal of Biological Chemistry 253, 4886–4891
Chanarin I, Lumb M, Deacon R, Perry J 1980 Vitamin B12 regulates folate metabolism by the supply of formate. Lancet 2, 505–507
Chang S, Kirksey A, Morre D M 1981 Effects of vitamin B12 deficiency on morphological changes in dendritic trees of Purkinje Cells in developing cerebellum of rats. Journal of Nutrition 111, 848–857
Chauhan M S, Dakshinamurti K 1981 Fluorimetric assay of B6 vitamin in biological material. Clinica Chimica Acta 109, 159–167
Chen M F, McIntyre P A, Kertcher J A 1978 Measurement of folates in human plasma and erythrocytes by a radiometric microbiological method. Journal of Nuclear Medicine 19, 906–912
Chen L H 1981 An increase in vitamin E requirement induced by high supplementation of vitamin C in rats. American Journal of Clinical Nutrition 34, 1036–1041
Combs G F 1981 Assessment of vitamin E status in animals and man. Proceedings of the Nutrition Society 40, 187–194
Connelly J L, Johnson W A 1975 Branched-chain α-ketoacid dehydrogenases. In: Gubler C J (ed) Thiamine. John Wiley, New York
Cooper J R, Pincus J H 1979 The role of thiamine in nervous tissue. Neurochemical Research 4, 223–229
DeLuca H F 1980 Vitamin D: revisited 1980. Clinics in Endocrinology and Metabolism 9, 3–26
Devgun M S, Fiabane A, Paterson C R, Zarembski P, Guthrie A 1981 Vitamin and mineral nutrition in chronic alcoholics including patients with Korsakoff's psychosis. British Journal of Nutrition 45, 469, 472
Drake J R, Fitch C D 1980 Status of vitamin E as an erythropoietic factor. American Journal of Clinical Nutrition 33, 2386–2393
Elliott J G, Lachance P A 1980 Effects of vitamin A and ascorbic acid on in vitro cholesterol biosynthesis in the rat. Journal of Nutrition 110, 1488–1496
England J M, Linnell J C 1980 Problems with the serum vitamin B12 assay. Lancet 2, 1072–1074
Fairney A, Turner C, Hanson S, Zambou M 1979 A simple micromethod for 25-hydroxy vitamin D estimation. Annals of Clinical Biochemistry 16, 106–110
Goldsmith G A (1975) Riboflavin deficiency. In: Rivlin R S (ed) Riboflavin. Plenum, London
Gould J 1954 The use of vitamins in psychiatric practice. Proceedings of the Royal Society of Medicine 47: 215–220
Greenwood J, Love E R, Pratt O E 1981 Carrier-mediated transport of thiamine across the blood-brain barrier. Journal of Physiology 310, 238
Griffiths W 1981 Assay for serum 25-hydroxyvitamin D and its clinical applications. MSc Thesis, University of Surrey
Gutteridge J M C, Wright E B 1970 A simple and rapid thin layer chromatographic technique for detection of methyl malonic acid in urine. Clinica Chimica Acta 27, 289–291
Haddad J G, Min C, Mendelsohn M, Slatoposky E, Hahn T J 1977 Competitive protein binding radioassay of 24, 25 dihydroxyvitamin D in sera from normal and anephric subjects. Archives of Biochemistry and Biophysics 182, 390–395
Hakim A M, Pappius H M 1981 The effect of thiamine deficiency on local cerebral glucose utilisation. Annals of Neurology 9, 334–339
Hall C A 1981 Vitamin B12 deficiency and early rise in mean corpuscular volume. Journal of the American Medical Association 245, 1144–1146
Halsted C H, Robles A, Mezey E 1973 Distribution of ethanol in the human gastrointestinal tract. American Journal of Clinical Nutrition 26, 831–834
Halsted C H 1980 Folate deficiency in alcoholism. American Journal of Clinical Nutrition 33, 2736–2740
Harper C 1979 Wernicke's encephalopathy . . . a more common disease. Journal of Neurology and Neurosurgery 42, 226–231

Hassan S S M 1980 Spectrophotometric determination of the K vitamins. Methods of Enzymology 67, 125–128
Heindel J J, Riggs T R 1978 Amino-acid transport in vitamin-B6 deficient rats: dependence on growth hormone supply. American Journal of Physiology 235, E316–E323
Herbert V, Zalusky R, Davidson C A 1963 Correlation of folate deficiency with alcoholism and associated macrocytosis, anaemia and liver disease. Annals of Internal Medicine 58, 977–988
Hermann W J, Ward K, Faucett J 1979 The effect of tocopherol on high-density lipoprotein cholesterol: a clinical observation. American Journal of Clinical Pathology 72, 848–852
Houts T M, Carney J A 1981 Radioassay for cobalamin (vitamin B12) requiring no pretreatment of serum. Clinical Chemistry 27, 263–267
Howard L, Wagner C, Schenker S 1974 Malabsorption of thiamine in folate deficient rats. Journal of Nutrition 104, 1024–1032
Hoyumpa A M, Breen K J, Schenker S, Wilson F A 1975 Thiamine transport across the rat intestine, II. Effect of ethanol. Journal of Laboratory and Clinical Medicine 86, 803–816
Hoyumpa A M 1980 Mechanisms of thiamine deficiency in chronic alcoholism. American Journal of Clinical Nutrition 33, 2750–2761
Ithakissios D A, Kubiatowicz D O, Wicks J H 1980 Room temperature radioassay for B12 with oyster toadfish (opsanus tau) serum as binder. Clinical Chemistry 26, 323–326
Jolliffe N 1941 Treatment of neuropsychiatric disorders with vitamins. Journal of the American Medical Association 117, 1496–1500
Karl A F, Griswold D 1980 Actions of insulin and vitamin A on sertoli cells. Biochemical Journal 186, 1001–1003
Kubasik N P, Graham M, Sine H E 1979 Storage and stability of folate and vitamin B12 in plasma and blood samples. Clinica Chimica Acta 95, 147–149
Kuo Y J, Shanbour L L 1978 Effects of ethanol on sodium, 3-O-methyl glucose and L-alanine transport in the jejunum. American Journal of Digestive Diseases 23, 51–56
Lane M, Alfred C P, Mengel C E, Doherty M A, Doherty J 1964 The rapid induction of human riboflavin deficiency with galactoflavin. Journal of Clinical Investigation 43, 357–373
Leathen J H 1970 Nutrition. In: Johnson A D, Gomer W R, Vandermark N L (eds) The testes. Academic Press, New York, vol 3, p 188–190
Leigh D, McBurney A, McIlwain H 1981 Erythrocyte transketolase activity in the Wernicke-Korsakoff syndrome. British Journal of Psychiatry 139, 153–159
Lindenbaum J 1980 Folate and B12 deficiencies in alcoholism. Seminars in Haematology 17, 119–129
Loo Y H 1980 Vitamin B6 effects on the developing brain. In: Tryfiates G P (ed) Vitamin B6: metabolism and role in growth. Food and Nutrition Press, Westport
Majumdar S K, Patel S, Shaw G K, O'Gorman P, Thomson A D 1981 Vitamin C utilisation status in chronic alcoholic patients after short-term intravenous therapy. International Journal for Vitamin and Nutrition Research 51, 274–278
Marcus M, Prabhudesai M, Wassef S 1980 Stability of vitamin B12 in the presence of ascorbic acid in food and serum: restoration by cyanide of apparent loss. American Journal of Clinical Nutrition 33, 137–143
McCormick D B 1975 Metabolism of riboflavin. In: Rivlin R S (ed) Riboflavin. Plenum Press, London
McLaren D S, Docherty M A, Boyd D H A 1981 Plasma thiamine pyrophosphate and erythrocyte transketolase in chronic alcoholism. American Journal of Clinical Nutrition 34, 1031–1033
Mezey E 1980 Alcoholic liver disease: roles of alcohol and malnutrition. American Journal of Clinical Nutrition 33, 2709–2718
Nutrition Reviews 1981 Genetic determination of coenzyme synthesis in red cells 39, 331–332
Oliver L K 1980 Colorimetric analysis of vitamin A and carotene. Methods in Enzymology 67, 199–203
Omaye S T, Turnbull J D 1980 Effect of ascorbic acid on heme metabolism in hepatic mecrosomes. Life Sciences 27, 441–449
Paltridge G, Rudzki Z, Ryall R G 1980 Validity of transcobalamin II band radioassay for

the determination of serum vitamin B12 concentrations. Annals of Clinical Biochemistry 17, 287–292
Pincus J H 1972 Subacute necrotizing encephalomyelopathy: (Leigh's disease): a consideration of clinical features and etiology. Developmental Medicine and Child Neurology 14, 87–101
Pitt G A J 1981 The assessment of vitamin A status. Proceedings of the Nutrition Society 40, 173–178
Powers H J, Thurnham D I 1980 Physiological effects of marginal riboflavin deficiency in young adults and geriatrics: a reduction in the in vivo survial time of erythrocytes. Proceedings of the Nutrition Society 39, 17A
Raisz L G 1980 Direct effects of vitamin D and its metabolites on skeletal tissue. Clinics in Endocrinology and Metabolism 9, 27–41
Robison W G, Kuwabara T, Bieri J G 1980 Deficiencies of vitamins E and A in the rat: retinal damage and lipofuscin accumulation. Investigations in Ophthalmology and the Visual Sciences 19, 1030–1037
Robson L C, Schwarz M R 1980 The effects of vitamin B6 deficiency on the lymphoid system and immune responses. In: Tryfiates G P (ed) Vitamin B6: metabolism and role in growth. Food and Nutrition Press, Westport
Rose M 1981 Editorial: clinical application of serum vitamin B12 assay. Journal of Clinical Pathology 34, 341–342
Russell R M 1980 Vitamin A and zinc metabolism in alcoholism. American Journal of Clinical Nutrition 33, 2741–2749
Schenker S, Henderson G I, Hoyumpa A M, McCaudless D W 1980 Hepatic and Wernicke's encephalopathies: current concepts of pathogenesis. American Journal of Clinical Nutrition 33, 2719–2726
Schmidt K H, Hagmaier V, Hornig D H, Vuilleumier J P, Rutishauser G 1981 Urinary oxalate excretion after large intakes of ascorbic acid in man. American Journal of Clinical Nutrition 34, 305–311
Schrijver J, Speek A J, Klosse J A, Van Rijn H J M, Schreurs W H P 1982 A reliable semiautomated method for the determination of total thiamine in whole blood by the thiochrome method with high-performance liquid chromatography. Annals of Clinical Biochemistry 19: 52–56
Schurah C J 1981 The level of vitamin C reserves required in man: towards a solution to the controversy. Proceedings of the Nutrition Society 40, 147–154
Schultz S G 1977 Sodium-coupled solute transport by small intestine: a status report. American Journal of Physiology 233, 249–254
Shane B, Tamura T, Stokstad E L R 1980 Folate assay: a comparison of radioassay and microbiological methods. Clinica Chimica Acta 100, 13–19
Sharma S K, Quastel J H 1965 Transport and metabolism of thiamine in rat brain cortex in vitro. Biochemical Journal 94, 790–800
Shouten H, Statius van Eps L W, Struyker Boudier A M 1964 Transketolase in blood. Clinica Chimica Acta 10, 474–476
Siddik Z H, Mimnaugh E G, Trush M A, Gram T E 1980 The effect of vitamin A deficiency on hepatic, renal and pulmonary glutathione-S-transferase activities in the rat. Biochemical Journal 188, 889–893
Smeets E H J, Muller H, De Wael J 1971 A NADH-dependent transketolase assay in erythrocyte haemolysates. Clinical Chimica Acta 33, 379–386
Sprince H, Parker C M, Smith G C, Gonzales L J 1975 Protective action of ascorbic acid and sulphur compounds against acetaldehyde toxicity: implications in alcoholism and smoking. Agents and Actions 5, 164–173
Tanaka K 1981 New light on biotin deficiency. New England Journal of Medicine 304, 839–840.
Tezuka I, Makino K 1959 Hyperglycaemia in pyridoxine deficient rats. Journal of Vitaminology 5, 304–306
Thomson A D 1978 Alcohol and nutrition. Clinics in Endocrinology and Metabolism 7, 405–428
Thomson A D 1982 Alcohol-related structural brain changes. British Medical Bulletin 38, 87–94
Thomson A D, Frank O, Baker H, Leevy C M 1971a Thiamine propyl disulphide:

absorption and utilisation. Annals of Internal Medicine 74, 529–534
Thomson A D, Baker H, Leevy C M 1971b Folate induced malabsorption of thiamine. Gastroenterology 60, 756–762
Thomson A D, Rae S A, Majumdar S K 1980 Malnutrition in the alcoholic. In: Clark P, Kricka L (eds) Medical consequences of alcohol abuse. Ellis Horwood, Chichester, ch 6, p 103–155
Thomson A D, Majumdar S K 1981 The influence of ethanol on intestinal absorption and utilisation of nutrients. Clinics in Gastroenterology 10, 263–293
Thurnham D I 1981 Red cell enzyme tests: do marginal deficiencies have any physiological significance? Proceedings of the Nutrition Society 40, 155–163
Victor M, Adams R D 1971 The Wernicke-Korsakoff syndrome. Davis, Philadelphia.
Whitehead C C 1981 The assessment of biotin status in man and animals. Proceedings of the Nutrition Society 40, 165–172
Williams D G 1976 Methods for the stimation of three vitamin dependent red cell enzymes. Clinical Biochemistry 9: 252–255
Williams R R 1976 Breast and thyroid cancer and malignant melanoma promoted by alcohol induced pituitary secretion of prolactin, TSH and MSH. Lancet 1, 996–999
Wood B, Breen K J, Penington D G 1977 Thiamine status in alcoholism. Australia and New Zealand Journal of Medicine 7, 475–484

SECTION TWO

The hospitalised alcoholic

(ii) Organ complications

11 G. Lake-Bakaar

Gastrointestinal complications of alcoholism

INTRODUCTION

The gastrointestinal system is exposed to much higher concentrations of alcohol than any other tissue in the body. Ingestion of alcohol at a dose of 0.8 g/kg body weight results in alcohol concentrations of 7–8 g/dl in the stomach and 1–4 g/dl in the jejunum (Halsted et al, 1973a). The intestinal epithelium has the capacity to metabolise small amounts of alcohol which presumably is normally produced by bacteria in the gut (Krebs & Parkins, 1970). The stomach and intestine contain low activities of alcohol dehydrogenase as well as the microsomal ethanol-oxidizing system (MEOS). Tissue injury might, therefore, result from:

1. direct toxic effect of alcohol or congeners present in the alcoholic beverage;
2. toxic effect of alcohol metabolites, acetaldehyde and acetate;
3. changes in cellular redox potential occurring as a consequence of alcohol metabolism.

Alcohol is absorbed by passive diffusion throughout the entire length of the gastrointestinal tract. Tissue damage might, therefore, occur anywhere along the length of the gastrointestinal tract. Absorption is more rapid from the duodenum and jejunum than from the stomach. Thus blood levels of alcohol in patients with gastrectomies rise faster and to higher maximal levels than in normal subjects (Elmslie et al, 1965). The rate of absorption varies directly with the concentration ingested (Cooke & Birchell, 1969); it is reduced when alcohol is taken following or together with a meal (Broitman et al, 1976) presumably as a result of the delay in gastric emptying; it is also dependent on the type of beverage consumed (Kalant, 1971). Sex differences in the rates of alcohol absorption have been observed in man. At a given dose of alcohol calculated on the basis of the body weight, women absorb alcohol faster and achieve significantly higher and earlier peak blood alcohol levels than men (Morgan & Morgan, 1976).

ORAL CAVITY AND SALIVARY GLANDS

Alcohol is excreted in saliva. The concentration of alcohol in saliva is similar to that in blood (Beazell & Ivey, 1940).

Local application of alcohol to the tongue or buccal mucosa in healthy volunteers stimulates the flow of saliva, whereas direct instillation into the stomach is without effect (Martin & Pangborn, 1971) suggesting the presence of a local reflex. In patients with chronic alcoholic cirrhosis, salivary flow rate in response to dilute citric acid is greater compared to controls. However, protein secretion is reduced (Durr et al, 1975).

Clinical enlargement of the parotid gland is present in 12 per cent of chronic alcoholics and in about 50 per cent of patients with alcoholic hepatitis or cirrhosis (Bode, 1981). The mechanisms underlying these changes in the parotid gland are obscure. However, it is of interest that salivary iso-amylase and the immunoreactive trypsin: amylase ratio (Lake-Bakaar et al, 1980) is increased in chronic alcoholic pancreatitis. The effect of alcohol on the salivary glands merits further study. Glossitis and stomatitis which are reported to be common in chronic alcoholics probably result from poor nutrition since they usually respond to vitamin supplements (Beazell & Ivey, 1940). The effect of alcohol on vitamin absorption is dealt with later in this chapter (see also Ch. 10).

OESOPHAGUS

Alcohol can affect the oesophagus in several ways. Its acute effects suggests that it might be a potent cause of oesophagitis. Following oral or intravenous ethanol administration in healthy volunteers a reduction in peristaltic activity in the distal third of the oesophagus as well as a decrease in the lower oesophageal sphincter resting pressure has been observed (Hogan et al, 1972). These changes may in part, be due to a direct effect on autonomic nerve function. Abnormalities in oesophageal motility have been described in patients with alcoholic neuropathy (Winship et al, 1968). There is also direct evidence that alcohol administered orally results in gastro-oesophageal reflux (Kaufman & Kaye, 1978). During continuous monitoring of distal oesophageal pH, a significant increase in intraluminal acidity was observed in response to oral alcohol in healthy volunteers.

Barrett's syndrome, a condition characterised by columnar cells lining the lower oesophagus, is thought to be due to longstanding reflux oesophagitis. Patients with this condition have an increased incidence of alcohol abuse (Messian et al, 1978). It would therefore, seem likely that alcohol might be a potent cause of chronic oesophagitis in man. However, there is little available clinical evidence for this, and the case remains unproven (Wienbeck & Berges, 1980).

Other changes which can occur in the oesophagus as a result of alcohol include Mallory-Weiss tears. These are found in the lower oesophageal mucosa in alcoholics and result from the vomiting which ethanol can induce.

Oesophageal varices can also occur in alcoholic cirrhosis as a result of portal hypertension. Rupture of these varices can result in massive haematemesis or melaena.

The relationship between alcohol and cancer of the oesophagus is considered at the end of this chapter.

STOMACH

Exposure of the gastric mucosa to alcohol results in the rapid development of structural changes. Patchy haemorrhages occur within 1 hour of exposure which resolve completely within 16–72 hours after withdrawal (Davenport, 1967). Ultrastructurally, there is a disruption of the cell membranes and their intercellular contact points. Gastric mucosal cells disintegrate with chronic exposure (Eastwood & Kirchner, 1974).

Gastric mucosal permeability is increased in animals (Kuo et al, 1974) and man (Gordon et al, 1974) in response to alcohol. This is accompanied by a rapid reduction in transmural gastric potential difference (Geall et al, 1970) and an increase in back-diffusion of acid (Davenport, 1967). The severity of mucosal injury correlates closely with the decrease in transmucosal potential difference (Eastwood & Erdmann, 1978). It is of interest that other fat soluble substances like acetylsalicylic acid, bile acids, and acetic acid which cause alterations in mucosal permeability also result in gastric erosion (Silen & Skillman, 1974).

Alcohol initially increases gastric mucosal blood flow, but with the appearance of back-diffusion of H^+ ions, mucosal blood flow decreases (Augur, 1970). A decrease in mucosal blood flow is a common factor in the development of gastric erosions and haemorrhage due to stress or drugs (Silen & Skillman, 1974).

It is generally accepted that the direct effect of alcohol on gastric mucosa is to stimulate gastric acid. Alcohol administered either orally or intravenously stimulates acid secretion (Beazell & Ivey, 1940; Davenport, 1967). However in these in vivo studies it is not possible to separate the direct effects of alcohol on parietal cells from the indirect effects occurring through neural or humoral factors. A linear relationship has been demonstrated between gastric acid output and the dose of intravenous alcohol in dog (Weise et al, 1961) and man (Hirschowitz et al, 1956).

There is now also evidence suggesting that the direct effect of alcohol might not be to stimulate acid secretion. Indeed, direct application of alcohol to an in vitro stomach preparation results in the inhibition of acid secretion (Shanbour, 1980). Alcohol affects several of the enzymes which are thought to be involved in the active transport of ions across the gastric mucosa. The active transport of sodium, hydrogen and chloride are inhibited by alcohol. The mechanisms whereby alcohol affects gastric acid secretion is probably multifactorial. It is of interest that alcohol (6 per cent) in a recent study was no more effective than an equal volume of water in stimulating acid output in man (Cooke, 1972).

Measurement of the changes in cyclic AMP (adenosine monophosphate) levels induced by alcohol in the gastric mucosa might be expected to resolve the question as to whether the effect of alcohol on acid secretion is stimulatory or inhibitory. Cyclic AMP is thought to be related to active secretion of ions; increased levels would therefore suggest stimulation rather than inhibition. However, the reported levels are too inconsistent to allow for satisfactory resolution of this problem.

The chronic effects of alcohol on gastric acid secretion are similarly inconsistent. Large daily doses of ethanol (4.4 g/kg) administered orally to dogs for a period of 12 months, more than doubled the mean daily acid secretion from Heidenhain pouches (Chey et al, 1972). The mean maximal acid output from the stomach also increased, suggesting an increase in the mean parietal cell mass. However, contrary results have been obtained in man. The mean basal and maximal acid outputs in a group of chronic alcoholics who drank for more than 5 years was significantly less than those of healthy controls (Chey et al, 1968). Acid hyposecretion has also been reported in alcoholic cirrhotics (Scobie & Summerskill, 1964).

Alcohol also has an effect on gastric motility. At concentrations between 5 per cent and 30 per cent, X-ray studies have shown a delay in gastric emptying in man (Beazell & Ivey, 1940). Similarly, alcohol before a balanced fat diet almost doubled gastric emptying time (Barboriak & Meade, 1970), and, in rats, the normal rhythmic opening of the pylorus is disturbed. The mechanisms underlying the effect of alcohol on gastric motility have not been satisfactorily elucidated (Cooke, 1972).

The association between alcohol abuse and acute erosive gastritis has often been reported (Beazell & Ivey, 1940). In a systemic endoscopic study, excessive alcohol ingestion was the aetiological factor in 44 per cent of patients with haemorrhagic erosive gastritis (Dagradi et al, 1973). Distinct lesions associated with bleeding occur as a result of alcohol in patients with atrophic gastritis (Dinoso et al, 1972). Superficial or atrophic gastritis is commoner in chronic alcoholics (Beazell & Ivey, 1940). Moderate amounts of alcohol significantly increase gastrointestinal blood loss in man (Granerus & Svensson, 1969), an effect not observed with buffered sodium-acetyl salicylate preparations in normal volunteers (Bouchier & Williams, 1968).

In addition to alcohol, congeners such as acetaldehyde and acetic acid present in some alcoholic beverages may also be involved in the pathogenesis of acute erosive gastritis (O'Keane et al, 1971).

Peptic ulceration does not appear to be associated with alcohol abuse. In a large questionnaire study, no association between alcohol consumption and the prevalence of peptic ulceration was found (Friedman et al, 1974). Furthermore the risk of developing an ulcer does not appear to be related to alcohol consumption.

Alcohol does not appear to affect the healing or relapse rates of gastric ulcers (Piper et al, 1978), nor does it affect ulcer site and size (Thomas et al, 1980). Although patients with alcohol-induced liver disease have a high incidence of peptic ulcers (Bode, 1980), this is probably not related to alcohol consumption.

SMALL INTESTINE

The small intestinal lumen, like the stomach, is also exposed to high concentrations of alcohol. Thus alcohol, its congeners and its metabolites acetaldehyde and acetate, can therefore all combine to produce structural changes in the small intestine.

Haemorrhagic lesions in the villous tips of the duodenum have been observed in human volunteers after ingestion of alcohol in doses as low as 1 g/kg body weight (Gottfried et al, 1976). In the rat, acute ingestion of alcohol produces lesions which are concentration dependent. Oral ingestion, therefore, produces lesions which are more severe proximally. They develop within 10 minutes of exposure to alcohol and disappear between 4–16 hours after stopping alcohol (Baroana et al, 1974). On the other hand, rats fed chronically with alcohol develop shortened villi, decreased numbers of villous cells and increased regenerative activity in the crypts; erosive lesions are not seen (Baroana et al, 1974). Ultrastructural changes also develop, such as swelling of the mitochondria, dilatation of the smooth endoplasmic reticulum and reduction in ribosomes (Rubin et al, 1972).

Alcohol and small intestinal absorption

Biological membranes consist of a bilayer of lipids with the hydrophilic moiety directed toward the outer surface and the non-polar hydrocarbon chains orientated towards the inner point of the membrane. Proteins and glycoproteins are present within this lipid bilayer. Interaction between the protein molecules and the polar and non-polar constituents of the lipids is of importance in maintaining the conformation of the proteins and therefore, their biological activity. The hydrocarbon chain of alcohol can interact with the hydrophobic region of membrane lipids and proteins, modifying the fluidity of the membrane. Evidence for a change in membrane fluidity due to alcohol has been obtained from spin-label studies using electron paramagnetic resonance techniques (Chin & Goldstein, 1977). This may affect the transport channels through the lipid bilayer or decrease the activity of membrane-bound enzymes such as lactase and of enzymes such as intestinal ATP-ase which play a role in active transport (Wilson & Hoyumpa, 1979).

Alcohol also alters intestinal permeability to macromolecules. Rats treated by daily gavage of ethanol for 4–8 weeks show increased intestinal permeability for horseradish peroxidase. Electron microscopy suggests an alteration in the apical junctions (Worthington-Roberts, 1980). In man, alcohol increases intestinal permeability to PEG 400, both in chronic alcoholics during intoxication and in non-alcoholics after acute alcohol ingestion. The changes in permeability in both groups return to normal within 103 hours after stopping alcohol (Robinson et al, 1981). One implication of this is that the simultaneous ingestion of alcohol and drugs might increase absorption of the drugs. There is evidence, for example, that alcohol may increase the absorption of diazepam (Hayes et al, 1977).

The effects of alcohol on the enterocyte membrane, which is primarily concerned with absorption, might be responsible for the interference with intestinal transport. Any alteration of the conformational structure of membrane-bound enzymes would inhibit the absorption of substances which are actively transported, whereas changes in the intercellular junctions would increase the transport of passively absorbed substances.

Monosaccharides

Alcohol inhibits D-glucose transport across the small intestine in a concentration-dependent manner. This inhibition does not appear to be related to an effect on the basolateral Na^+/K^+-ATPase activity since in in vitro experiments, alcohol reduced glucose uptake when placed in the mucosal compartment, but had no effect via the serosal compartment. Uptake across the brush border thus appears to be selectively affected by alcohol (Dinda & Beck, 1977). However, the precise mechanisms by which alcohol inhibits glucose transport has not been fully elucidated. Glucose transport inhibition appears unrelated to changes in osmolality induced by alcohol (Dinda & Beck, 1977). Information on the effect of alcohol on glucose absorption in man is lacking.

D-xylose, like D-glucose appears to be actively absorbed in animals. The mechanism of transport in man has not been fully elucidated. Results of the effect of alcohol on D-xylose absorption in man are inconsistent. Decreased absorption is frequently observed in chronic alcoholics. However, the degrees of malabsorption reported vary widely (zero to 76 per cent). This may reflect differences in the group of patients studied. The presence or absence of cirrhosis or portal hypertension, the mean daily alcohol intake, ascites and disturbed renal function will all influence the distribution and excretion of xylose. The nutritional state is also of relevance. In one study, improvement in the nutritional state of a group of chronic alcoholics increased their mean D-xylose absorption (Mezey, 1975). Oral, but not intravenously administered alcohol reduces D-xylose absorption in chronic alcoholics (Mezey, 1975). The mechanism for this is not fully explained.

Amino-acid transport

Alcohol markedly inhibits active transport of L-phenylalanine, L-leucine, L-glycine, L-alanine, L-methionine and L-valine in animals. In man, ethanol (0.4 mol/l) in jejunal perfusates more than halved L-methionine absorption (Israel et al, 1969). Inhibition is considered to be via an effect on Na^+/K^+-ATPase. It is possible that this might contribute to the state of clinical malnutrition common in chronic alcoholics.

Vitamin absorption

Folic acid. Acute alcohol ingestion suppressed H^3-pteroylglutamic acid in only 1 of 5 healthy subjects (Halsted et al, 1967). On the other hand, serum folic acid levels are frequently lowered in alcoholics and are closely related to histological alterations of the jejunal mucosa. Folic acid deficiency in alcoholics is probably multifactorial. It may be due to inadequate dietary intake, decreased storage in a cirrhotic liver, increased hepatic synthesis of inactive polyglutamates or decreased absorption. Alcohol has also been shown to interrupt the enterohepatic circulation of folate by imparing its secretion into bile (Steinbart et al, 1980). At low physiological concentration (<1.0 μmol/l) folic acid is absorbed from the small intestine by an active transport process which may involve a binding protein; at high concentrations absorption is largely passive. Folic acid absorption at physiological concentrations is reduced in chronic alcoholics. However, it is improved after two weeks of adequate nutrition despite continuing alcohol (Halsted et al, 1973b). Impaired folate absorption in chronic alcoholics may thus be a function of malnutrition per se rather than of alcoholism.

Thiamine. Thiamine deficiency is common in alcoholics. The absorption of this vitamin in animals is similar to that of folate, being actively transported at low concentrations (<1 mmol/l) and passively absorbed by simple diffusion at high concentrations ($<$ 1mmol/l). Alcohol decreases movement of thiamine across the basolateral membrane; however, mucosal border uptake by the enterocytes remains normal (Hoyumpa et al, 1975). Alcohol might, therefore, reduce active thiamine transport by inhibiting Na^+/K^+-ATPase activity (Wilson & Hoyumpa, 1979). In man, two studies have shown conflicting results. In one, no change was observed, and in the other, there was a decrease in thiamine absorption in response to alcohol.

Vitamin B_{12}. Deficiency of this vitamin is not uncommon in chronic alcoholics. Alcohol substituted isocalorically for carbohydrate in normal adults with a history of alcoholism reduced ^{57}C-vitamin B_{12} urinary excretion by 41 per cent after 3–8 weeks (Lindenbaum & Lieber, 1969). Studies in the rat suggest that alcohol might decrease gastric intrinsic factor secretion and reduce the uptake of intrinsic factor-B_{12} complex.

Vitamins A, D and E. Oral administration of alcohol to normal human subjects resulted in decreased vitamin A levels. However, a pathological vitamin A test was obtained in only 8 per cent of chronic alcoholics (Small et al, 1959). Low serum levels of 25-hydroxycholecalciferol in alcoholics is assumed to be due to dietary insufficiency and reduced exposure to sunshine (Lund et al, 1977).

Low plasma levels of vitamin E have been reported in alcoholics in spite of normal faecal fat excretion (Losowsky & Leonard, 1967).

Effect on iron, calcium and trace elements

Increased amounts of iron are found in the liver in about one-third of alcoholics. It has been suggested that this may be due to increased absorption of iron from the intestine. However, the effect of alcohol on iron absorption is an unsettled issue (Wilson & Hoyumpa, 1979). In one study, alcohol taken as whisky or brandy increased the obsorption of ferric iron in man, but not ferrous or haemoglobin iron (Charlton et al, 1964). Acute alcohol studies in animals suggest either decreased or unchanged ferrous iron absorption.

In a recent study (Chapman et al, 1982) nonhaem ^{59}Fe absorption measured by whole body counter was significantly increased in alcoholics with anaemia. However iron absorption was not increased in alcoholics with normal haemoglobin. Thus chronic alcoholism per se does not appear to affect iron absorption. Similarly, acute alcohol had no significant effect on iron absorption irrespective of whether the alcohol was administered orally or intravenously. It has been suggested in the studies where ferric iron absorption was increased by alcohol, that this might have been via an indirect effect on gastric acid stimulation. Gastric acid facilitates chelation of ferric salts with ascorbic acid and other exogenous agents; the chelates remain soluble in the alkaline milieu of the small intestine, enhancing iron absorption.

Intestinal calcium transport is an active Vitamin D-dependent process which depends on the presence of Ca^{2+}-ATPase and a soluble calcium binding protein.

The effect of alcohol on ^{59}calcium absorption has been studied in rats using an in vitro everted sac preparation after acute and chronic alcohol ingestion. Acute alcohol ingestion produced no significant change in ^{59}calcium absorption from either the duodenum or the ileum compared to controls. ^{59}Calcium absorption from the duodenum, but not the ileum was significantly decreased in chronic alcohol-fed rats compared to controls (Krawitt, 1973). Acute alcohol ingestion does not appear to affect calcium absorption in non-alcoholic human subjects (Verdy & Caron, 1973).

Decreased calcium absorption in alcoholics might be expected because of steatorrhoea from pancreatic disease or cholestasis, with consequent failure of vitamin D absorption. However, the studies in rat suggest that the effect of alcohol on calcium absorption is not wholly dependent on vitamin D. Administration of vitamin D or 1, 25-dihydroxycholcalciferol did not alter the effect of alcohol on calcium transport (Krawitt, 1974).

Zinc is actively transmitted across the rat jejunum. Infusion of alcohol to normal or chronic alcoholic patients however, does not affect urinary zinc excretion. In contrast, manganese absorption has been shown to be increased by ethanol.

Water and electrolytes

In studies using a triple lumen perfusion system, the mean absorption of water and sodium in volunteers ingesting alcohol for 2 weeks was reduced by approximately 70 per cent compared to healthy controls. Acute intestinal perfusion with alcohol however, had no effect on sodium transport (Mekhijian & May, 1977).

However, it can be argued that luminal perfusion studies do not distinguish between reduced absorption and increased secretion. Cholera enterotoxin stimulates intestinal fluid secretion by receptor-mediated activation of adenylate cyclase. Activation of this enzyme results in increased production of cylic AMP. In vitro addition of alcohol to rabbit jejunal mucosa in organ culture significantly increased cyclic AMP levels (Wilson & Hoyumpa, 1979). The effect of alcohol on water and electrolyte transport may be to increase secretion via cyclic AMP rather than to reduce absorption.

Fat absorption

Alcohol administered simultaneously with corn oil delayed the absorption of the oil. The primary effect of the alcohol, however, is probably to reduce gastric emptying (Barboriak & Meade, 1969).

Steatorrhoea is a common finding in chronic alcoholics. However, this is frequently the result of pancreatic disease. The daily ingestion of alcohol in five alcoholics on a normal hospital diet with vitamin supplements did not increase faecal fat excretion (Lindenbaum & Lieber, 1975).

Alcohol ingested chronically in rats enhances fatty acid incorporation into triglycerides; this effect is associated with an increase in the activity of the enzyme system responsible for fatty acid esterfication (Carter et al, 1971).

Diarrhoea occurs in about one-third of 'binge' drinkers. Possible causes of this diarrhoea include pancreatic and hepatic dysfunction; the effects of alcohol on intestinal motility; lactase deficiency; and altered water and electrolyte absorption or secretion. There is no evidence that this is related to alcohol induced malabsorption of fat.

ALCOHOL AND CANCER OF THE GASTROINTESTINAL TRACT

Schwartz et al (1962) in an analysis of almost 4000 patients with cancer, demonstrated a significant correlation between daily alcohol consumption and the frequency of cancers of the tongue, hypopharynx and larynx. Since heavy drinkers in general are heavy smokers, the effect of smoking per se needs to be isolated. However, even after standardisation of their data for smoking habits a higher incidence of cancer of the larynx and pharynx was still apparent. The ratio of the observed to expected frequency of cancers of the upper digestive tract in a sample of alcoholics was 3.4 for cancer of the pharynx and oral cavity and 9 for cancer of the larynx (Schmidt & Delint, 1972). Alcohol and smoking independently increase the risk of development of the tumours of the tongue, larynx and pharynx (Halsted et al, 1971).

The relationship between oesophageal cancer and alcohol abuse has also been demonstrated in several studies. People in high-risk alcohol exposure groups such as barmen and waiters show an increased mortality from this disease (Wynden & Bross, 1961). The mean daily alcohol intake in a group of patients with cancer of the oesophagus was significantly greater than age and sex matched controls. Furthermore, beverages containing greater amounts of alcohol appear to carry an increased risk. In heavy whisky drinkers the risk was 25 times, whereas for heavy beer drinkers it was 10 times that of control subjects drinking less than 30 g of alcohol daily. These data were also standardized for tobacco consumption (Wynden & Bross, 1961). The high incidence of cancer of the oesophagus in China is thought to be due to the strong drink, pai kan, which contains over 60 per cent alcohol.

The mechanism by which alcohol promotes upper gastrointestinal tract cancers is unknown. It might, by inducing microsomal enzymes, enhance the biotransformation of many carcinogenic compounds. It might also act by promoting deficiencies in essential nutrients and inhibiting cell mediated and humoral immune reactions. Finally, by promoting reflux, it might lead to chronic oesophagitis and stenosis both of which can lead to oesophageal cancer.

CONCLUSION

The gastrointestinal tract is exposed to much greater concentrations of alcohol than any other tissue in the body. Direct structural damage to the mucosal lining of the intestine is therefore not uncommon in alcoholism. Interactions also take place between the hydrocarbon chain of alcohol and the hydrophobic regions of both lipids and protein of the small intestinal epithelial cell membrane. This produces changes in the transport channels across the mucosal cell membrane and also alters the orientation of membrane-bound enzymes. Several of the absorptive functions of the small intestine can thus be affected by alcohol.

A significant correlation exists between daily alcohol consumption and the frequency of cancers of the upper digestive tract. This association exists independently of smoking.

Alcohol thus inflicts severe morbidity on the gastrointestinal tract. Elucidation of the mechanisms whereby many of these changes are produced remains one of the more interesting challenges for the future.

REFERENCES

Augur N A 1970 Gastric mucosal blood flow following damage by ethanol, acetic acid or aspirin. Gastroenterology 58: 311–320

Barboriak J J, Meade R C 1970 Effect of alcohol on gastric emptying in man. American Journal of Clinical Nutrition 23: 1151–1153

Baraona E, Pirola R C, Lieber C S 1974 Small intestinal damage and changes in cell population produced by ethanol ingestion in the rat. Gastroenterology 66: 226–234
Beazell J M, Ivey A C 1940 The influence of alcohol on the digestive tract. Journal of Studies on Alcohol 1: 45
Bode J C H 1980 Alcohol and the gastrointestinal tract. In: Frick P, Von Harnack G-A, Martins G A, Prader A (eds) Advances in internal medicine and paediatrics. Springer Verlag, Berlin
Bouchier I A D, Williams H S 1969 Determination of faecal blood-loss after combined alcohol and sodium-acetylsalicylate intake. Lancet 1: 178–180
Broitman S A, Gottlieb L S, Vitale J J 1976 Augmentation of ethanol absorption by mono- and disaccharides. Gastroenterology 70: 1101–1107
Carter E A, Drummey G D, Isselbacher K J 1971 Ethanol stimulates triglyceride synthesis by the intestine. Science 174: 1245–1247
Chapman R W, Morgan M Y, Boss A M, Sherlock S 1982 Acute and chronic effects of alcohol on iron absorption. Digestive Diseases and Sciences, in Press
Charlton R W, Jacobs P, Seftel H, Bothwell T H 1964 Effect of alcohol on iron absorption. British Medical Journal 2: 1427–1429
Chey W Y, Kosay S, Lorber S H 1972 Effects of chronic administration of ethanol on gastric secretion of acid in dogs. American Journal of Digestive Diseases 17: 153–159
Chey W Y, Kusakcioglu O, Dinosa V, Lorber S H 1968 Gastric secretion in patients with chronic pancreatitis and in chronic alcoholics. Archives of Internal Medicine 122: 399–403
Chin J H, Goldstein D B 1977 Effects of low concentrations of ethanol on the fluidity of spin-labelled erythrocyte and brain membranes. Molecular Pharmacology 13: 435–441
Cooke A R 1972 Ethanol and gastric function. Gastroenterology 62: 501–502
Cooke A R, Birchall A 1969 Absorption of ethanol from the stomach. Gastroenterology 57: 269–272
Dagradi A E, Lee E R, Bosco D L, Stempien St J 1973 The clinical spectrum of hemorrhagic erosive gastritis. American Journal of Gastroenterology 60: 30–46
Davenport H W 1967 Ethanol damage to canine oxyntic glandular mucosa. Proceedings of the Society for Experimental Biology and Medicine 126: 657–662
Denis P H, Galmiche J P 1980 Alcohol induced changes in esophageal motility. In: Stock C, Sarles H (eds) Alcohol and the gastrointestinal tract. Inserm, Paris, vol 95, p 377–390
Dinda P K, Beck I T 1977 On the mechanism of the inhibitory effect of ethanol on intestinal glucose and water absorption. American Journal of Digestive Diseases 22: 529–533
Dinoso V P, Meskinpour H, Lorber S H 1972 Studies on the acute effects of ethanol on the gastric mucosa in man. Gastroenterology 62: 843
Dürr H K, Bode J C, Gieseking R, Haase R, v. Arnim I, Beckmann B 1975 Anderungen der exokrinen Funktion der Glandula parotis und des Pankreas bei Patienten mit Leberzirrhose und chronischem Alkoholismus. Munchen Medizin Wochenschrift 117: 841
Eastwood G L, Erdmann K R 1978 Effect of ethanol on canine gastric epithelial ultrastructure and transmucosal potential difference. American Journal of Digestive Diseases 23: 429–435
Eastwood G L, Kirchner J P 1974 Changes in the fine structure of mouse gastric epithelium produced by ethanol and urea. Gastroenterology 67: 71–84
Elmslie R G, Davis R A, Magee D F, White T T 1964 Absorption of alcohol after gastrectomy. Surgery, Gynecology and Obstetrics 119: 1256–1258
Friedman G D, Siegelaub A B, Seltzer C C 1974 Cigarettes, Alcohol, coffee and peptic ulcer. New England Journal of Medicine 290: 469–473
Geall M G, Phillips S F, Summerskill W H J 1970 Profile of gastric potential difference in man. Effects of aspirin, alcohol, bile and endogenous acid. Gastroenterology 58: 437–443
Gordon M J, Skillman J J, Edwards B G, Silen W 1974 Effects of ethanol, acetylsalicyclic acid, acetaminophen, and ferrous sulfate on gastric mucosal permeability in man. Surgery 76: 405–412
Gottfried E B, Korsten M A, Lieber C S 1976 Gastritis and duodenitis induced by alcohol: an endoscopic and histologic assessment. Gastroenterology 70: 890
Granerus G, Svensson S-E, Wetterqvist H 1969 Histamine in alcoholic drinks. Lancet 1: 1320
Gray J P, Hoyumpa A M, Dunn G D, Henderson G I, Wilson F A, Swift L L 1980 Effect

of ethanol on fluidity of enterocyte membranes. In: Stock C, Sarles H (eds) Alcohol and the gastrointestinal tract. Inserm, Paris, vol 95, p 469–476
Green P H R, Tall A R 1979 Drugs, alcohol and malabsorption. American Journal of Medicine 67: 1066–1076
Halsted C H, Griggs R C, Harris D W 1967 The effect of alcoholism on the absorption of folic acid (H^3-PGA) evaluated by plasma levels and urine excretion. Journal of Laboratory and Clinical Medicine 69: 116–131
Halsted C G, Robles E A, Mezey E 1971 Decreased Jejunal uptake of labelled folic acid (H^3-PGA) in alcoholic patients: roles of alcohol and nutrition. New England Journal of Medicine 285: 701–706
Halsted C H, Robles E A, Mezey E 1973a Distribution of ethanol in the human gastrointestinal tract. American Journal of Clinical Nutrition 26: 831–834
Halsted C H, Robles E A, Mezey E 1973b Intestinal malabsorption in folate-deficient alcoholics. Gastroenterology 64: 526–532
Hayes S L, Pablo G, Radomski T, Palmer R F 1977 Ethanol and oral diazepam absorption. New England Journal of Medicine 296: 186–189
Hirschowitz B I, Pollard H M, Hartwell S W, London J 1956 The action of ethyl alcohol on gastric secretion. Gastroenterology 30: 244–256
Hogan W J, Viegas de Andrade S R, Winship D H 1972 Ethanol-induced acute oesophageal motor dysfunction. Journal of Applied Physiology 32: 755–760
Hoyumpa A M, Breen K J, Schencker S, Wilson F A 1975 Thiamine transport across the rat intestine. II Effect of ethanol. Journal of Laboratory and Clinical Medicine 86: 803–816
Israel Y, Valenzuela J E, Salazar I 1969 Alcohol and amino acid transport in the human small intestine. Journal of Nutrition 98: 222–224
Morgan Jones B, Morgan M K 1976 Women and Alcohol: intoxication, metabolism and the menstrual cycle. In: Greenblatt M, Schukit M A (eds) Alcoholism problems in women and children. Grune & Stratton, New York
Kalant H 1971 Absorption, distribution and elimination of ethanol: effects on biological membranes. In: Kissin B, Begleiter H (eds) The biology of alcoholism. Plenum Press, New York
Kaufman S E, Kaye M D 1978 Induction of gastro-oesophageal reflux by alcohol. Gut 19: 336–338
Krawitt E L 1973 Ethanol inhibits intestinal calcium transport in rats. Nature 243: 88–89
Krawitt E L 1975 Effect of ethanol ingestion on duodenal calcium transport. Journal of Laboratory and Clinical Medicine 85: 665–671
Krebs H A, Perkins J R 1970 The physiological role of liver alcohol dehydrogenase. Biochemical Journal 118: 635–644
Kuo Y S, Shanbour L L, Sernka T J 1974 Effect of ethanol on permeability and iron transport in the isolated dog stomach. American Journal of Digestive Diseases 19: 818–824
Lake-Bakaar G, McKavanagh S, Gatus B, Summerfield J A 1980 The relative values of serum immuno-reactive trypsin concentration and total amylase activity in the diagnosis of mumps, chronic renal failure and pancreatic disease. Scandinavian Journal of Gastroenterology 15: 97–107
Lindenbaum J, Lieber C S 1969 Alcohol-induced malabsorption of vitamin B^{12} in man. Nature 224: 806
Lindenbaum J, Lieber C S 1975 Effects of chronic ethanol administration on intestinal absorption in man in the absence of nutritional deficiency. Annals of the New York Academy of Science 252: 228–234
Losowsky M S, Leonard P J 1967 Evidence of Vitamin E deficiency in patients with malabsorption or alcoholism and the effects of therapy. Gut 8: 539–543
Lund B, Sørensen O H, Hilden M, Lund B 1977 The hepatic conversion of vitamin D in alcoholics with varying degrees of liver affection. Acta Medica Scandinavica 202: 221–224
Martin S, Pangborn R M 1971 Human parotid secretion in response to ethyl alcohol. Journal of Dental Research 50: 485
Mekhjian H S, May E S 1977 Acute and chronic effects of ethanol on fluid transport in the human small intestine. Gastroenterology 72: 1280–1286
Messian R A, Hermos J A, Robbins A H, Friedlander D M, Schimmel E M 1978 Barrett's esophagus. Clinical review of 26 cases. American Journal of Gastroenterology 69: 458–466

Mezey E 1975 Intestinal function in chronic alcoholism. Annals of the New York Academy of Science 252: 215–227
O'Keane M, Smith S, Goldberg A 1971 Gastric erosions caused by home-brewed lager. Lancet 2: 795–797
Piper D W, Shinners J, Greig M, Thomas J, Waller S L 1978 Effect of ulcer healing on the prognosis of chronic gastric ulcer — four year follow-up. Gut 19: 419–424
Robinson G M, Orrego H, Israel Y, Devenyi P, Kapur B M 1981 Low-molecular-weight polyethylene glycol as a probe of gastrointestinal permeability after alcohol ingestion. Digestive diseases and Sciences 26: 971–977
Rubin E, Rybak B J, Lindenbaum J, Gerson C D, Walker G, Lieber C S 1972 Ultrastructural changes in the small intestine induced by ethanol. Gastroenterology 63: 801–814
Schmidt W, De Lint J 1972 Causes of death of alcoholics. Journal of Studies on Alcohol 33: 171–185
Schwartz D, Lellouch J, Flamant R, Denoix P F 1962 Alcool et cancer. Résultats d'une enquête retrospective. Revue Francaise d'Etudes Cliniques et Biologiques 7: 590
Scobie B A, Summerskill W H J 1964 Reduced gastric acid output in cirrhosis: quantitation and relationships. Gut 5: 422–428
Shanbour L L 1980 Effect of alcohol on acid secretion and ion transport in the gastric mucosa. In: Stock C, Sarles H (eds) Alcohol and the gastrointestinal tract. Inserm, Paris, vol 95, p 391–404
Silen W, Skillman J J 1974 Stress ulcer, acute erosive gastritis and the gastric mucosal barrier. Advances in Internal Medicine 19: 195–212
Small M, Longarini A, Zamcheck N 1959 Disturbances of digestive physiology following acute drinking episodes in 'skid-row' alcoholics. American Journal of Medicine 27: 575–585
Steinbert S, Campbell C, Hillman R 1980 Disruption of folate metabolism by alcohol. Alcoholism. Clinical and experimental Research 4: 229
Thomas J, Greig M, McIntosh J, Hunt J, McNeil D, Piper D W 1980 The location of chronic gastric ulcer: a study of the relevance of ulcer size, age, sex, alcohol, analgesic intake and smoking. Digestion 20: 79–84
Verdy M, Caron D 1973 Ethanol et absorption du calcium chez l'humain. Biologie et Gastroenterologie (Paris) 6: 157
Weise R E, Schapiro H, Woodward E R 1961 Effect of parenteral alcohol on gastric secretion. Surgical forum 12: 281
Wienbeck M, Berges W 1980 Does alcohol cause oesophagitis and oesophageal cancer. In: Stock C, Sarles H (eds) Alcohol and the gastrointestinal tract. Inserm, Paris, vol 95, p 405–414
Winship D H, Calflisch C R, Zboralske F F, Hogan W J 1968 Deterioration of esophageal peristalsis in patients with alcoholic neuropathy. Gastroenterology 55: 173–178
Worthington-Roberts B 1980 Changes in intestinal passive permeation induced by alcohol. In: Stock C, Sarles H (eds) Alcohol and the gastrointestinal tract. Inserm, Paris, vol 95, p 507–518
Wynder E L, Bross I J 1961 A study of etiological factors in cancer of the esophagus. Cancer 14: 389–413

12

Odette Guy Henri Sarles

Pancreatic disorders in alcoholism

INTRODUCTION

Alcoholic pancreatitis

Alcoholic pancreatitis may be either chronic or acute.

Alcoholic chronic pancreatitis belongs to the pathological group of calcifying chronic pancreatitis (CCP) which also includes chronic pancreatitis secondary to hypercalcaemia, familial pancreatitis and the tropical form. This group is characterized by pancreatic lesions (Nakamura et al, 1972; Payan et al, 1972) which will be described below. The patchy distribution of the lesions explains why, in the first stages of the disease, clinical symptoms may be evident and pancreatic function may remain normal, the only biological effects being a short-lasting increase of the level of pancreatic enzymes in blood after each attack of pain, and an increased concentration of lactoferrin in pancreatic juice. The lesions of the duct epithelium permit the transudation of serum proteins into pancreatic juice, and explain the increased serum concentration of calcium and albumin, which is not a specific character of CCP. Obstruction of the ducts by precipitates, stones and scars is probably responsible for the attacks of acute pancreatitis superimposed on chronic lesions, for the progressive pancreatic insufficiency and for the frequent formation of cysts and retention pseudocysts (Sarles et al, 1979). Studies which will be described below, carried out on pure pancreatic juice, showed that even in fairly advanced cases, the secretion of protein is normal or increased in those territories which are still functioning. This explains why pancreatic insufficiency is more evident in duodenal juice, which is a mixture of a reduced quantity of a normal juice and of other secretions (bile, duodenal juice), than in pure pancreatic juice collected by endoscopic catheterisation.

Alcoholic acute pancreatitis is mostly observed in chronic alcoholics after paroxysmal increase of consumption (Kager et al, 1972). It is possible that this is only a complication of the chronic form.

Chronic alcohol consumption or associated dietary disorders may lead to other pancreatic disturbances. In the United States of America (Pitchumoni et al, 1980), in contrast to Europe (Sarles, 1973), it is frequently associated with a low protein diet, and pancreatic insufficiency reversed by giving a well-balanced diet may be observed (Mezcy & Potter, 1976). Similarly, in predisposed subjects, alcohol consumption may lead to hyperlipidemia, which is sometimes responsible for acute attacks of pancreatitis (Cameron et al, 1971). These problems will not be studied in this chapter, which will be concerned only with chronic and acute alcoholic pancreatitis.

Human pancreatic secretion

This has been extensively studied. Most of the digestive enzymes have been isolated in their secretory form, active enzymes for lipase, amylase and carboxyl ester hydrolase and inactive precursors or zymogens for chymotrypsinogens, trypsinogens, proelastases and prophospholipase A_2. Procarboxypeptidases A and B have been characterized only in their active forms. The properties of these proteins are well documented in the review of Desnuelle & Figarella (1979). Moreover, for most of them, their concentrations in pancreatic secretion are known (Guy & Figarella, 1981). The determination of their molecular properties using a variety of techniques: DEAE-cellulose chromatography (Figarella et al, 1969), polyacrylamide gel electrophoresis (De Caro et al, 1975), or two dimensional isoelectric focusing/sodium dodecyl sulphate gel electrophoresis (Scheele et al, 1981), now permits an accurate view of the composition of pancreatic juice. Measurement of their specific activities, i.e. the number of enzyme units per mg of protein, is also a good approach to the determination of enzyme levels in pancreatic juice. Besides digestive enzymes, which account for at least 80 percent of secretory proteins, a low level of some non-digestive proteins has been characterized in normal pancreatic secretion. These include serum albumin, immunoglobulins, lactoferrin, 'stone protein' and lysosomal enzymes. Information obtained on normal exocrine pancreatic secretion permits evaluation of the modifications induced by alcohol consumption.

METHODS

Collection of duodenal juice

The simplest way to collect duodenal juice is to use a Lagerlof-type double-lumen tube allowing gastric and duodenal suction at a low pressure. If the tube is provided with a metal gauge, it can be rapidly positioned under fluoroscopic control. To prevent gastric juice from passing down into the duodenum, we use a double-lumen tube provided with a small inflatable balloon which occludes the gastric side of the pylorus. The patient is placed on his left side and a marker injected into the stomach. Contamination of duodenal juice by gastric juice was found in only one third of cases or less (Sarles et al, 1968; Multigner et al, 1981). This technique is absolutely necessary if lactoferrin has to be estimated, because saliva has a high lactoferrin content.

One has to keep in mind that duodenal juice is a mixture of pancreatic juice, bile, gastric juice and sometimes saliva. Though the only source of pancreatic enzymes is the exocrine pancreas, water and bicarbonate originate also from the other sources, especially bile. This explains the results of authors who found an increased secretion of water and bicarbonate in the 'early stage' of chronic pancreatitis (Dreiling et al, 1973), when in pure pancreatic juice in the same patients bicarbonate secretion is decreased (Sahel & Sarles, 1979). Bicarbonate hypersecretion probably originates from the alcoholic liver, as it has been shown that, in such cases, biliary secretion of water and bicarbonate is increased.

Collection of pure pancreatic juice

In our studies, pure pancreatic juice has been collected by two methods, either by cannulation of the main pancreatic duct during the course of biliary or pancreatic surgery, or by endoscopic retrograde catheterization of the main pancreatic duct (ERCP) (Sahel & Sarles, 1979). The patients submitted to ERCP were sedated with diazepam (10 mg intravenously) immediately before the procedure. A side-viewing gastroduodenoscope (JFB_2 Olympus) was inserted, with the patients lying in the prone position. After observation of the papilla of Vater, a standard Teflon catheter, 1.7 mm in diameter with four additional lateral holes close to the tip, was deeply inserted into the main pancreatic duct (25–30 mm). The correct position of the catheter in the pancreatic duct was verified by the aspiration of clear colourless juice. Secretin (0.5 clinical unit/kg) was then injected intravenously as a rapid bolus. Pure pancreatic juice samples were collected by gentle manual aspiration for up to 10 min. At the end of this first 10-min period, cholecystokinin-pancreozymin (CCK-PZ) (3 Crick-Harper-Raper units/kg) was injected intravenously and pancreatic juice was collected as before for an additional 10 min. Secretin and CCK-PZ were purchased from the Gastrointestinal Research Unit, Karolinska Institutet, Stockholm. Each sample of pancreatic juice was collected in an ice-chilled tube. Every sample contaminated with bile or blood was discarded. Protein concentrations were determined by spectrophotometry using an extinction coefficient of $E_{1\,cm}^{1\%}$ = 20 at 280 nm. Bicarbonate concentration was estimated by the Van Slyke method.

Estimation of lactoferrin

Quantitative measurements of lactoferrin were performed by radial immunodiffusion (Figarella et al, 1978; Multigner et al, 1980). Immunoplates LC (low concentration) Partigen lactoferrin, and pure standard lactoferrin (concentration 4 mg/dl) were from Behring Institute, Marburg. The immunoplates contained 12 wells. The wells were filled twice with 20 μl of diluted lactoferrin standard or test sample. Three wells were used for standard lactoferrin (20 μg/ml, 10 μg/ml and 5 μg/ml, respectively). The nine other wells were used for pancreatic juice, diluted with 0.9 per cent isotonic saline up to 10–30 mg of protein/ml. After diffusion for 48 h at room temperature, the immunoplates were washed with isotonic saline for three days. Then the plates were stained for two hours in a solution of 0.1 per cent amidoschwarz (Merck) and then destained with 10 per cent acetic acid. A standard curve was constructed by plotting the square of the diameters of the precipitation rings against lactoferrin concentration, and lactoferrin concentrations of samples of pancreatic juice were read off from this standard curve. The range of visualization of lactoferrin concentrations was about 2–25 μg/ml. When the estimation of lactoferrin was made on duodenal juice, prior protein concentration was necessary and was performed according to Lundh's technique. 9 ml cold (–15°C) absolute alcohol was added to 1 ml duodenal juice. The mixture was kept in crushed ice for 30 minutes and then centrifuged in a refrigerated centrifuge for 15 minutes at 7000 rpm. The supernatant was discarded and the precipitate was dissolved with 0.1 ml isotonic saline solution. This solution was used for lactoferrin assay.

MODIFICATIONS OF EXOCRINE PANCREATIC FUNCTION

In 1978, Renner et al reported an interesting study of three profiles of pure pancreatic secretion collected by ERCP in one patient with a history of chronic alcoholism. When admitted to hospital with acute pancreatitis, the secretory profile of protein differed markedly from that of healthy volunteers, with a high concentration of protein throughout the period of secretin stimulation and the sporadic appearance of free proteolytic activity. After 10 weeks of abstention from alcohol, an apparent recovery to an almost normal protein secretion was observed, but 6 months later, after the patient had resumed drinking alcohol, a new increase in protein concentration was observed, especially during CCK-PZ stimulation. The changes in the three secretory profiles appeared to correlate closely with the stages of the initial disease, remission and resumption of alcohol consumption, and were in agreement with the claimed increase of protein concentration induced by alcohol consumption (Palasciano & Sarles, 1977).

A more extensive study of the modifications of exocrine pancreatic function induced by chronic alcohol consumption was performed by Sahel & Sarles (1979) on pure pancreatic juice collected from 25 patients by ERCP. Patients who never consumed more than a daily mean of 40 g ethanol were called 'non-alcoholic controls' and patients who consumed more than 100 g/day ethanol for at least 5 years were called alcoholic patients. Out of this group, some patients presented with chronic pancreatitis and were called 'alcoholic chronic pancreatitis' and some patients presented with neither clinical symptoms nor radiological or biological signs of chronic pancreatitis and were called 'alcoholic controls'. Differences were observed in protein and bicarbonate concentrations. As shown in Figure 12.1, in two

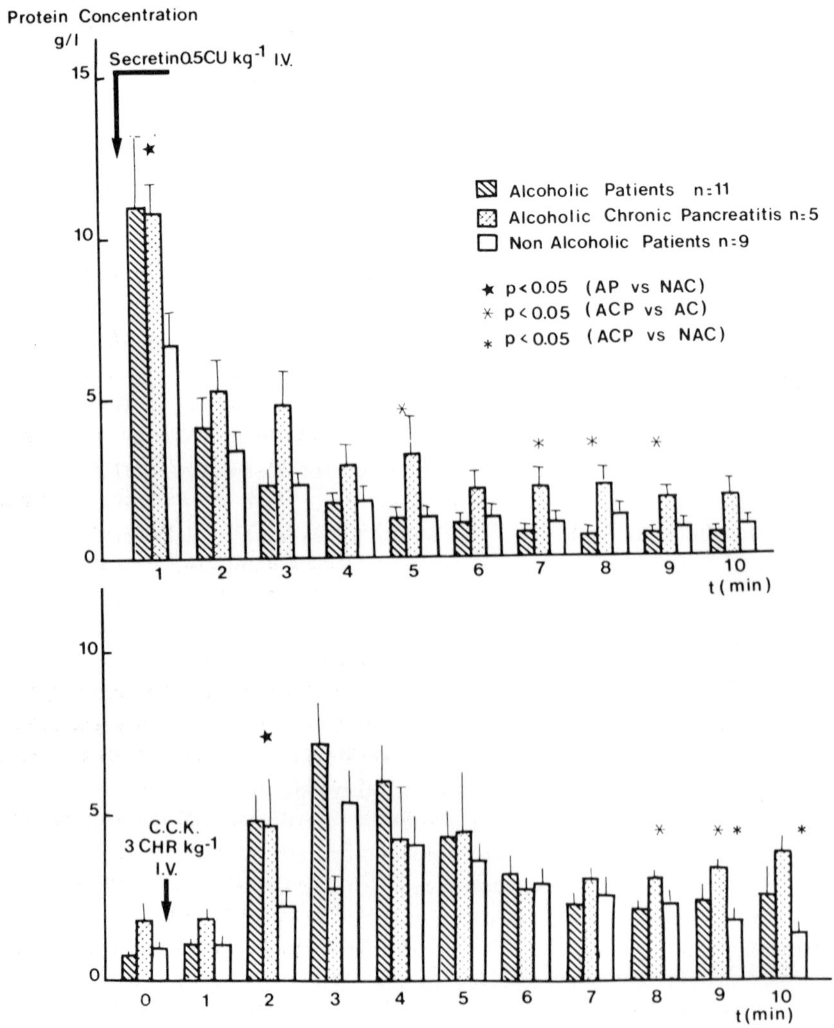

Fig. 12.1 Protein concentration of pancreatic juice collected by ERCP. Columns represent means ± SEM. AC : alcoholic controls; NAC: non-alcoholic controls; AP : alcoholic patients; ACP : alcoholic chronic pancreatitis. Probability, p, was calculated by t-test.

1 minute samples, in the first sample following secretin and in the second sample following CCK stimulation, protein concentration was significantly higher in all alcoholic patients (control and chronic pancreatitis) than in non-alcoholics. The first sample corresponds to the resting secretion and the second one to the hormone effect. These two samples often contain precipitates. In the other samples, the difference between alcoholic and non-alcoholic patients was no longer significant, but in all samples after secretin, protein concentration was higher in alcoholic chronic pancreatitis than in alcoholic controls. When pancreatic secretion had returned to resting rates,

protein concentration was significantly greater in alcoholic chronic pancreatitis than in alcoholic controls in six samples and than in non-alcoholic controls in two samples. Flow rates were similar in alcoholic and non-alcoholic controls, which demonstrates that protein hyperconcentration in alcoholic versus non-alcoholic controls is not due to a decreased secretion of water. Bicarbonate concentration was significantly lower in alcoholic versus non-alcoholic controls in two samples after secretin. This could be due to a direct action of ethanol on duct cells. However, bicarbonate output was not significantly different between alcoholic and non-alcoholic controls. In conclusion, in alcoholic patients the hyper-concentration of protein is not compensated for by a hyper-secretion of water and bicarbonate, but on the contrary, protein and bicarbonate concentrations vary in the opposite direction. The significant increase in protein concentration of alcoholics after CCK stimulation is confirmed by the recent results of Renner et al (1980), but the latter found no statistical difference after secretin stimulation. The differences found by Sahel & Sarles (1979) in protein and bicarbonate concentrations have been observed for pancreatic basal secretion of dogs between animals alcohol-fed for 12–15 months and normal animals (Noel-Jorand et al, 1981).

Since meal-stimulated secretion cannot be studied in man by ERCP, basal and meal-stimulated secretions have been studied after collection of duodenal juice (Planche et al, 1982). After a 30 min basal period a modified Lundh meal (12 per cent protein, 12 per cent carbohydrate and 6 per cent fat in 250 ml of water) was admininistered intragastrically. Chymotrypsin concentration and output were estimated during the basal period and in four 30 min periods following administration of the meal. Chymotrypsin concentration was significantly higher in alcoholics when compared with non-alcoholic patients during the basal state. This difference progressively disappears after a test meal, although in all collections the means of chymotrypsin output remain higher in alcoholics. Therefore, chronic alcohol consumption modifies more basal than meal-stimulated pancreatic secretion, which would not completely agree with the results obtained with hormone-stimulated secretion collected by ERCP. The effect on basal secretion would confirm the modifications induced by secretin stimulation, but the pancreatic secretory response to meal would be different from response to CCK-stimulation.

MODIFICATIONS OF THE COMPOSITION OF PANCREATIC JUICE

Some modifications in the composition of pancreatic juice are induced by alcohol consumption, modifications which become more important in alcoholic chronic pancreatitis. The enzyme activities are modified and the levels of some proteins considered as minor components of normal pancreatic secretion are strongly increased.

Effect of alcohol consumption on enzyme activities

The activities of enzymes in pancreatic juice are not significantly different in alcoholic pancreatitis compared to non-alcoholic controls. Lipase activity was measured directly and potential activities of chymotrypsinogen and trypsinogen were determined after trypsin activation (Colomb et al, 1979a).

Table 12.1 Specific activities of human pancreatic juice (μmol substrate hydrolyzed/min/mg protein)

Enzymes	Non-alcoholic controls n = 8	Alcoholic chronic pancreatitis n = 19
Chymotrypsinogen	50 (42–60)	57 (20–85)
Trypsinogen	36 (30–43)	38 (19–82)
Lipase	247 (130–302)	217 (48–382)

As shown in Table 12.1, specific activities seem similar if the *mean* values are considered. But in fact, in contrast to the pancreatic juice of non-alcoholic patients, which exhibits almost constant specific activities, in pancreatic juice of patients with alcoholic chronic pancreatitis, the values obtained are very dispersed. The same differences are observed in lyophilized pancreatic juice collected from surgery and kept at –20°C and in freshly collected pancreatic juice obtained by ERCP. This eliminates the possibility of a degradation during lyophilisation and storage. These differences can be interpreted as the result of differences in the relative proportions of enzymes or as the result of a more or less selective denaturation of enzymes.

The first hypothesis is supported by Rinderknecht et al (1979a) who found a specific effect of chronic alcohol abuse on the secretory profile of trypsinogens. Human pancreatic juice contains two trypsinogens (Figarella et al, 1969) differing in their isoelectric point but with very close molecular properties (Guy et al, 1978). Trypsinogen 1, the major form, is present in a quantity twice that of trypsinogen 2, which is more anionic and has been often called anionic trypsinogen. The proportion of the two trypsinogens is fairly constant in normal secretion. Rinderknecht et al (1979a) have studied the distribution of the two trypsinogens in the pancreatic juices of 14 healthy normal subjects, 11 chronic alcoholics without detectable pancreatic disease and 15 patients with pancreatitis. The experiment was performed by polyacrylamide gel electrophoresis at pH 8.2 of the one-minute sample showing the highest concentration of trypsinogen after CCK-PZ administration. Trypsinogen was assayed in each gel segment of 0.5 cm section after activation by human enterokinase. As reported by Figarella et al (1969), the proportion of trypsinogen 1 to trypsinogen 2 averaged about 2 in healthy normal subjects, with widely dispersed values. In chronic alcoholics, total trypsinogen concentration of pancreatic juice was much higher than in normal subjects, which is in good agreement with the increase of total protein concentration found in the pancreatic juice of alcoholics. However, these authors also reported a selective increase of trypsinogen 2, leading to a very low ratio trypsinogen 1 to trypsinogen 2 (0.5) in the pancreatic juice of alcoholics. In patients with alcoholic chronic pancreatitis, the results were different, the ratio remained low, close to 0.5, but the increase of trypsinogen 2 lacked statistical significance and, by contrast, trypsinogen 1 was significantly decreased. These results on chronic alcoholics are difficult to explain by the author's suggestions: first an unequal enzyme induction from chronic alcohol abuse with no significant increase of chymotrypsin, elastase and trypsin inhibitor; second, a selective stimulation of the gene coding for trypsinogen 2.

By contrast the results obtained on alcoholic chronic pancreatitis can be supported by the second hypothesis which explains variations of specific activities by a more or less selective denaturation. Chromatography of pancreatic juice on DEAE-cellulose at pH 8.0 in conditions which separate perfectly the two forms of trypsinogen (Figarella et al, 1969), and in the presence of benzamidine, a competitive trypsin inhibitor to prevent any activation during chromatography, give support to this hypothesis. The analysis of pancreatic juice of patients with alcoholic chronic pancreatitis showed a non-selective increase of trypsinogen 2 (Colomb et al, 1981). Some samples gave the same ratio trypsinogen 1 to trypsinogen 2 as normal, equal to 2, some samples gave a decrease of trypsinogen 1 and other samples a decrease of trypsinogen 2. The most important modification in the behaviour of these proteins of pancreatic juice from alcoholic chronic pancreatitis was evidence of a strong association between proteins which were eluted in large peaks with poor separation and a low activity. This abnormal behaviour indicates a partial denaturation of some enzymes. Trypsinogen 1 appeared to be the most sensitive enzyme and, of course, in these conditions, the ratio trypsinogen 1 to trypsinogen 2 decreased strongly below 1, which is in agreement with Rinderknecht's results. But by contrast with the latter, other enzymes seemed easily denaturated: chymotrypsinogen, procarboxypeptidase A and even trypsinogen 2. In addition, the peculiar instability of trypsinogens is well known. On one hand, trypsinogen 1 activates very rapidly (Colomb & Figarella, 1979b) and in the absence of calcium it can be converted into inert proteins devoid of activity. On the other hand, if trypsinogen 2 activates less rapidly, the absence of this form of trypsinogen in 23 pancreatic juices out of 34 studied samples (Robinson et al, 1972) suggests a peculiar instability of this enzyme rather than genetic variation. Therefore, it is reasonable to think that the large variations in enzyme activities, and particularly in trypsinogen activity, are due to a more or less selective denaturation or activation. Of course, these variations are related to the degree of pancreatic pathology and samples from alcoholic chronic pancreatitis are probably those submitted to the most important modifications. However, the hypothesis of a specific effect on one enzyme during alcohol consumption before the onset of pancreatitis remains improbable.

Effect of alcohol consumption on the level of some minor components of pancreatic juice

Serum-type proteins (albumin, immunoglobulins A, G and M)

These represent 1.8 per cent of total proteins in normal pancreatic juice, and are increased to 12.5 per cent in pancreatic juice of patients with chronic calcifying pancreatitis (Clemente et al, 1971). The major serum protein, albumin, is significantly increased in all pancreatic diseases which may be ascribed to lesions of the duct epithelium and transudation of interstitial fluids (Multigner et al, 1980). However, in human pancreatic juices (normal and pathological) the ratio albumin to IgA differs significantly from that in human serum, suggesting a local synthesis of IgA, which has been confirmed by the finding of rare IgA plasma cells in pancreatic tissue (Desnuelle & Figarella, 1979).

Lactoferrin

The presence of lactoferrin was first described in pancreatic juice of patients with CCP (Colomb et al, 1974). Lactoferrin is an iron-binding protein discovered in milk and then found in many external secretions such as mammary, bronchial, nasal, salivary and lachrymal secretions. It is also present in specific granules of neutrophil leukocytes. Lactoferrin has been demonstrated to be present in acinar cells of human pancreas and localized at the ultrastructural level in the zymogen granules and endoplasmic reticulum cisternae (Lechêne et al, 1981a). Lactoferrin concentration is specifically increased in pancreatic juice of patients suffering from CCP; in these patients, the concentration range is from 0.03 to 0.5 per cent of total proteins, approximately ten times higher than in normal subjects or in patients suffering from other pancreatic diseases, whose concentration is below 0.03 per cent. Lactoferrin concentration was measured by radial immunodiffusion, and the results of the analysis of pure pancreatic juice collected from 81 patients make this test valuable for diagnosis of pancreatic disease and in the differentiation of chronic calcifying pancreatitis even in the earliest stage (Multigner et al, 1980). The same diagnostic value was obtained by radioimmunoassay of lactoferrin (Fedail et al, 1978). Less clear cut differences have been obtained from the measurement of lactoferrin in duodenal juice (Multigner et al, 1981). However, it is important to notice that among the CCP patients there is no correlation between the quantity of alcohol ingested and the amount of lactoferrin. Lactoferrin is increased as early as the first clinical stage of the disease. Moreover, 11 patients without CCP and drinking more than 100 g alcohol per day did not present an increase in lactoferrin concentration, which indicates that the increase is linked to the disease and not to alcoholism.

Lysosomal enzymes

The presence of lysosomal enzymes in pure pancreatic juice was reported first by Rinderknecht et al (1979b), who showed that the secretion of lysosomal enzymes follows that of digestive enzymes and is mediated by the same hormone, CCK-PZ. In normal subjects the concentration is low. The most prominent lysosomal enzyme is N-acetyl-β-D glucosaminidase, followed by N-acetyl-β D-galactosaminidase, arylsulfatase, α-L-fucosidase, α-D-mannosidase and β-D-glucuronidase. α-D-glucosidase is in barely detectable amount. In alcoholics, increases as high as 60-fold were observed for arylsulfatase, N-acetyl-β-D-glucosaminidase, β-D-glucuronidase, and leucine naphthylamidase. Recently, Figarella et al (1982) have confirmed the normal presence of these hydrolases in human pancreatic juice. In addition, these authors observed the normal presence of alkaline and acid phosphatases and demonstrated the significant increase of most of the lysosomal enzymes in the juice of men suffering from chronic calcifying pancreatitis. To explain the increased release of lysosomal enzymes in pancreatic juice, a leakage from necrotic cells due to tissue damage, as evoked for serum proteins, seems unlikely since lysosomal enzymes increase both in levels of enzyme and in specific activities (Figarella et al, 1982). Therefore, both results on alcoholics and CCP patients support the hypothesis of a general hyperactivity, an increased synthesis and secretion of lysosomal proteins from pancreatic acinar cells of chronic alcoholics and patients with pancreatitis.

Calcium, citrate, carbohydrates

It has been shown that calcium concentrations in pancreatic juice were not different in alcoholic and non-alcoholic normal people but were increased in alcoholic patients with chronic pancreatitis (Sarles et al, 1980). However, the ratio calcium to protein concentration was not modified, which indicates, as already assumed by Gullo et al (1974) from experiments on duodenal juice, that the increased concentration of calcium is a consequence of pancreatic lesions.

Citrate is normally present in human pancreatic juice and the ratio citrate to protein concentration is decreased in alcoholics, but not significantly (Sarles et al, 1980).

An increase of hexosamine concentration in pure pancreatic juice of chronic pancreatitis (calcifying or non-calcifying) patients during wash-out and secretin phases has been shown by a group of Japanese (Harada et al,

1980), and the increase was significantly higher in alcoholics than non-alcoholics in suspected chronic pancreatitis. The authors supposed that the increase of mucosubstance could cause an increase in viscosity, leading to protein plug formation in the pancreatic ducts.

PANCREATIC LESIONS

Characterization of pancreatic lesions

Pancreatic lesions have been characterized in alcohol-induced pancreatitis. Serial sections of pancreas from the Wirsung duct to the most peripheral acini have permitted a three-dimensional reconstruction of the pancreatic ducts (Nakamura et al, 1972). The observed lesions are not different from those of chronic pancreatitis secondary to hyperparathyroidism, hereditary, idiopathic or tropical chronic pancreatitis. One significant feature is the patchy lobular distribution of the lesions, with the presence of normal lobules in the middle of pathological lobules and the intensity of lesions varying from one lobule to the other. A morphometric study of the fragments devoid of lesions has shown, at the ultrastructural level, some modifications compatible with a hypersecretion of acinar cells compensating for the destroyed inactive cells. The number of zymogen granules is decreased, but the number of prozymogen granules and condensing vacuoles is increased; the number of lysosomes is not significantly changed and residual bodies are decreased. Mitochondria are not modified and the rough endoplasmic reticulum and Golgi apparatus are significantly more dilated (Tasso et al, 1973).

The lesions are characterized by alterations of interlobular ducts with dilatation of the ducts and epithelium atrophy and by the frequency of protein plugs in the ductal lumen. Every possible transitional form of protein precipitate may be present. At one extreme, there is the protein film corresponding to a normal highly concentrated juice, and at the other end of the spectrum there are the mature protein plugs, concentric laminar concentrations of protein, often calcified forming stones. It is reasonable to think that intraductal protein plugs are the first lesion, and it seems evident that they are the first step of stone formation. The characterization of the same protein in precipitates and stones is a convincing argument in favour of this evolution of pancreatic disorders in alcoholic pancreatitis.

Pancreatic plugs and stones

Protein plugs may be found in the pure human pancreatic juice collected by endoscopic retrograde catheterisation of the main pancreatic duct. They are present in basal and/or CCK-stimulated secretion, which shows that they are probably preformed in the ducts and washed out by stimulated juice. In most cases, precipitates are light and very tiny but they often block the

Table 12.2 Frequency of precipitates in pancreatic juice

	Pancreatic juice with precipitates		
Patients (n)	number	%	significance*
Controls (52)	2	3.85	
Alcoholics (33)	7	21.20	<0.05 <0.001
Chronic calcifying pancreatitis			<0.01
alcoholics (15)	10	59.10	
non-alcoholics (7)	3		

*significance was determined by chi² test

flow of juice, making it difficult to collect basal juice. The frequency of precipitates was studied in 107 patients and the results given in Table 12.2 are highly significant (Guy et al, 1982). In normal controls, precipitates are present only in some rare cases (3.8 per cent), which could explain the lesions frequently observed during ageing and resembling those of chronic calcifying pancreatitis. This frequency is considerably increased in chronic patients without pancreatic lesions (21.2 per cent), and the incidence is much higher in patients with CCP (59.1 per cent). It could reach 66 per cent taking into account only alcoholic chronic pancreatitis, but the number of patients is too low to consider the results as significant. Solubilization of these precipitates is not easy. After saline extraction, which contains most proteins of pancreatic juice, the insoluble material is extracted by sodium citrate which has been shown to dissolve pancreatic stones (Lohse et al, 1981). This citrate-soluble fraction contains a small number of proteins (2 to 4 according to the sample) which can be separated by isoelectric focusing. They all have the same molecular weight determined by sodium dodecyl-sulphate gel electrophoresis (13 500) and the isoelectric points are very close, located between 6.3 and 6.8. Inside this family of proteins, the main protein component of pancreatic stone, the 'stone protein' is present. The

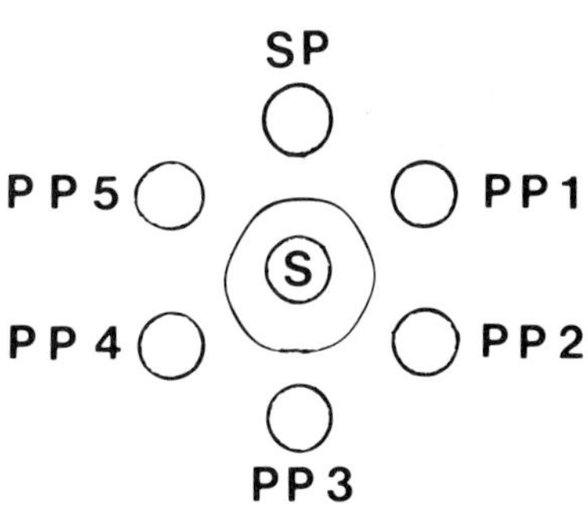

Fig. 12.2 Immunological cross-reactions between stone protein (SP) and proteins extracted from 5 different precipitates (PP). S represents the antiserum against stone protein.

similarity in molecular weight and isoelectric point had suggested its presence, and its immunological identity has been demonstrated using an antiserum to the stone protein (Fig. 12.2). Only the protein content of pancreatic plugs has been studied (Guy et al, 1982).

In pancreatic stones, the presence of calcium carbonate in the form of calcite was first characterized (95.5 per cent by weight) (Périnet et al, 1972). Later, the stone protein was isolated from pancreatic stones obtained at surgery from patients suffering from chronic calcifying pancreatitis (De Caro et al, 1979). The same major protein was found in all stones following extensive extraction by isotonic saline or sodium citrate. It is a glycoprotein rich in aspartic and glutamic acid with a molecular weight of 13 500. Immunological reactions between this protein and different antisera, either to normal or to CCP pancreatic juice, have demonstrated that this protein is a component of normal and CCP pancreatic juices. Immunocytochemical localization using an antiserum to the stone protein has shown that the protein is stored in zymogen granules and secreted by acinar cells, like all pancreatic enzymes (Lechêne et al, 1981b). The protein has not been identified as a known protein of pancreatic juice. It has no enzymatic activity and is immunologically different from chymotrypsinogens, trypsinogens, lipase, phospholipase, amylase and carboxyl ester hydrolase (De Caro et al, 1981).

Possible mechanisms of precipitation

The important modifications observed in the exocrine pancreatic secretion suggest some mechanisms to explain precipitate formation. If some changes are probably a secondary event in the course of the disease and a consequence of lesions (increase of albumin, calcium), some other modifications can play a role in the phenomenon of precipitation. Different mechanisms have been proposed. The raised concentration of mucosubstance has been considered to contribute to precipitate formation (Harada et al, 1980). Partial activation of zymogen has been evoked by Allan & White (1974) as the probable event initiating protein precipitation, and Renner et al (1978) have supported this view. It is well known that activation and hyperconcentration of pancreatic juice are closely related, since the rate of trypsinogen activation increases with trypsinogen concentration and it is not surprising to find free chymotryptic activity in hyperconcentrated samples of pancreatic juice. However, the results obtained until now do not indicate whether obstruction of ductules follows activation of zymogen or activation is secondary to precipitate formation. The importance of lactoferrin, which is known to associate strongly with acidic macromolecules to form complexes (Heckman, 1971), cannot be completely eliminated.

However, the most important factor is certainly the hyperconcentration of proteins, which has been proposed for many years and demonstrated by Sahel & Sarles (1979) and Rinderknecht et al (1979a). The presence of partly denatured enzymes in pancreatic juice also favours the association and aggregation of proteins leading to precipitation. The origin of these structural modifications is not clear, but some variations in the ionic equilibrium, suggested by the decrease of bicarbonate concentration, can play an important part. The role of the 'stone protein' which is present in the first step of lesion formation, precipitates, cannot be omitted. Until now, no quantitative assay of this protein has been performed and no relation can be established between the stone protein concentration in pancreatic juice and the frequency of precipitates. However, it is important to note that we have observed in some Sephadex filtrations of proteins of pancreatic juice a specific precipitation of the low molecular weight protein fraction containing the stone protein after storage for 24 hours at pH 8.0 and +4°C (Figarella & Guy, unpublished data). This result underlines the importance of the stone protein in precipitate formation. Moreover, the same protein content found in precipitates from alcoholics and CCP patients indicates that the mechanism of precipitation is the same in both cases and that only the modifications of pancreatic secretion induced by alcohol consumption may be responsible for pancreatic lesions in chronic calcifying pancreatitis.

BIOCHEMICAL DIAGNOSIS OF ALCOHOLIC PANCREATITIS

There is no specific biological effect of alcoholic pancreatitis. Biochemical methods are necessary to make the diagnosis of chronic (calcifying) pancreatitis or of acute pancreatitis associated with chronic ethanol consumption. It has been shown that there is no statistical threshold of toxicity of alcohol, but a continuous series of individual thresholds, from the lowest ones in predisposed patients who will develop a CCP with alcohol consumption lower than 20 ml of pure alcohol a day, to the highest tolerances (Durbec & Sarles, 1979). Therefore, the frontier between alcoholic pancreatitis and the so called 'idiopathic pancreatitis' is not precise and most 'idiopathic' cases are in reality alcoholic pancreatitis in patients with low ethanol tolerance.

Alcoholic chronic pancreatitis generally presents with irregular recurrent episodes of pain located in the upper half of the abdomen, radiating to the back and lasting more than one day. It begins generally in males, 30 to 45 years old having a large alcoholic intake (Sarles et al, 1979).

As indicated above, during the first months or years of the disease, pancreatic function test may be normal. In that case, some biological consequences are diagnostically useful: (i) a transient increase of any pancreatic enzyme (amylase, pancreatic isoamylases, lipase, trypsin, phospholipase) estimated in serum 24, 48 and 72 hours after the beginning of an attack, (2) an increased concentration of lactoferrin in pancreatic juice (Multigner et al, 1980; Fedail et al, 1978), (sensitivity 80 per cent, specificity 99 per cent) rather than in duodenal juice (sensitivity 52 per cent, specificity 89 per cent) can suggest the existence of CCP. When lactoferrin is normal and serum albumin raised, CCP is not probable, and it is necessary to search for a cause of acute recurrent pancreatitis (gallstones, hyperlipidemia, pancreas divisum, etc.), (3) an increased level of albumin in pure pancreatic juice (Multigner et al, 1980) indicates active pancreatic lesions, either acute or chronic pancreatitis or cancer; when normal, an extrapancreatic cause of pain must be searched for, (4) an abnormal increase of serum pancreatic enzymes after injection of submaximal doses of secretin and CCK-PZ (evocative test) (Howat & Braganza, 1979), may be found months or years before the appearance of clinical pancreatic insufficiency.

Later, during the course of the disease, pancreatic insufficiency demonstrated by duodenal aspiration is a good test. Its sensitivity varies in different centres according to the relative frequency of incipient or of overt forms. It is frequently around 90 per cent (Sarles et al, 1979; Howat & Braganza, 1979), but it is not specific for chronic pancreatitis, being abnormal in pancreatic cancer, transiently after an attack of acute pancreatitis, in diabetes, malnutrition, etc. At this stage, lactoferrin estimation is less useful because pancreatic calcifications are visible frequently on plain X-ray films. Latent diabetes must be searched for by a glucose tolerance test. When pancreatic insufficiency is mild or moderate, it is absolutely useless to estimate steatorrhea. An abnormal fecal fat excretion is only observed in the case of extreme lipase insufficiency (Sarles et al, 1963; Di Magno et al, 1977).

In the late stages, it may be useful to control the efficiency of pancreatic extract therapy by repeated measurement of fecal fat excretion. Steatorrhea must be determined from three days' collections. When the lipid content of diet averages 70–110 g total fat a day, it is not useful to relate fecal fat to ingested fat, since, in this range, fat excretion is not dependent on the quantity of dietary fat (Planche et al, 1961, 1966). As fat excretion continues to decrease for some weeks after the beginning of pancreatic extracts, the effect of treatment must be evaluated after at least 6 weeks.

Different screening tests have been proposed to replace duodenal intubation. As these are generally less sensitive than a careful clinical examination associated with plain X-ray films of the abdomen and an estimation of pancreatic enzymes in serum, they are of little interest. Nevertheless, measurement of the uptake of ^{11}C methionine (Syrota et al, 1981), a safe, easy test, might be a method of the future.

The biochemical diagnosis of alcoholic acute pancreatitis is not different from the biochemical diagnosis of any other types of acute pancreatitis.

CONCLUSION

In conclusion, chronic ethanol consumption modifies exocrine pancreatic secretion. The most important effect is an increased concentration of total proteins and a parallel increased concentration of some minor components of the exocrine pancreatic secretion. This is compatible with a hypersecretion of acinar cells. These modifications are probably the origin of the protein precipitates which may be found in the pancreatic juice of alcoholics and contain, besides a small amount of all secretory proteins, mainly the 'stone protein' isolated from pancreatic stones of patients with chronic calcifying pancreatitis. The frequency of precipitates is considerably increased in the pancreatic juice of patients who develop an alcoholic chronic pancreatitis after many years of alcoholism. At this stage, pancreatic lesions and obstruction of ducts by plugs or calcified stones are responsible for some additional modifications of the exocrine pancreatic secretion. If some of them are non-specific and can be found in other pancreatic diseases, the increase of lactoferrin seems to be specific for chronic calcifying pancreatitis.

REFERENCES

Allan J, White T T 1974 An alternate mechanism for the formation of protein plugs in chronic calcifying pancreatitis. Digestion 11: 428–431

Cameron J L, Crisler C, Margolis S, Demester T R, Zuidema G D 1971 Acute pancreatitis with hyperlipemia. Surgery 70: 53–61

Clemente F, Ribeiro T, Colomb E, Figarella C, Sarles H 1971 Comparaison des protéines de sucs pancreatiques humains normaux et pathologiques. Dosage des protéines sériques et mise en évidence d'une protéine particulière dans la pancréatite chronique calcifiante. Biochimica Biophysica Acta 251: 456–466

Colomb E, Guy O, Sarles H, Figarella C 1979a Activités enzymatiques du suc pancréatique de malades atteints de pancréatite chronique calcifiante. Gastroentérologie Clinique et Biologique 3: 763–768

Colomb E, Figarella C 1979b Comparative studies on the mechanism of activation of the two human trypsinogens. Biochimica Biophysica Acta 571: 343–351

Colomb E, Adrich Z, Guy O, Sarles H, Figarella C 1981 Etude par chromatographie des enzymes de la sécrétion pancréatique de malades atteints de pancréatite chronique calcifiante. Gastroentérologie Clinique et Biologique 5: 12A.

De Caro A, Guy O, Crotte C, Figarella C 1975 Identification des enzymes du suc pancréatique humain sur gel de polyacrylamide. Archives Françaises des Maladies de l'Appareil Digestif 64: 115–123

De Caro A, Lohse J, Sarles H 1979 Characterization of a protein isolated from pancreatic calculi of men suffering from chronic calcifying pancreatitis. Biochemical Biophysical Research Communication 87: 1176–1182

De Caro A, Guy O, Adrich Z, Sarles H 1981 Pancreatic lithogenesis. Gastroenterology 80: 1133

Desnuelle P, Figarella C 1979 Biochemistry. In: Howat H T, Sarles H (eds) The exocrine pancreas. Part I, The normal pancreas. Saunders, Philadelphia, p 86–125

Di Magno E P, Malagelada J R, Go V L N, Amsertel G 1977 Fate of orally ingested enzymes in pancreatic insufficiency. New England Journal of Medicine 296: 1318–1322

Dreiling D A, Greenstein A, Bordalo O 1973 The hypersecretory state of the pancreas. American Journal of Gastroenterology 59: 505–511

Durbec J P, Sarles H and the International Group for the Study of Pancreatic Diseases 1979 A multicentric survey on the etiology of pancreatic diseases. Relationship between the relative risk of developing chronic pancreatitis and alcohol, protein and lipid consumption. Digestion 18: 337–350

Fedail S S, Harvey R F, Salmon P R, Read A E 1978 Radio-immunoassay of lactoferrin in pancreatic juice as a test for pancreatic diseases. Lancet 1: 181–182

Figarella C, Clemente F, Guy O 1969 On zymogens of human pancreatic juice. FEBS Letters 3: 351–353

Figarella C, Estevenon J P, Sarles H 1978 Measurement of lactoferrin in pancreatic juice. Lancet 1: 1105–1106

Figarella C, Vogt E, Hosli P 1982 Alkaline phosphatase and acid lysosomal hydrolases in pancreatic juice and fibroblast cell cultures of patients with chronic calcifying pancreatitis. 28 European Journal of Clinical Investigation. In press

Gullo L, Sarles H, De Barros Mott C, Tiscornia O, Pauli A M, Pastor J 1974 Pancreatic secretion of calcium in healthy subjects and various diseases of the pancreas. Rendiconti Romani di Gastroenterologia 6: 35–44

Guy O, Lombardo D, Bartelt D C, Amic J, Figarella C 1978 Two human trypsinogens. Purification, molecular properties and N-terminal sequences. Biochemistry 17: 1669–1675

Guy O, Figarella C 1981 The proteins of human pancreatic external secretion. Journal of Gastroenterology 16: 59–61

Guy O, Robles-Diaz G, Adrich Z, Sahel J, Sarles H 1982 Protein content of precipitates present in pancreatic ducts. Pancreatic lithogenesis. Submitted to Gastroenterology

Harada H, Takeda M, Yabe H, Hanafusa E, Hayashi T, Kunichika K et al 1980 The hexosamine concentration and output in human pure pancreatic juice in chronic pancreatitis. Gastroenterologica Japonica 15: 520–526

Heckman A M 1971 Association of lactoferrin with other proteins as demonstrated by changes in electrophoretic mobility. Biochimica Biophysica Acta 251: 383–387

Howat H T, Braganza J M 1979 Assessment of pancreatic dysfunction in man. In: Howat H T, Sarles H (eds) The exocrine pancreas. Part II, Investigation of pancreatic disease. Saunders, Philadelphia, p 129–175

Kager L, Lindberg S, Agren G 1972 Alcohol consumption and acute pancreatitis in men. Scandinavian Journal of Gastroenterology 7: 15

Lechêne de la Porte P, Figarella C, Sarles H 1981a Immunocytochemical localization of lactoferrin in human pancreas. Hoppe Seyler's Zeitfehrift fuer Phisiologifche Chemie 362: 1293–1296

Lechêne de la Porte P, De Caro A, Amouric M, Sarles H 1981b Localisation immunocytochimique de la protéine majoritaire des calculs pancréatiques humains. La Nouvelle Presse Médicale 10: 3851

Lohse J, Vérine H, Sarles H 1981 Studies on pancreatic stones, I. In vitro dissolution. Digestion 21: 125–132

Mezey E, Potter J J 1976 Changes in exocrine pancreatic function produced by altered dietary protein intake in drinking alcoholics. Johns Hopkins Medical Journal 138: 7–12

Multigner L, Figarella C, Sahel J, Sarles H 1980 Lactoferrin and albumin in human pancreatic juice: a valuable test for diagnosis of pancreatic diseases. Digestive Diseases and Sciences 25: 173–178

Multigner L, Figarella C, Sarles H 1981 Diagnosis of chronic pancreatitis by measurement of lactoferrin in duodenal juice. Gut 22: 350–354

Nakamura K, Sarles H, Payan H 1972 Three dimensional reconstruction of the pancreatic ducts in chronic pancreatitis. Gstroenterology 62: 942–949

Noel-Jorand M C, Colomb E, Astier J P, Sarles H 1981 Pancreatic basal secretion in alcohol-fed and normal dogs. Digestive Diseases and Sciences 26: 783–789

Palasciano G, Sarles H 1977 Chronic alcoholism and human pancreatic secretion. Irish Journal of Medical Science suppl, October: 34

Payan H, Sarles H, Demirdjian M, Gauthier A P, Cros R C, Durbec J P 1972 Study of the histological features of chronic pancreatitis by correspondance analysis. Identification of chronic calcifying pancreatitis as an entity. Biomedicine 18: 663–670

Perinet G, Vérine H, Lafont R, Haladjian J 1972 Etude thermique de calculs pancréatiques humains et bovins. Comptes Rendus de l'Académie des Sciences 274: 3303–3305

Pitchumoni C S, Sonnenshein M, Candido S M 1980 Nutrition in the pathogenesis of alcoholic pancreatitis. American Journal of Clinical Nutrition 33: 631–636

Planche N E, Delmont J, Sarles H, Greusard C 1961 Action de la quantité des graisses ingérées sur l'excrétion quotidienne moyenne des graisses fécales et l'absorption de la trioléine marquée au ^{131}I. Comptes Rendus des séances de la Société de Biologie 65: 1343–1345

Planche N E, Crotte C, Mulé A, Sarles H 1966 Effets des variations des lipides alimentaires sur l'excrétion fécale des graisses chez le rat. Revue Française d'Etudes Cliniques et Biologiques 11: 931–934

Planche N E, Palasciano G, Meullenet J, Laugier R, Sarles H 1982 Effects of intravenous alcohol on pancreatic and biliary secretion in man. Digestive Diseases and Sciences. In press.

Renner I G, Rinderknecht H, Douglas A P 1978 Profiles of pure pancreatic secretions in patients with acute pancreatitis. The possible role of proteolytic enzymes in pathogenesis. Gastroenterology 75: 1090–1098
Rinderknecht H, Renner I G, Carmack C 1979a Trypsinogen variants in pancreatic juice of healthy volunteers, chronic alcoholics and patients with pancreatitis and cancer of the pancreas. Gut 20: 886–891
Rinderknecht H, Renner I G, Koyama H H 1979b Lysosomal enzymes in pure pancreatic juice from normal healthy volunteers and chronic alcoholics. Digestive Diseases and Sciences 24: 180–186
Renner I G, Rinderknecht H, Valenzuela J E, Douglas A P 1980 Studies of pure pancreatic secretions in chronic alcoholic subjects without pancreatic insufficiency. Scandinavian Journal of Gastroenterology 15: 241–244
Robinson L A, Kim Won J, White T T, Hadorn B 1972 Trypsins in human pancreatic juice. Their distribution as found in 34 specimens. Scandinavian Journal of Gastroenterology 7: 43–45
Sahel J, Sarles H 1979 Modifications of pure human pancreatic juice induced by chronic alcohol consumption. Digestive Diseases and Sciences 24: 897–905
Sarles H, Pastor J, Pauli A M, Barthelemy M 1963 Determination of pancreatic function. Gastroenterologia 99: 279–300
Sarles H, Dani R, Prezelin G, Souville C, Figarella C 1968 Cephalic phase of pancreatic secretion in man. Gut 9: 214–221
Sarles H 1973 An international survey on nutrition and pancreatitis. Digestion 9: 389–403
Sarles H, Sahel J, Staub J L, Bourry J, Laugier R 1979 Chronic pancreatitis. In: Howat H T, Sarles H (eds) The exocrine pancreas. Part III, Diseases of the pancreas. Saunders, Philadelphia, p 402–439
Sarles H, Sahel J, Palasciano G, Capitaine Y, Meullenet J 1980 Alcohol consumption and the human pancreas. Colloque de l'INSERM, Alcohol and the Gastrointestinal Tract 95: 289–314
Scheele G, Bartelt D, Bieger W 1981 Characterization of human exocrine pancreatic proteins by two dimensional isoelectric focusing/sodium dodecyl sulfate gel electrophoresis. Gastoenterology 80: 461–473
Syrota A, Dop-Ngassa M, Cerf M, Paraf A 1981 ^{11}C-L-methionine for evaluation of pancreatic exocrine function. Gut 22: 907–915
Tasso F, Stemmelin N, Sarles H, Clop J, Durbec J P, Cros R C Cornee J 1973 Comparative morphometric study of the human pancreas in its normal state and in primary chronic calcifying pancreatitis. Biomedicine 18: 134–144

13

William Jenkins

Liver disorders in alcoholism

The association between chronic alcohol abuse and cirrhosis has long been recognised, but it is only comparatively recently that ethanol itself, rather than other associated features such as malnutrition, has been regarded as responsible for the liver damage. Evidence incriminating ethanol as the major aetiological factor has come from epidemiological surveys and experimental studies in animals and man.

EPIDEMIOLOGICAL SURVEYS

There is a close correlation between the mortality rate from cirrhosis in different countries and the per capita consumption of ethanol (Schmidt, 1977; Fig. 13.1) but not the nutritional status of the population. Furthermore, the death rate from cirrhosis within a country changes as the alcohol consumption varies. Thus, deaths from cirrhosis fell dramatically in France during the period of wine rationing in the war years (Péquignot, 1974), and in the United States during prohibition. Conversely the mortality rate from cirrhosis increased by 350 per cent in Ontario as alcohol consumption rose from 1.8 litres in 1933 to 8.9 litres in 1967 (Rankin et al, 1975). Because only a minority of alcoholics (8–15 per cent) have cirrhosis on liver biopsy at any given time (Klatskin, 1961), it has been suggested that many alcoholics are protected against the development of cirrhosis (Galambos, 1974). However, the studies of Lelbach (1975) indicate that there is a combined cumulative risk factor for the development of cirrhosis in alcoholics given by the average daily alcohol consumption multiplied by the time of consumption at that level. Above a daily intake of 80 g alcohol the probability of an individual developing cirrhosis increases linearly with time. These studies suggest that all alcoholics are at risk of developing cirrhosis, though the time of heavy consumption required to develop it varies.

EXPERIMENTAL STUDIES

In humans

Daily administration of non-inebriating doses of ethanol to volunteers over a period of 1–3 weeks consistently produces fat accumulation in the liver

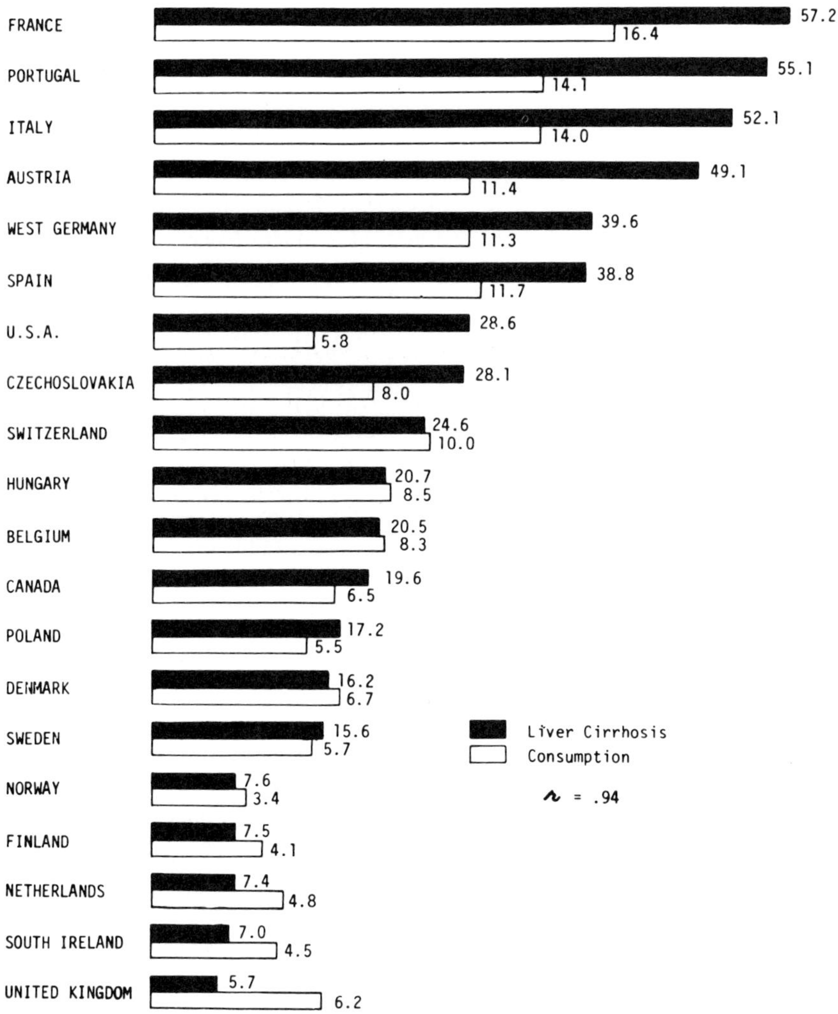

Fig. 13.1 Cirrhosis mortality per 100 000 population 25 years of age and older and alcohol consumption per capita (from Schmidt, 1977).

despite an otherwise nutritionally adequate diet (Rubin & Lieber, 1968). Thus, ethanol ingestion itself, rather than malnutrition, can cause hepatic steatosis, but attempts to produce more advanced alcoholic liver disease in volunteers are obviously not justified, so further studies depend on animal models.

In animals

Chronically ethanol-fed rats were first used to demonstrate the development of fatty liver after 2–3 weeks despite adequate nutrition, so implicating ethanol as the major factor in its pathogenesis (Lieber, Jones & de Carli, 1965). Continuing the ethanol feeding does not cause more serious alcoholic liver damage in rats, possibly because their lifespan is too short for cirrhosis to develop. However, chronically ethanol-fed baboons, which are more comparable to human alcoholics, develop not only fatty liver, but inflammation and cirrhosis as well (Lieber, de Carli & Rubin, 1975). Thus, the whole spectrum of alcoholic liver disease seen in man can be reproduced in baboons by prolonged ethanol feeding. This unequivocally incriminates ethanol rather than malnutrition as the major causal factor.

MECHANISMS OF ALCOHOLIC LIVER DAMAGE

If alcoholic cirrhosis is the result of a single process, it is difficult to understand why it takes several years to develop, since the injurious agent is ingested daily at a constant rate. It is possible that alcoholic liver damage is the result of several processes in series, each with a long half-life, or that the liver damage is produced by a combination of the effects of ethanol and a precipitating factor, which occurs at random independently of alcohol consumption (Orrego, Israel & Blendis, 1981). It is unlikely that the universal changes which occur after ethanol consumption for a very short time, such as fatty liver or mitochondrial enlargement, can be the single cause leading to cirrhosis.

ACUTE METABOLIC EFFECTS OF ETHANOL

The bulk of ethanol ingested has to be metabolised because there is no storage mechanism for ethanol in the body, and because only 2–10 per cent of ethanol consumed is excreted by the lungs and kidneys. Alcohol dehydrogenase (ADH) located in the hepatocyte cytosol is the major enzyme catalysing the oxidation of ethanol to acetaldehyde coupled with the conversion of NAD to $NADH^+$. Reoxidation of $NADH^+$ to NAD is normally the rate-limiting stop in the oxidation of ethanol. As a result there is an accumulation of H^+ and disturbance of the redox potential of the hepatocyte during alcohol metabolism. This is partly counteracted by a shift in a number of secondary reactions in which $NAD/NADH^+$ are also involved. Thus, the lactate/pyruvate ratio shifts in favour of lactate and hyperlactacidaemia results (Lieber et al, 1962a); there is increased lipogenesis (Lieber & Schmid, 1961); and preferential utilisation of ethanol instead of fatty acids as the main fuel for the hepatocytes' mitochondria, and consequently decreased fatty acid oxidation (Ontko, 1973). Many of the metabolic abnormalities seen in alcoholics can be explained by the change in redox potential of the hepatocyte during the metabolism of ethanol:

1. Secondary hyperuricaemia is due to impaired renal excretion of uric acid as a result of lactacidosis (Lieber et al, 1962b). It is well known that excessive alcohol consumption may aggravate or precipitate attacks of gout (Newcombe, 1972).

2. Hypoglycaemia may follow an alcoholic binge in fasted individuals whose liver glycogen stores are depleted (Arky & Freinkel, 1966). This probably occurs because of the shift in the lactate/pyruvate ratio in favour of lactate, so inhibiting one of the initial steps in gluconeogenesis.

3. Acidosis is due to a combination of the hyperlactacidaemia and increased production of ketones because fatty acid oxidation is decreased (Levy et al, 1973).

4. Hepatic steatosis occurs because the availability of both fatty acids and α-glycerophosphate, which are the precursors of triglyceride, increases as a result of the redox potential change during ethanol oxidation.

METABOLIC CHANGES FOLLOWING CHRONIC ETHANOL CONSUMPTION

Proliferation of the smooth endoplasmic reticulum is a striking feature seen on electron microscopy of hepatocytes from either chronically ethanol-fed animals (Iseri, Lieber & Gottlieb, 1966) or human subjects (Lane & Lieber, 1966). The biochemical counterpart of this morphological change is an increase in many microsomal enzymes including cytochrome P_{450} (Rubin, Hutterer & Lieber, 1968), microsomal γ-glutamyltransferase (Ishii et al, 1976), and various drug-detoxifying enzymes (Joly et al, 1973). Ohnishi and Lieber (1977) have described a combination of cytochrome P_{450} reductase and phospholipids in vitro which has the characteristics of the microsomal ethanol-oxidising system (MEOS) in vivo. Stimulation of such microsomal enzyme systems by chronic alcohol intake may have several clinically important consequences.

1. Ethanol tolerance is increased after chronic ethanol intake. This is partly due to adaptation of the central nervous system (Noble & Tewari, 1977), but the rate of ethanol metabolism also increases by up to 100 per cent (Hawkins, Kalant & Khanna, 1966). It falls to normal again within 14 days of alcohol withdrawal. The cause of the increased rate of ethanol metabolism is controversial. Lieber & DeCarli (1970) have suggested that it is due to an increase in microsomal mass and MEOS activity, whereas other studies suggest that it is a result of increased reoxidation of $NADH^+$ and greater oxygen utilisation by mitochondria (Videla, Bernstein & Israel, 1973). This is thought to be brought about by an increase in ATP hydrolysis at the hepatocyte plasma membrane, so increasing the availability of ADP for phosphorylation in the mitochondria permitting oxidation of of more $NADH^+$.

2. Chronic alcoholics are often resistant to the effects of drugs such as the tranquilisers and sedatives. This is at least partly due to an increase in the rate of their metabolism by microsomal enzymes induced by ethanol. Conversely these drugs may be potentiated in the presence of alcohol, because it inhibits their metabolism by competing with them. Other compounds are converted to toxic metabolites by the liver microsomes, and microsomal enzyme induc-

tion by alcohol may explain the increased toxicity of carbon tetrachloride (CCl_4) and paracetomol (acetaminophen) in chronic alcoholics.

3. An increase in triglyceride synthesis results partly from the increased availability of fatty acids and α-glycero-phosphate during ethanol metabolism, but alcohol also appears to stimulate lipid synthesis by the induced microsomes (Baraona et al, 1973). Hepatic L-α-glycerophosphate acyltransferase activity increases after chronic ethanol consumption.

4. The microsomal oxidation of ethanol is not linked to phosphorylation of ADP but only generates heat. If this exceeds that needed to maintain body temperature, the energy released by ethanol oxidation is wasted. This led to the concept of the 'empty' calories of alcohol, and may explain why volunteers fed 2000 kcal daily as alcohol as well as their normal diet failed to gain weight.

ROLE OF ACETALDEHYDE

The first product of ethanol oxidation in the liver is acetaldehyde, which is further oxidised to acetate by hepatic aldehyde dehydrogenase. Since $NADH^+$ is also generated by this reaction, the oxidation of acetaldehyde may potentiate the redox changes produced during ethanol oxidation as discussed previously.

Since it is a highly reactive toxic compound, acetaldehyde has been incriminated in the pathogenesis of alcohol-induced liver damage. Several mechanisms have been postulated. Acetaldehyde binds non-enzymatically to phospholipids (Kenney, 1980), amino groups of amino acid residues and sulfhydryl groups (Lindros, 1978). By binding with constituent proteins acetaldehyde may produce neoantigens and activate cytotoxic lymphocytes directed against the liver (Kakumu & Leevy, 1977).

Lipid peroxides and free radicals, which are thought to cause the liver damage in CCl_4 and paracetamol (acetaminophen) poisoning, are also generated during ethanol metabolism. Glutathione normally serves as a free radical scavenger and protects against such damage. However, large doses of ethanol reduce hepatic glutathione levels. This is probably due to acetaldehyde complexing with L-cysteine to form a hemiacetal. Thus, in alcohol-fed animals large amounts of free radicals may be produced because of increased microsomal mass which, when combined with reduced glutathione levels, may result in hepatotoxicity.

Another effect of ethanol, which is probably mediated by acetaldehyde, is the alteration in synthesis and secretion of liver proteins. The secretion of newly synthesised glycoproteins and albumin is inhibited by alcohol in vitro and in vivo (Tuma, Zetterman & Sorell, 1980). Acetaldehyde is thought to be responsible since this effect is abolished by pyrazole, which inhibits acetaldehyde formation, and is mimiced by the addition of acetaldehyde. It appears that acetaldehyde does this through an effect on the micro-tubules, which facilitate protein export from the hepatocyte. The microtubules have been reported to be shorter and thicker after ethanol administration (Matsuda et al, 1979).

IMMUNOLOGICAL MECHANISMS

The hypothesis that the immune response plays a part in the production of perpetuation of alcoholic liver disease rests on the concept that lymphocytes are sensitised to antigenic components in the liver. Mallory's hyaline may be one of several neoantigens, which activate a humoral and cellular immune reaction (Leevy et al, 1976). However, the role of Mallory's hyaline or other immune mechanisms as the initial cause of liver damage is not established. The immunological abnormalities seen in alcoholic liver disease may be epiphenomena. Mallory's hyaline is not specific for alcoholic liver disease, and its presence does not appear to be related to the severity or prognosis of the disease. Nevertheless, immunological mechanisms may perpetuate the alcohol-induced liver injury, particularly in alcoholic hepatitis where circulating lymphocytes, which are cytotoxic against autologous liver cells, are frequently found (Paronetto & Lieber, 1976).

HISTOLOGY OF ALCOHOLIC LIVER DISEASE

Fatty liver

This is the single most common lesion. It may also be seen with the more advanced lesions of alcoholic hepatitis, fibrosis and cirrhosis. The hepatocytes are swollen not only because of the accumulation of fat, but also because of retention of export proteins and water, which contribute to the hepatomegaly. Fatty liver alone is a benign lesion, and is readily reversible on abstinence (Rubin & Lieber, 1968). Its presence usually indicates recent drinking.

Alcoholic hepatitis

This is characterised by hepato-cellular necrosis and in infiltration with polymorphonuclear leucocytes. It may be superimposed on an established cirrhosis. The lesions are usually concentrated in the centribolbular areas around the hepatic veins, where the oxygen tension is lowest, but they may be more diffuse in severe cases. Mallory's hyaline is often seen within some hepatocytes, but its presence is not pathognomonic of alcoholic hepatitis. In some cases, sclerosis around the central vein and obliteration of the lumen is seen, and this may cause some portal hypertension even before cirrhosis has developed (Goodman & Ishak, 1982).

Cirrhosis

This represents an irreversible stage in the spectrum of alcoholic liver disease. The features which suggest but do not prove an alcoholic aetiology are concomitant fatty infiltration, haemosiderosis and Mallory's hyaline.

Primary hepatocellular carcinoma

This is a late complication of alcoholic cirrhosis. The incidence has been reported to be as high as 30 per cent (Krasner et al, 1976). Hepatomas develop most often in male alcoholics, who have abstained and so survived long enough to develop neoplastic change. Recently it has been suggested that hepatitis B virus infection may play a part in the pathogenesis of hepatomas in alcoholic cirrhosis. In a French series (Bréchot et al, 1982) of 20 patients, hepatitis B virus DNA was integrated into the genome of the neoplastic liver cells in all cases, though only 9 of the 16 tested had serological markers of hepatitis B virus infection.

THE PROGRESSION OF ALCOHOLIC LIVER DISEASE

Although the risk of developing alcoholic cirrhosis is related to the total amount of alcohol consumed (Lelbach, 1975), it is estimated that only about one third of alcoholics will do so. Other factors which may increase the susceptibility to develop cirrhosis have been invoked. A genetic predisposition has been suggested, perhaps mediated via differences in alcohol and acetaldehyde metabolism (Jenkins & Thomas, 1981), or by variations in the immune response associated with certain HLA antigens, which could perpetuate liver damage initiated by alcohol. However, despite extensive polymorphism of alcohol dehydrogenase and acetaldehyde dehydrogenase, no particular isozyme or group of isozymes has been shown to be associated with a predisposition to develop alcoholic liver disease. Furthermore, the numerous studies of association between certain HLA antigens and alcoholic cirrhosis have given conflicting results, and later larger surveys with better control populations have not confirmed that any such association exists (Faizallah et al, 1982). Thus, no biochemical or immunological marker which will identify alcoholics particularly at risk of developing serious liver damage has yet been demonstrated, so this largely depends on the early recognition of precirrhotic lesions.

Alcoholic hepatitis has long been thought to be a necessary precursor of cirrhosis (Schaffner & Popper, 1970), and it has been claimed that it may rapidly progress to cirrhosis even though patients have abstained (Galambos, 1972). Sclerosis around the terminal hepatic vein is thought to predict progression to cirrhosis if drinking continues, even in the absence of overt alcoholic hepatitis (Nakano, Warner & Lieber, 1982), though this latter suggestion is controversial.

CLINICAL FEATURES OF ALCOHOLIC LIVER DISEASE

Symptoms and clinical signs in alcoholic liver disease are extremely variable, but they tend to increase as liver injury progresses. In patients with alcoholic fatty liver, smooth hepatomegaly is often the only abnormal finding on clinical examination.

The diagnosis of alcoholic hepatitis was originally restricted to severely ill patients with tender enlarged livers often with an audible bruit, fever, jaundice, ascites, anorexia and encephalopathy frequently progressing to coma and death (Beckett et al, 1961). However, it was quickly realised that the typical histological changes of alcoholic hepatitis, which were believed to predict progression to cirrhosis, were often found in patients with minimal and non-specific clinical symptoms such as anorexia, nausea and lethargy. Although severe symptoms are usually associated with marked histological changes, the converse is not always true, and extensive necrosis may also be seen in patients with minimal clinical abnormalities. Thus, the clinical picture of alcoholic hepatitis ranges from a nearly asymptomatic disorder to a fulminant fatal disease.

Patients with established cirrhosis may present for the first time with one or more of its complications such as bleeding from oesophageal varices secondary to portal hypertension, or with ascites without acute alcoholic hepatitis ever having been recognised histologically or clinically. The picture resembles other types of end-stage liver disease. Only the history of alcohol abuse, hepatomegaly and other associated features of alcoholism point to the aetiology. These include bilaterally enlarged parotids, testicular atrophy and muscle wasting. Dupuytren's contracture of the palmar fascia is related to the alcoholism rather than to cirrhosis. Loss of memory and concentration, irritability, hallucinations, convulsions and tremor may also be stigmata of alcoholism, but it is important to distinguish this picture from that of early hepatic precoma.

BIOCHEMICAL TESTS IN THE DIAGNOSIS OF ALCOHOLIC LIVER DISEASE

Although a history of regular consumption of more than 80 g alcohol daily in men and 60 g daily in women suggests alcohol as a possible cause of liver disease, drinking histories are notoriously unreliable and many alcoholics will exceed these amounts without developing serious liver damages. Thus, biochemical tests are needed which will identify alcohol as the cause of liver disease; detect liver damage in alcoholics; and stage alcoholic liver disease and the extent of liver cell necrosis, as these are important prognostic factors. Unfortunately no specific biochemical test of identifying alcoholic liver disease exists. The plasma ratio of α-amino-n-butyric acid to leucine is raised in many chronic alcoholics (Shaw, Stimmel & Lieber, 1976) and was thought to be diagnostic, but a later study (Morgan, Milson & Sherlock, 1977) showed that it was a relatively non-sensitive index of hepatocellular damage rather than of alcoholism.

The serum aspartate transaminase (AST, GOT) and alanine transaminase (ALT, GPT) are common screening tests indicating liver damage. Both are frequently raised in alcoholic liver disease, but they are relatively insensitive, and are a poor reflection of liver cell necrosis as shown on liver biopsy

(Kallai et al, 1964). The serum AST may be elevated in alcoholics even when hepatic steatosis is the only histological abnormality (Kontinnen, Hartel & Louhija, 1970). Conversely in alcoholic hepatitis the serum transaminases are only moderately elevated, and normal values are occasionally found (Beckett, Livingstone & Hill, 1961). It is possible that the elevated serum AST found in alcoholics with fatty liver may not simply be a result of enzyme leakage from damaged hepatocytes, but may at least partly be due to an increased specific activity of AST in the liver mitochondria (Jenkins & Peters, 1978). In alcoholic cirrhosis with or without alcoholic hepatitis lower than normal specific activities of AST and particularly ALT have been found in liver biopsies (Matloff, Selinger & Kaplan, 1980). This may explain why the serum AST/ALT ratio is often greater than two in alcoholic hepatitis and cirrhosis (Cohen & Kaplan, 1979), and is thought to distinguish alcoholic liver damage from other causes of liver injury.

Serum γ-glutamyltransferase (GGT) is a more sensitive marker for alcoholic liver disease (Rosalki & Rau, 1972), but again it is neither specific nor a reliable marker of liver cell necrosis (Wu et al, 1976). The elevation of serum GGT in chronic alcoholics may reflect enzyme induction (Rosalki et al, 1972; Ishii et al, 1976) as well as liver cell damage.

The serum level of glutamate dehydrogenase (GDH) might be expected to provide a more reliable index of liver damage in alcoholics, since its activity in the liver is very much higher than in other organs (Schmidt & Schmidt, 1962). Also, it is concentrated in the centrilobular zones of the liver, where alcohol exerts its greatest toxic effects (Guder et al, 1975), and within the hepatocytes it is found exclusively in mitochondria, which are thought to be damaged early in the course of alcoholic liver disease (Svoboda & Manning, 1964). In a study of 100 alcoholic patients, Van Waes & Lieber (1977) claimed that the serum activity of GDH reliably reflects liver cell necrosis, and that a serum value two and a half times the normal value indicates alcoholic hepatitis. For these reasons they suggested that serum GDH activity should be estimated routinely in alcoholics. However, the

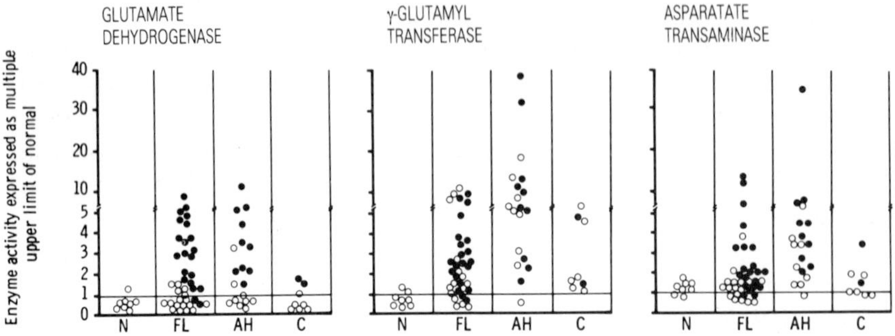

Fig. 13.2 Serum GDH, GGT and AST in alcoholic patients grouped by liver biopsy histology (● > 80 g ethanol/day before biopsy; ○ < 80 g ethanol/day before biopsy) (from Jenkins et al, 1982).

possibility that recent alcohol consumption may increase the serum GDH independently of the histological change was not investigated. GDH activity is considerably raised in liver biopsies from recently drinking patients with alcoholic steatosis (Jenkins & Peters, 1978), and a subsequent study (Jenkins et al, 1982) showed that recent heavy alcohol consumption increased the serum activity of GDH independently of the hepatic histological change (Fig. 13.2). Since a high serum activity of GDH in alcoholics may result not only from liver cell necrosis, but also from recent alcohol excess, it is not a reliable marker of the former. In addition its lower sensitivity compared with serum AST and serum GGT limits its value for identifying and monitoring the progress of alcoholic liver disease.

Thus, assay of the activities of these enzymes in serum does not permit an accurate diagnosis or staging of alcoholic liver disease, which depends on a combination of characteristic clinical and histological features as well as consistent changes in serum biochemical tests. Perhaps the most important diagnosis to make is that of alcoholic hepatitis, where the combination of fever, jaundice, right upper quadrant pain, with moderately elevated serum transaminases, a leucocytosis and high serum alkaline phosphatase may mimic extrahepatic obstruction (Mikkelsen et al, 1968). The distinction between alcoholic hepatitis, a medical condition, and extrahepatic obstruction, a surgical entity, is important since the mortality of laparotomy in patients with alcoholic hepatitis is high (Greenwoodet al, 1972). An ultrasound examination of the liver and gallbladder to look for a dilated biliary system is probably the investigation of choice to exclude extrahepatic obstruction, but evidence of hepatic dysfunction, such as a low serum albumin and a prolonged prothrombin time not corrected by systemic vitamin K administration also helps to exclude extra-hepatic obstruction, and is more consistent with alcoholic hepatitis. Other non-specific serum changes in acute and chronic alcoholism include elevations in uric acid, lactate, triglyceride and reduction in glucose, phosphate and magnesium.

In alcoholic cirrhosis the most striking biochemical abnormalities are elevations of the serum proteins particularly in the β-γ fraction on electrophoresis, and elevation of the immunoglobulins particularly IgA (Aron et al, 1971). Conventional serum tests of liver function are altered to a variable extent depending on the degree of hepatic dysfunction, but again are not specific for an alcoholic aetiology of the cirrhosis. However, an elevated alkaline phosphatase without evidence of cholestasis, and continuous presence of α-fetoprotein in the blood are suggestive of the development of a hepatoma (Van Waes et al, 1976).

REFERENCES

Arky R A, Freinkel N 1966 Alcohol hypoglycaemia, V. Alcohol infusion to test gluconeogenesis in starvation with special reference to obesity. New England Journal of Medicine 274: 426–433

Aron E, Lamy J N, Lamy L, Weill J D 1971 Le depistage de la cirrhose alcoohique du foie par le dosage immunologique des IgA et de la transferrine. Presse Medicale 79: 357–358

Baraona E, Pirola R C, Lieber C S 1973 Pathogenesis of postprandial hyperlipemia in rats fed ethanol-containing diets. Journal of Clinical Investigation 52: 296–303

Beckett A G, Livingstone A V, Hill K R 1961 Acute alcoholic hepatitis. British Medical Journal 2: 1113–1119

Bréchot C et al 1982 Evidence that hepatitis B virus has a role in liver cell carcinoma in alcoholic liver disease. New England Journal of Medicine 306: 1384–1387

Cohen J A, Kaplan M M 1979 The SGOT/SGPT ratio — an indicator of alcoholic liver disease. American Journal of Digestive Diseases 24: 835–838

Faizallah R, Woodrow J C, Krasner N K, Walker R J, Morris A I 1982 Are HLA antigens important in the development of alcohol-induced liver disease? British Medical Journal 285: 533–535

Galambos J T 1972 Natural history of alcoholic hepatitis. 3. Histological changes. Gastroenterology 63: 1026–1035

Galambos J T 1974 Alcoholic hepatitis. In: Schaffner F, Sherlock S, Leevy C M (eds) The liver and its diseases. Intercontinental Medical Book Corporation, New York, p 255–267

Goodman Z D, Ishak K G 1982 Occlusive venous lesions in alcoholic liver disease. A study of 200 cases. Gastroenterology 83: 786–796

Greenwood S M, Leffler C T, Minkowitz S 1972 The increased mortality rate of open liver biopsy in alcoholic hepatitis. Surgery, Gynaecology and Obstetrics 134: 600–604

Guder W G, Habicht A, Kleissl J et al 1975 The diagnostic significance of liver cell inhomogeneity: serum enzymes in patients with central liver necrosis and the distribution of glutamate dehydrogenase in normal liver. Zeitschrift fur Klinische Chemie und Klinische Biochemie 4: 70–75

Hawkins R D, Kalant H, Khanna J M 1966 Effects of chronic intake of ethanol on rate of ethanol metabolism. Canadian Journal of Physiology and Pharmacology 44: 241–257

Iseri O A, Lieber C S, Gottlieb L S 1966 The ultrastructure of fatty liver induced by prolonged ethanol ingestion. American Journal of Pathology 48: 535–555

Ishii et al 1976 Hepatic gamma glutamyl transpeptidase (GGTP) activity: its activation by chronic ethanol administration. Gastroenterology 71: 913

Jenkins W J, Peters T J 1978 Mitochondrial enzyme activities in liver biopsies from patients with alcoholic liver disease. Gut 19: 341–344

Jenkins W J, Thomas H C 1981 Genetic factors in determining susceptibility to alcohol dependence and development of alcohol-induced liver disease. Clinics in Gastroenterology 10: 307–314

Jenkins W J, Rosalki S B, Foo Y, Scheuer P J, Nemesanszky E, Sherlock S 1982 Serum glutamate dehydrogenase is not a reliable marker of liver cell necrosis in alcoholics. Journal of Clinical Pathology 35: 207–210

Joly J G, Ishii H, Teschke R, Hasumura Y, Lieber C S 1973 Effect of chronic ethanol feeding on the activities and submicrosomal distribution of reduced nicotinamide adenine dinucleotide phosphate-cytochrome P-450 reductase and the demethylases for aminopyrine and ethylmorphine. Biochemical Pharmacology 22: 1532–1535

Kakumu S, Leevy C M 1977 Lymphocyte cytotoxicity in alcoholic hepatitis. Gastroenterology 72: 594–597

Kallai L, Mahn A, Roder V, Zupanic V 1964 Correlation between histological findings and serum transaminase values in chronic diseases of the liver. Acta Medica Scandinavica 175: 49–56

Kenney W C 1980 Interaction of acetaldehyde with phospholipids. Gastroenterology 79: 1030

Klatskin G 1961 Alcohol and its relation to liver damage. Gastroenterology 41: 443–451

Kontinnen A, Hartel G, Louhija A 1970 Multiple serum enzyme analyses in chronic alcoholics. Acta Medica Scandinavica 188: 257–264

Krasner N, Johnson P, Bomford A, Eddleston A L W F, Williams R 1976 Hepatoma in chronic liver disease. Gut 17: 390

Lane B P, Lieber C S 1966 Ultrastructural alterations in human hepatocytes following ingestion of ethanol with adequate diets. American Journal of Pathology 49: 593–603

Leevy C M, Chen T, Luisada-Opper A, Kanagasundaram N, Zetterman R 1976 Liver disease of the alcoholic: role of immunologic abnormalities in pathogenesis, recognition,

and treatment. In: Popper H, Schaffner F (eds) Progress in liver diseases. Grune & Stratton, New York, vol 5, p 516–530
Lelbach W K 1975 Cirrhosis in the alcoholic and its relation to the volume of alcohol abuse. Annals of the New York Academy of Sciences 252: 85–105
Levy L J, Duga J, Girgis M, Gordon E E 1973 Ketoacidosis associated with alcoholism in nondiabetic subjects. Annals of Internal Medicine 78: 213–219
Lieber C S, Schmid R 1961 The effect of ethanol on fatty acid metabolism; stimulation of hepatic fatty acid synthesis in vitro. Journal of Clinical Investigation 40: 394–399
Lieber C S Leevy C M, Stein S W, George W S, Chemick G R, Abelmann W H, Davidson C S 1962a Effect of ethanol on plasma free fatty acids in man. Journal of Laboratory and Clinical Medicine 59: 826–832
Lieber C S, Jones D P, Losowsky M S, Davidson C S 1962b Interrelation of uric acid and ethanol metabolism in man. Journal of Clinical Investigation 41: 1863–1870
Lieber C S, Jones D P, DeCarli L M 1965 Effects of prolonged ethanol intake: production of fatty liver despite adequate diets. Journal of Clinical Investigation 44: 1009–1021
Lieber C S, DeCarli L M 1970 Hepatic microsomal ethanol-oxidising system in vitro characteristics and adaptive properties in vivo. Journal of Biological Chemistry 245: 2505–2512
Lieber C S, DeCarli L M, Rubin E 1975 Sequential Production of fatty liver, hepatitis and cirrhosis in sub-human primates fed ethanol with adequate diets. Proceedings of the National Academy of Sciences 72: 437–441
Lindros K O 1978 Acetaldehyde: its metabolism and role in the actions of alcohol. In: Israel Y et al (eds) Research advances in alcohol and drug problems. Plenum, New York, vol 4, p 111–176
Matloff D S, Selinger M J, Kaplan M M 1980 Hepatic transaminase activity in alcoholic liver disease. Gastroenterology 78: 1389–1392
Matsuda Y, Baraona E, Saluspuro M, Lieber C S 1979 Effects of ethanol on liver microtubules and Golgi apparatus. Possible role in altered hepatic secretion of plasma proteins. Laboratory Investigation 41: 455–463
Mikkelsen W P, Turrill F L, Kern W H 1968 Acute hyaline necrosis of the liver. A surgical trap. American Journal of Surgery 116: 266–272
Morgan M Y, Milson J P, Sherlock S 1977 Ratio of plasma alpha amino-n-butyric acid to leucine as an empirical marker of alcoholism: diagnostic value. Science 197: 1183–1185
Nakano M, Worner T M, Lieber C S 1982 Perivenular fibrosis in alcoholic liver injury: ultrastructure and histological progression. Gastroenterology 83: 777–785
Newcombe D S 1972 Ethanol metabolism and uric acid. Metabolism 21: 1193–1203
Noble E P, Tewari S 1977 In: Lieber C S (ed) Metabolic aspects of alcoholism. University Park Press, Baltimore, p 149
Ohnishi K, Lieber C S 1977 Reconstitution of the microsomal ethanol-oxidising system. Journal of Biological Chemistry 252: 7124–7131
Ontko J A 1973 Effects of ethanol on the metabolism of free fatty acids in isolated liver cells. Journal of Lipid Research 14: 78–86
Orrego H, Israel Y, Blendis L M 1981 Alcoholic liver disease: information in search of knowledge? Hepatology 3: 267–283
Paronetto F, Lieber C S 1976 Cytotoxicity of lymphocytes in experimental alcoholic liver injury in the baboon. Proceedings of the Society for Experimental Biology and Medicine 153: 495–497
Péquignot 1974 Les problemes nutritionnelles de al societee industrielle. Vie Medicale au Canada Francais 3: 216–225
Rankin J G, Schmidt W, Popham R E, De Lint J E 1975 Epidemiology of alcoholic liver disease: Insights and problems. In: Khanna J M, Israel Y, Kalant H (eds) Alcoholic liver pathology. Addiction Research Foundation, Toronto, p 31–41
Rosalki S B, Rau D 1972 Serum γ-glutamyl transpeptidase activity in alcoholism. Clinica Chimica Acta 39: 41–47
Rosalki S B, Rau D, Tarlow, D, Baylis E M 1972. Gamma glutamyl transpeptidase elevation in alcoholics and in patients receiving enzyme — inducing drugs Scandinavian Journal of Clinical and habiratory investigation 29, Supplement 126. Abstract 2-.15
Rubin E, Hutterer F, Lieber C S 1968 Ethanol increases hepatic smooth endoplasmic reticulum and drug-metabolizing enzymes. Science 159: 1469–1470

Rubin E, Lieber C S 1968 Alcohol-induced hepatic injury in non alcoholic volunteers. New England Journal of Medicine 278: 869–876
Schaffner F, Popper H 1970 Alcoholic hepatitis in the spectrum of ethanol-induced liver injury. Scandinavian Journal of Gastroenterology Suppl 7: 69–78
Schmidt E, Schmidt F W 1962 Methods and value of determination of glutamic acid dehydrogenase activity in the serum. A contribution to the importance of examination of enzyme relations in the serum. Klinische Wochenschrift 40: 962–969
Schmidt W 1977 The epidemiology of cirrhosis of the liver. In: Fisher M M, Rankin J G (eds) Alcohol and the liver. Plenum, New York, pl
Shaw S, Stimmel B, Lieber C S 1976 Plasma alpha amino n-butyric acid to leucine ratio: an empirical biochemical marker of alcoholism. Science 194: 1057–1058
Svoboda D J, Manning R T 1964 Chronic alcoholism with fatty metamorphosis of the liver. Mitochondrial alterations in hepatic cells. American Journal of Pathology 44: 645–652
Tuma D J, Zetterman R K, Sorrell M F 1980 Inhibition of glycoprotein secretion by ethanol and acetaldehyde in rat liver slices. Biochemical Pharmacology 29: 35–38
Van Waes L, Van Holder R, Van Maele V, Demeulenaere L 1976 Hepatocellular carcinoma. Evaluation of different diagnostic procedures in 13 cases, with a special note on alpha 1-fetoprotein. Acta Clinica Belgica 31(1): 9–15
Van Waes L, Lieber C S 1977 Glutamate dehydrogenase: a reliable marker of liver cell necrosis in the alcoholic. British Medical Journal 2: 1508–1510
Videla L, Bernstein J, Israel Y 1973 Metabolic alterations produced in the liver by chronic ethanol administration. Increased oxidative capacity. Biochemical Journal 134: 507–514
Wu A, Slavin G, Levi A J 1976 Elevated serum gamma-glutamyl-transferase (transpeptidase) and histological liver damage in alcoholism. American Journal of Gastroenterology 65: 318–323

Richard Fink

The effects of alcohol on endocrine function

In this chapter, effects of alcohol of clinical importance will be emphasised. For information concerning the effects on human and animal endocrine physiology, the review of Gordon & Southern (1977) should be consulted.

ADRENO-CORTICAL FUNCTION

Generally, chronic excess alcohol consumption is associated with adreno-cortical overactivity, although some studies have reported impaired function resulting from either primary or secondary adreno-cortical disorder. This spectrum of abnormal function will be considered under the following headings:

1. Adreno-cortical overactivity
2. Pseudo-Cushing's syndrome of alcoholism
3. Adreno-cortical insufficiency.

Adrenocortical overactivity

The association between hypercortisolaemia and alcohol excess was demonstrated by two interesting studies in which hospitalised alcoholics were investigated during prolonged, supervised, alcohol ingestion. Mendelson, Ogata & Mello (1971) investigated 4 well-nourished alcoholics over an 18 day period during which they consumed 86 per cent proof bourbon whisky every 4 hours day and night in doses averaging 4g/kg body weight/day. Before inception of drinking, plasma cortisol values were within the normal reference range, but during alcohol ingestion values increased by approximately 300 per cent. Stokes (1973) carried out a similar study in 18 alcoholics, reporting increased plasma 17-corticosterioids during programmed drinking, but when the alcoholics were encouraged to drink to the point of intoxication, steroid levels were generally lower.

Following publication of the studies by Mendelson, Ogata & Mello (1971) and by Stokes (1973), many workers reported similar findings, but claimed, in addition, that sustained alcohol consumption produced a separate clinical entity called the pseudo-Cushing's syndrome of alcoholism.

The pseudo-Cushing's syndrome of alcoholism

Alcoholic patients, on clinical examination, are frequently obese, hypertensive, bruised and show proximal muscle wasting. As these physical signs are those of true Cushing's syndrome, a Cushingoid alcoholic can be clinically indistinguishable from a patient with the 'true' syndrome. To complicate matters further, are claims that the two conditions are also inseparable on biochemical evaluation, as the Cushingoid alcoholic, like the patient with true Cushing's syndrome, is reported to show hypercortisolaemia, abnormal responses to dexamethasone and diminution of the diurnal cortisol rhythm (Smals et al, 1976; Rees et al, 1977; Smals et al, 1977; Frajria & Angela; 1977). Evidently, the only way to prove that alcohol excess is responsible for the features of Cushing's syndrome is to demonstrate that the alcoholic reverts to normal, both clinically and biochemically, on abstinence from alcohol (Smals et al, 1977; Rees et al, 1977). This reversible form of Cushing's syndrome associated with alcohol excess has been named the pseudo-Cushing's syndrome of alcoholism (PCSA). Other workers have questioned whether the pseudo Cushings syndrome is a separate clinical entity. Fink et al (1981) carried out intravenous dexamethasone suppression tests on ten alcoholic patients on the day following admission to an alcohol treatment unit. Three of the patients were clinically Cushingoid, while the remaining seven were normal on clinical examination. Four of the patients failed to show the expected diminution in plasma cortisol levels, and it is of interest that only one of the clinically Cushingoid alcoholics were among the abnormal responders. A further point of note was that none of the patients showed hypercortisolaemia, and this was attributed to the fact that all patients had received on admission the necessary medication (epanutin, chlormethiazole) for suppression of the withdrawal syndrome. Significantly, none of the reports describing the PCSA indicate that medication was administered for suppression of the withdrawal reaction, despite the fact that most of the patients were studied shortly after admission to hospital. As Merry & Marks (1972) have shown, significant elevation of plasma cortisol is found in alcoholics during the acute phase of abstinence.

It therefore seems probable that cortisol resistance to the suppressive effect of dexamethasone is a non-specific finding in alcoholics, and that the PCSA could represent the coincidental occurrence in the same individual of stress related hypercortisolaemia, and the physical features of Cushing's syndrome (simple obesity, alcohol induced proximal muscle wasting, etc.).

Adreno-cortical insufficiency

Primary adreno-cortical insufficiency occurs in alcoholic patients, although the incidence of this is unknown. Magraf et al (1967) described 4 such subjects who demonstrated, in response to injected adreno-corticotrophin, significantly lower increases of plasma cortisol and urinary 17-oxogenic steroid concentrations than normal controls. This was attributed to depletion of adrenal gland precursor substrates (ascorbic acid, cholesterol), a phenomenon previously shown in the experimental animal fed excess alcohol (Smith, 1951).

This evidence of primary adreno-cortical insufficiency was thought to be of some clinical importance (Magraf et al, 1967), as the operative mortality rate in alcoholics, which is several times that of non-alcoholics may reflect such suboptimal responses to stress.

Secondary adreno-cortical insufficiency in alcoholics is also documented, with Wright (1974) reporting that in 25 per cent of cases, cortisol response to insulin-induced hypologlycaemia is either absent or reduced. The mechanism is unclear but may involve abnormal synthesis and release of corticotrophin-releasing factor at the hypothalamic level.

EFFECT OF ALCOHOL ON GONADAL FUNCTION

Sexual dysfunction is common amongst male alcoholics, with diminished libido, impotence and sterility. Initially, these were attributed entirely to concomitant liver disease and the consequent failure to detoxify oestrogenic compounds, but more recently the toxic effect of alcohol on the testis and the hypothalamic-pituitary axis has been recognised. The following review will generally consider the clinical biochemistry of alcohol induced sexual dysfunction in pre-cirrhotic males and females. The effect of cirrhosis on sexual function is reviewed in two recent articles (Van Thiel & Lester, 1979; Baker et al, 1976).

General clinical pathology

Male patients presenting with alcohol-induced sexual dysfunction show varying results, presumably because of different drinking histories, nutritional status and degree of liver injury. In general, total plasma testosterone concentration is below the reference range in 13–50 per cent of subjects, while in 60 per cent the plasma concentration of sex-hormone binding globulin is elevated, giving rise to subnormal values for 'free' biologically active testosterone. Basal serum gonadotrophin levels may be normal, but are low in relation to suppressed testosterone in more than 65 per cent of patients, and do not show the expected 50 per cent increment after administration of clomiphene. Testicular biopsy reveals severe reduction in germinal elements and peritubular fibrosis. Interestingly, Leydig cells may be normal on microscopic examination (Van Thiel, Lester & Sherins, 1974; Lindholm et al, 1978a; Lindholm et al, 1978b).

Pathogenesis

As pointed out by Van Thiel (Van Thiel, Lester & Sherins, 1974), the above abnormal results may arise as a result of single or combined lesions of the pituitary-gonadal axis, or as a result of enhanced peripheral metabolism of sex steroids. Pathogenesis will therefore be considered under the headings shown below.

The effect of alcohol on testicular function

Normal gonadal function in the male requires optimal intratesticular concentrations of testosterone and vitamin A. As already shown, testosterone levels are low in 13–50 per cent of alcoholics and recent work has also revealed an abnormality of intratesticular metabolism of vitamin A (Van Thiel, Gavaler & Lester, 1974), in which vitamin A in its absorbed state, retinal, is not oxidised to the biological active metabolite retinol. The reason for this is that both alcohol and vitamin A (retinal) share the same intratesticular enzyme, alcohol dehydrogenase, which preferentially oxidises alcohol. Whether these biochemical abnormalities account for the injury to the tubules seen on histological examination is unknown, and it remains a possibility that this is also due to the direct toxic effect of alcohol and its metabolite, acetaldehyde.

With regard to the Leydig cells, it has been shown above that they may be normal on histological examination in alcoholics and that, therefore, the failure of testosterone synthesis is probably at the molecular level. For example, Leydig cell receptor sites may function abnormally as a result of the fluidising effect of alcohol on cell membranes (Chin & Goldstein, 1977). Supporting evidence for this derives from reports (Cicero et al, 1980) that ethanol markedly inhibited gonadotrophin — stimulated production of testosterone in enzymatically dispersed rat cell testis preparations, and that 50 per cent of heavy drinkers did not show the expected increment in testosterone after administration of human chorionic gonadotrophin (HCG) (Van Thiel, Lester & Sherins, 1974).

Alcohol might also interfere with testosterone biosynthesis, and Van Thiel & Lester (1976) have suggested that the increased NADH: NAD ratio generated by the metabolism of alcohol many inhibit the activity of enzymes such as 4, 5 isomerase, 3α hydroxysteroid reductase and 17β reductase. Whatever the mechanism, the deleterious effect of alcohol on testosterone synthesis is rapid, and Glikahri et al (1978) have shown a 20 per cent reduction in plasma testosterone in normal volunteers during hangover after excess alcohol consumption.

The effect of alcohol on hypothalamic pituitary dysfunction

There is ample evidence that gonadotrophin release is abnormal during and after alcohol ingestion in normal individuals (Gordon & Southern, 1976) and in alcoholic subjects (Van Thiel, Lester & Sherins, 1974). The principal abnormalities are the absence of the normal pulsatile release of gonadotrophins, and the failure of luteining hormone (LH) and follicle-stimulating hormone (FSH) to show compensatory increases in the presence of primary testicular disease (Cicero et al, 1979), or following stress-testing with clomiphene citrate (Van Thiel, Lester & Sherins, 1974).

These disorders of hypothalamic-pituitary neurobiochemistry have not been completely elucidated: Chapin, Briese & Mueller (1980) showed that the inhibitory effect of alcohol on LH release is not inhibited by haloperidol (a dopamine agonist), suggesting that this inhibition was not mediated by dopamine deficiency. These workers also showed that inhibition of LH release was independent of hyperprolactinaemia and was not due to the toxic effect of acetaldehyde, as the non-metabolisable alcohol n-butanol exerted similar inhibitory effects on gonadotrophin release. One possibility which has received experimental support is that alcohol interferes with the synthesis or release of luteinising-hormone releasing hormone (LHRH) in the hypothalamus. Cicero et al (1979), for example, restored alcohol-inhibited LH release by administering synthetic LHRH.

The effect of alcohol on the peripheral metabolism of sex steroids

Measurement of testosterone A ring reductase activity in hepatic biopsy material before and after 21 days excess alcohol consumption showed gradually increasing activity of this enzyme (Gordon et al, 1976). This was associated with a 17–42 per cent increase in testosterone breakdown.

The effect of alcohol on reproductive function in women

Mendelson, Mello & Ellingboe (1981) studied 6 normal females and observed no abnormality of gonadotrophin or oestradiol levels during both the follicular and luteal phases of the menstrual cycle, when blood ethanol concentrations were maintained at 88 mg/dl.

On the other hand, alcoholic women frequently complain of loss of libido, menstrual irregularity and infertility (Borhamanesh & Haghighi, 1970). The endocrine changes in such patients were recently investigated by Hughes et al (1980), who showed that in 13 women of reproductive age, hypothalamic amenorrhoea was found in 3, anovulation in 2 and inadequate luteal phase in 6. This is consistent with histological study of ovarian tissue from alcoholic women which shows normal findings in respect of follicular and stromal morphology, although in some cases absence of the luteal phase was seen (Barr & Summers, 1957).

EFFECT OF ALCOHOL ON THYROID FUNCTION

Assessment of thyroid function in alcoholics is not straightforward, as varying degrees of liver damage interfere with the diagnostic performance of routine thyroid function tests.

In alcoholic cirrhotics protein synthetic activity is impaired, with the result that the production of thyroid binding proteins (thyroid binding globulin, albumin and pre-albumin) will be reduced. As thyroid function tests carried out in the routine laboratory measure both bound and free hormone, and because the bound moiety is greater than the free, subnormal values will be observed for total thyroxine (T4). However, values in respect of free T4 are generally normal, although 'free' triiodothyronine (T3) values have also been found to be low (Chopra et al, 1974), suggesting that the peripheral conversion of T4 to T3 is impaired in these patients (Chopra et al, 1974; Green et al, 1977).

Alcoholic cirrhotics, and indeed alcoholic patients with moderate hepatic damage (steatosis) also show abnormal hypothalamic control of thyroid gland function. The incidence of this is surprisingly high, with Green et al (1977) reporting that the thyroid-stimulating hormone (TSH) response to thyrotropin-releasing hormone (TRH) was delayed and therefore diagnostic of hypothalamic dysfunction (Hall et al, 1972) in 8 of 12 alcoholics with varying degrees of liver damage. Presumably also reflecting hypothalamic or pituitary disorder is the finding by Kallner (1981) that the TSH response to TRH was 'blunted' in 4 of 10 alcoholics on admission to hospital.

Although evaluation of thyroid function is rarely indicated in patients with alcoholic hepatitis, one interesting case report (Stuart & Schultz, 1978) describes a 25 year old male alcoholic with prominent eyes, diffusely enlarged thyroid, increased radio-iodine uptake and evidence on liver biopsy of alcoholic hepatitis. Serum values for T4 and FTI (free thyroxine index) were all in the thyrotoxic range, providing biochemical evidence in support of Graves disease, but on abstinence and resolution of hepatitis, both the clinical and biochemical features of thyroid overactivity disappeared. The authors' suggestion is that with progressive liver disease peripheral conversion of T4 to T3 was reduced, resulting in a compensatory rise of TSH which produced excess T4 and clinical signs of thyrotoxicosis. Other workers (Kallner, 1981) have also drawn attention to the problem created by the alcoholic who, during the acute phase of withdrawal, closely stimulates the clinical signs of thyrotoxicosis (tachycardia, tremor, sweating, agitation). In view of the unreliability of routine thyroid function tests in such patients, Kallner suggests that a rise in plasma T3 concentration, 3 hours after TRH injection will distinguish the alcoholic with normal thyroid gland function from similar patients with genuine thyrotoxicosis.

Alcoholics without clinical evidence of severe hepatic disease generally show normal values in respect of thyroid function tests. In 33 alcoholics on the day of admission to an alcohol unit, normal values were found for plasma 'free' T3 and T4 concentrations and basal TSH concentrations (Fink & Guest, 1980 — unpublished). Similarly in 41 alcoholics investigated, 7 days after admission to an alcohol unit, all thyroid function tests were within the reference range, although on admission low levels were observed for plasma T3 and T4 concentrations in 2 and 9 patients respectively (Wright, 1978).

EFFECT OF ALCOHOL ON PROLACTIN RELEASE

Plasma prolactin values are slightly elevated in 40 per cent of chronic alcoholic patients (Lindholm et al, 1978a) and this finding may relate to gonadal dysfunction these patients experience. In normal individuals acutely exposed to alcohol (1.5 g/kg) no effect was observed on basal prolactin values (Glikahri et al, 1978). However, the expected increment of prolactin after TRH was not observed during hangover. This suggests enhanced dopamine activity during this time, although this theory is in conflict with hypotheses suggested by other workers (Chapin et al, 1980) and discussed above.

EFFECT OF ALCOHOL ON VASOPRESSIN (ANTI-DIURETIC HORMONE) RELEASE

It is common knowledge that alcohol ingestion causes diuresis, and this has been attributed to suppression of vasopressin release from the posterior pituitary. Recently this hypothesis was tested (Linkola et al, 1978), and although alcohol ingestion produced diuresis it was, surprisingly, assoated with a marked rise in the plasma concentration of vasopressin. This result suggests that other factors are responsible for alcohol-induced diuresis (see also Ch. 6). For instance, alcohol is osmotically active and its presence in urine may generate an osmotic diuresis. Another explanation for the association of vasopressin increase and diuresis during alcohol ingestion is that catecholamines, which are released during such occasions, may counteract the cellular actions of vasopressin at the level of cyclic AMP (adenosine monophosphate) synthesis (Beck et al, 1972).

THE EFFECT OF ALCOHOL ON THE RENIN-ANGIOTENSIN AXIS

The realisation that regular alcohol consumption is a risk factor hypertension has focussed attention on alcohol-induced changes in the renin-angiotensin axis. In a preliminary study of 5 normal males, Linkola et al (1976) found that after consuming between 1.5–2.3 g ethanol/kg body weight these subjects showed suppressed plasma aldosterone levels during intoxication, while during hangover both plasma aldosterone concentration and plasma renin activity were significantly increased. In a later study (Linkola, Fyhrquist & Glikahri, 1979) it was found that the greatest rise in plasma renin activity occurred in subjects experiencing nausea and vomiting, and that there was no correlation between plasma renin activity and plasma aldosterone concentration. The clinical significance of these results is unknown, as concurrent blood pressure readings were not taken.

EFFECT OF ALCOHOL ON THE ADRENAL MEDULLA

Early workers (Perman, 1960) observed increases in the urinary concentration of adrenalin following alcohol consumption. A valid criticism of this and previous studies was that no allowance had been made for the effect of alcohol-induced diuresis on observed catecholamine levels. This necessary adjustment was made by Anton (1965) who reported increased levels of noradrenalin, dopamine and metadrenalin in 20 normal males consuming 0.7 g alcohol per kg body weight. Why increases in urinary adrenalin were observed by the previous workers while Anton found increases in noradrenalin is not clear. One possibility is that subjects studied by the latter were more active. Physical activity is associated with increased release of noradrenalin.

Whereas the above workers studied normal subjects, Ogata et al (1971) investigated 4 male chronic alcoholics under 'laboratory' conditions and measured urinary catecholamine in relation to urinary creatinine concentration. During free access to alcohol, when mean blood alcohol levels were 191 mg/dl, a significant increase over baseline values was found for adrenalin and metadrenalin. During programmed drinking, when mean blood alcohol levels were 86 mg/dl, this elevation, although present, was not significantly increased. An interesting feature of this study was that despite consuming alcohol every 4 h for 20 days, catecholamine release did not diminish, suggesting that the sympathetic system and adrenal medulla did not develop alcohol tolerance. Further, catecholamine production appeared to be closely related, with amine levels during free choice drinking exceeding those during programmed drinking by a factor of 2.

With regard to plasma levels, Carlsson & Häggendal (1967) measured arterial noradrenalin levels using a fluorometric technique in 36 alcoholics after alcohol withdrawal. Maximal rises were seen after 13–24 h when levels were × 4 that of baseline. In three subjects, increments were greater than this and were associated with more pronounced withdrawal symptoms.

Alterations in the metabolism of catecholamines and other biogenic amines by alcohol

Inhibition of aldehyde dehydrogenase

In 1957, a patient with carcinoid disease, who had been given an alcoholic drink to provoke a flushing episode, was noted to excrete less 5-hydroxyindoleacetic acid (5-HIAA), the major metabolite of 5 hydroxytryptamine (Smith et al, 1957). This acute effect of alcohol was confirmed by later workers (Davis et al, 1967) and also subsequently demonstrated in chronic alcoholics (Olsen, Gursey & Vester, 1966).

The biochemical pathway altered by alcohol is as follows: under normal physiological conditions the immediate aldehyde derivative of the oxidative deamination of 5-hydroxytryptamine is largely oxidised further by aldehyde dehydrogenase to 5HIAA. Following alcohol ingestion, this enzyme is competitively inhibited by the alcohol metabolite acetaldehyde (Walsh, Truitt & Davis, 1970) with the production of the intermediate indole-aldehyde. Because cellular redox potential is also altered during alcohol ingestion with production of excess NADH, further metabolism favours reductive pathways, and increased amounts of the alcohol 5 hydroxytryptophol is formed.

A similar alteration of catecholamine metabolism is also observed during alcohol consumption. Davis et al (1967) administered 60 ml of ethanol to normal subjects and within 8 h noted a decrease in urinary 3-methoxy-4-hydroxymandelic acid and an increase in 3-methoxy-4-hydroxyphenylglycol. These amine alcohols are non-polar and would be expected to cross the blood-brain barrier, but the clinical significance of this is presently unknown.

The Picket-Spengler and other condensation reactions

Acetaldehyde generated from alcohol may also, at neutral pH condense with phenolic amines to form tetra-isoquinolines (TIOs) (Fig. 14.1). Acetaldehyde also complexes with native catecholamines to form cyclic derivatives which may combine with the parent compound to form tetrahydropapaveroline compounds (THPs) (Fig. 14.2). This is known as the Picket-Spengler reaction (Walsh, Truitt & Davis, 1970; Cohen & Collins, 1970; Sandler et al, 1973).

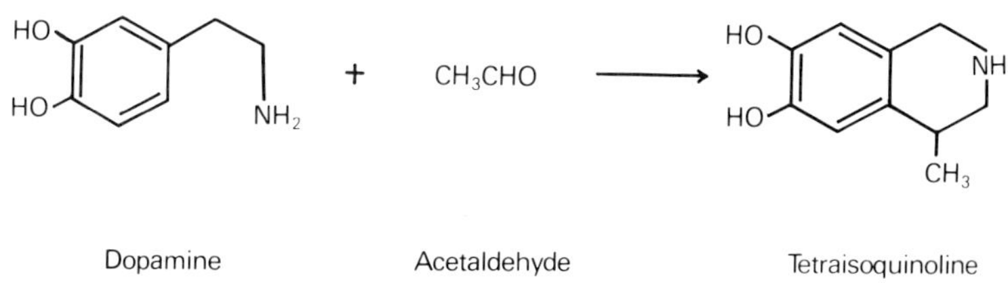

Fig. 14.1 Formation of tetraisoquinolines.

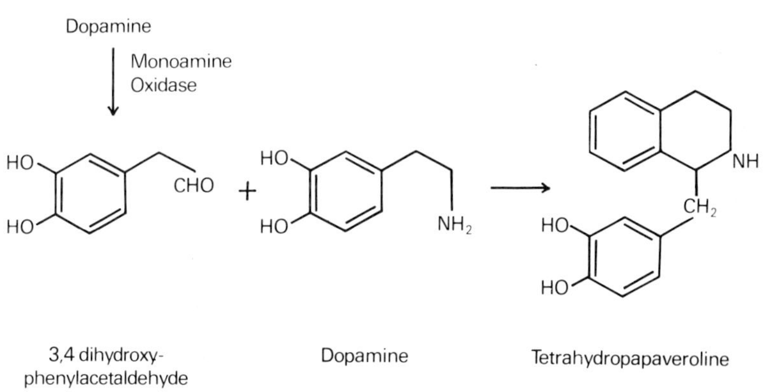

Fig. 14.2 Formation of tetrahydropapaveroline.

TIQs, THP — are they related to a biochemical basis of addiction?

Structurally, THP compounds resemble plant alkaloids (morphine) and some workers have suggested that these molecules form the biochemical basis of addiction to alcohol (Cohen & Collins, 1970; Walsh, Truitt & Davis, 1970). Support for this hypothesis has come from studies (Myers & Melchior, 1977) which showed that after the instillation of THP into cerebral ventricles of rats, these animals consumed excess alcohol in free choice situations where water was also available. Furthermore, this was observed in animals normally showing an aversion to alcohol. Unfortunately, other workers have failed to confirm these results (Brown, Amit & Smith, 1980). The current situation is reviewed by Duncan et al (1980).

Borg et al (1980) measured TIQ levels in blood and CSF in chronic alcoholics 1 and 14 days after withdrawal of alcohol. These compounds were always found in urine but the level did not show any consistent change in relation to time of sampling. TIQs were found in CSF in 6 patients: one at first sampling, 4 at both sampling and one on the final sampling occasion only. The significance of these changes is not clear.

THE EFFECT OF ALCOHOL ON GASTRO-INTESTINAL HORMONE SECRETION (see also Chs 11,12)

Secretin and pancreozymin

Alcohol excess is the second most common cause of pancreatitis in the UK, but its role in the pathogenesis of this disorder is unclear. One explanation suggests that alcohol ingestion increases both pancreatic exocrine secretion as well as spasm of the Sphincter of Oddi leading to increased pressure and ultimately the disruption of pancreatic ducts and acini.

Stimulation of pancreatic exocrine secretion presupposes that alcohol ingestion releases secretin and pancreozymin. With regard to the former, controversy reigns. Straus, Urbach & Yalow (1975) reported that in normal male subjects, 2 oz of 86° proof alcohol produced increase in plasma secretin values from a basal 100 pg/ml to 265 pg/ml within 10 minutes of ingestion. This rapid effect led the authors to believe that alcohol directly stimulates secretin release. In a later study of six normal subjects, Llanos et al (1977) also showed a stimulatory effect of alcohol ingestion on secretin release, but this was delayed until 60 minutes after ingestion. In view of this later increase, Llanos suggested that secretin release is mediated by gastrin, which in his study rose from a basal value of 52 pg/ml to 64 pg/ml after alcohol ingestion. However, as Chang, Chang & William (1980) pointed out, such an increment in plasma gastrin is less than that observed after a meal, and, therefore, more unlikely to stimulate gastrin release. The situation is further complicated by other workers, Hacki, Greenberg & Bloom (1978), who failed to observe plasma secretin release after oral ingestion of alcohol.

These various studies have been reviewed by Chang, Chang & William (1980) who attribute their divergent results to differing methodology and suggest further, that, in the studies reporting elevated secretin values, the assays were carried out in the presence of interference. The nature of these non-specific interfering substances could be plasma proteins and lipids.

Few studies are available reporting the effect of alcohol on pancreozymin release. In one involving dogs (Palasciano et al, 1974), pancreatic exocrine function was maximally stimulated by constant infusion of secretin. No significant quantitative or qualitative change was observed in pancreatic exocrine secretions following intraduodenal instillation of oleic acid, but a significant (650 per cent) increase in protein output was detected after installation of alcohol. This suggests that alcohol ingestion either sensitises the pancreas to pancreozymin or that endogenous production and release of this hormone is increased.

Gastrin

Although the stimulatory effect of ethanol ingestion on gastric acid production was reported many years ago, the mechanism responsible for this phenomenon is not entirely clear. Some workers believe that alcohol directly stimulates parietal cells (Irving, Watkins & Williams 1960), while others claim that local contact of alcohol with antral mucosa releases gastrin (Elwin, 1969) (Becker et al, 1974) and therefore acid indirectly.

With the advent of radio-immunoassay Becker, Reeder & Thompson (1974) showed that ingestion of 80 ml of 80 per cent alcohol by non-alcoholics was followed by a significant increase in plasma gastrin levels from 99 to 109 pg/ml, although the increment after 80 ml of 18 per cent alcohol was not statistically significant. Llanos et al (1977) confirmed that immunoreactive gastrin increased in normal subjects gastrin is not the only mediator in ethanol induced gastric secretion as this could also result from the local release of histamine (Irvine et al, 1960).

The clinical significance of both increased gastric secretion and elevated plasma gastrin levels following alcohol ingestion is obscure, as epidemiological studies have not shown that chronic ingestion is associated with an increased risk of peptic ulceration (Paffenberger, Wing & Hyde, 1974). This may be related to the fact that both basal and post-prandial gastrin levels in alcoholics fall to reference levels once alcohol is withdrawn.

Pancreatic polypeptide (PP)

In a recent study of PP in alcoholics (Fink et al, 1983), interesting results were obtained which may prove to be of some clinical importance.

Nine chronic alcoholic men without clinical evidence of disease were studied 1 and 14 days after admission to an alcohol unit. Basal blood

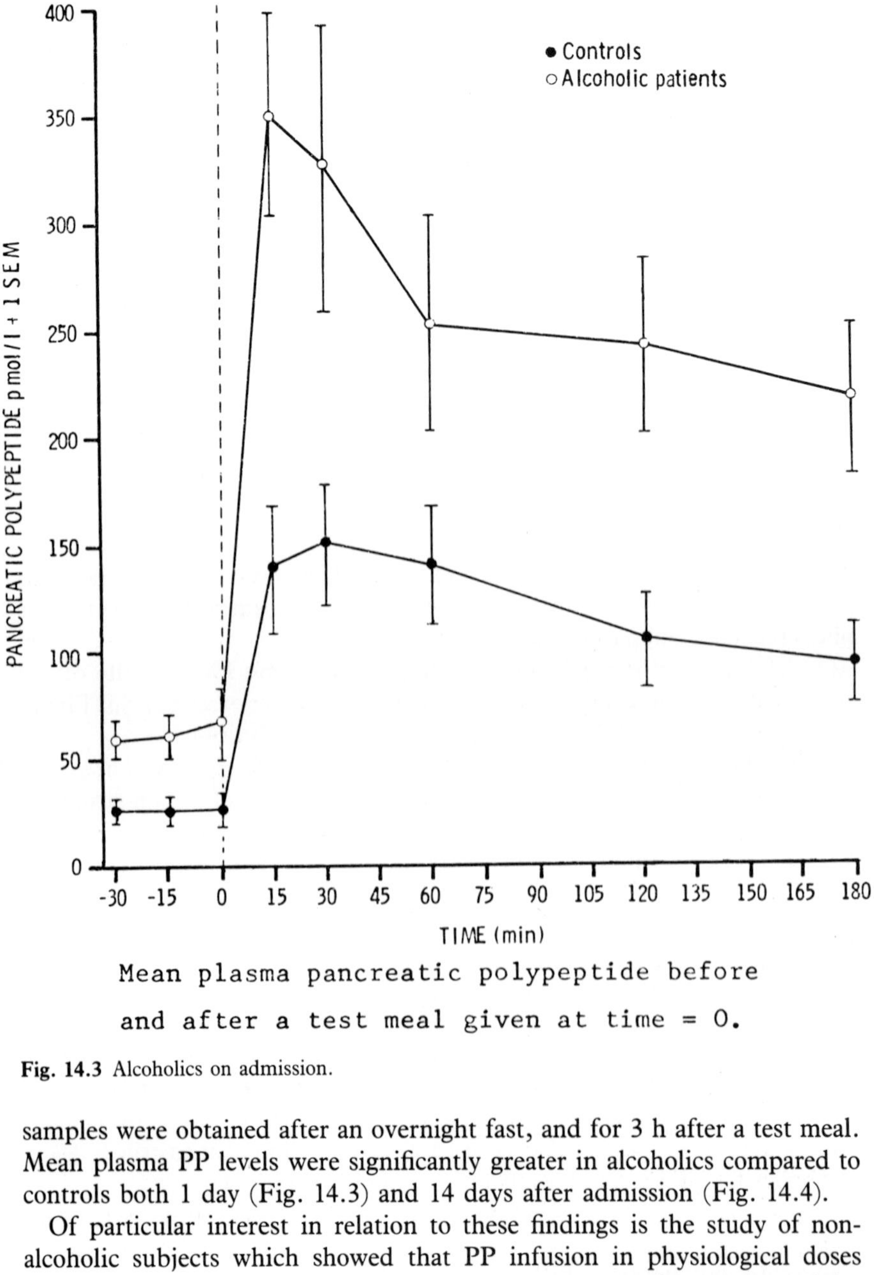

Fig. 14.3 Alcoholics on admission.

samples were obtained after an overnight fast, and for 3 h after a test meal. Mean plasma PP levels were significantly greater in alcoholics compared to controls both 1 day (Fig. 14.3) and 14 days after admission (Fig. 14.4).

Of particular interest in relation to these findings is the study of non-alcoholic subjects which showed that PP infusion in physiological doses caused a fourfold decrease in the stimulated post-prandial trypsin activity in pancreatic juice (Greenberg et al, 1978). This suggests that PP release could be responsible for inhibiting pancreatic exocrine function on completion of food ingestion. A further possibility is that sustained PP elevation could also be responsible for the subnormal pancreatic exocrine function reported in 30 per cent of alcoholic subjects. Evidence in support

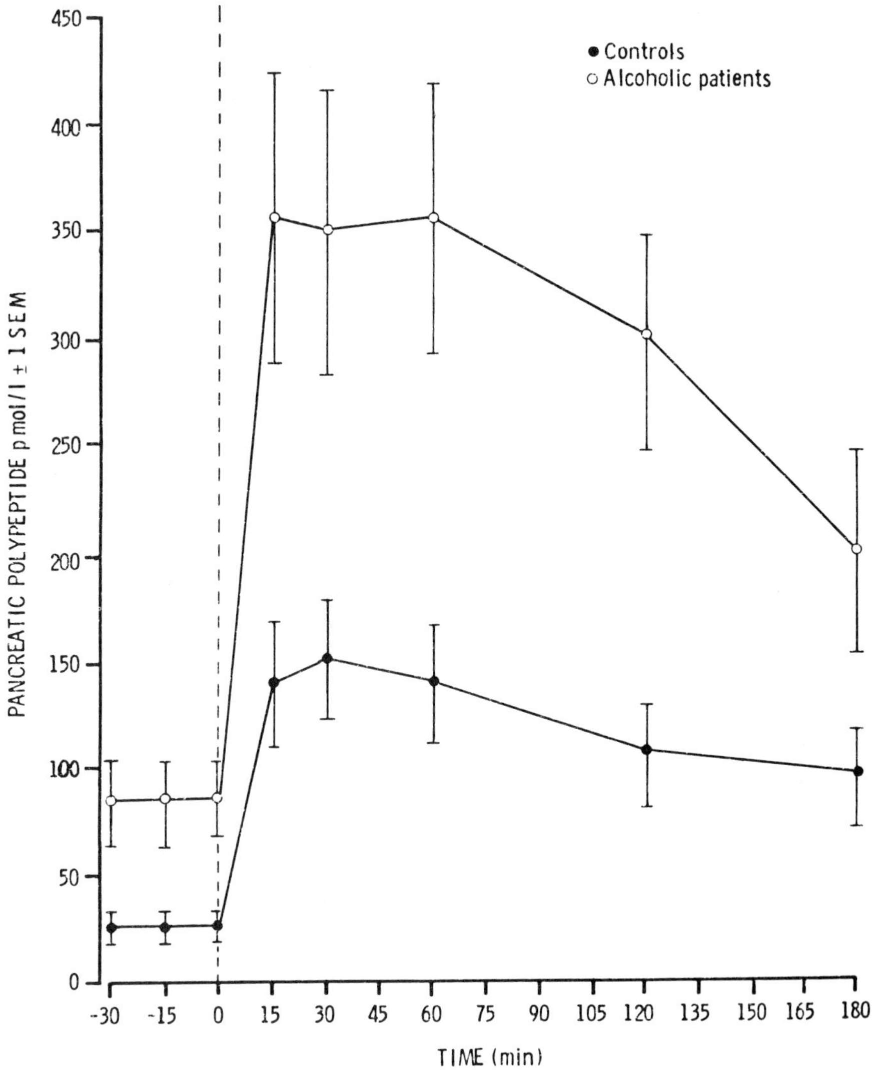

Mean plasma pancreatic polypeptide before and after a test meal given at time = 0

Fig. 14.4 Alcoholics 2 weeks after admission.

of this is not reported, although Sarles et al (1980) have shown that in non-alcholics receiving alcohol intravenously, a rise in plasma PP concentration is associated with a reciprocal fall in trypsin activity in biliary secretions.

THE EFFECT OF ALCOHOL ON BONE

As mineralisation of bone is under endocrine control, it is appropriate to consider in this chapter the effects of alcohol on bone.

Clinical features

The alcoholic is frequently involved in traumatic accidents, and experiences more bone fractures than moderate drinkers (Nilsson & Westlin, 1973). Of especial interest are further observations that alcoholics show reduced bone density (Saville, 1965; Nilsson & Westlin, 1973), and consequently a significantly increased incidence of 'metabolic' type fracture (Nilsson, 1970).

Routine bone biochemistry in alcoholic patients shows hypocalcaemia, (corrected for hypoalbuminaemia) in 5–15 per cent (Rosalki, 1974; Igbramov, 1967), and subnormal values for serum 25-hydroxyvitamin D and vitamin-D binding globulin, in 15 per cent and 13 per cent respectively (Fink & Rosalki, 1980 — unpublished). Other workers have documented increased secretion of glycosaminoglycans and hydroxyproline in the urine of rats fed alcohol, which is further evidence of bone dissolution in the presence of alcohol excess (Mezey, Potter & Marchant, 1979).

Pathogenesis

Hypocalcaemia could result from dietary insufficiency, malabsorption or increased urinary loss of calcium. With regard to malabsorption, two mechanisms are possible. Krawitt (1975) using everted duodenal and rat preparations, showed that the movement of Ca^{45} across the endothelial barrier was significantly inhibited by the presence of luminal alcohol, and this abnormality occurred despite normal serum levels of vitamin D. The second mechanism is steatorrhoea which occurs in some 30 per cent of alcoholics (Mezey et al, 1970). This may result from intestinal endothelial damage, intestinal hurry or pancreatic exocrine insufficiency (Roggin et al, 1972; Roginsky, Zanzi and Cohn, 1976).

In addition to enteral wastage, urinary loss of calcium, phosphorus and magnesium is found during alcohol induced diuresis (Kalbfleisch et al, 1963). The mechanism responsible for calcium loss is unknown but the failure to reabsorb phosphorus is probably mediated by PTH release which is significantly increased 30 minutes after alcohol ingestion (Williams et al, 1978). A possible reason for magnesium loss in alcoholics is the presence of lactic acidosis which interferes with the tubular absorption of this ion (Heaton et al, 1962). Accumulation of lactic acid following alcohol ingestion reflects the generation of excess NADH during the production of acetaldehyde from alcohol by alcohol dehydrogenase. Low serum levels of 25-OH vitamin D may also reflect poor diet and malabsorption. An important additional consideration, particularly in the UK, is insufficient exposure to sunlight.

Diminished bone ground substance could reflect the negative nitrogen balance which is documented in alcoholics (McDonald & Margin, 1976). Gonadal dysfunction could also contribute to loss of bone density, as sex steroids exert an anabolic effect on bone metabolism.

CONCLUSION

The effects of alcohol on endocrine function are wide-ranging. They include changes in the hypothalamic-pituitary axis and in endocrine glands under pituitary control such as the adrenal cortex, gonads and thyroid gland. In addition, alcohol produces effects on the posterior pituitary gland, the adrenal medulla, the renin-angiotensin system, gastro-intestinal hormones and the parathyroids. Such changes produce diverse clinical effects.

REFERENCES

Anton A H 1965 Ethanol and urinary catecholamines in man. Clinical Pharmacology & Therapeutics 6: 462–469

Baker H W G, Burger H G, Kretser D M, Dulmanis A et al 1976 A study of the endocrine manifestations of hepatic cirrhosis. Quarterly Journal of Medicine 45: 145–179

Barr R W, Summers S C 1957 Endocrine abnormalities accompanying hepatic cirrhosis and hepatoma. Journal of Clinical Investigation 51: 939–944

Beck N P, Reed S W, Murdaugh H V, Davis B B 1972 Effects of catecholamines and their interaction with other hormones on 3′, 5′ AMP of the kidney. Journal of Clinical Investigation 51: 939–944

Becker H O, Reeder D D, Thompson J C 1974 Gastrin release by ethanol in man and in dogs. Annals of Surgery 179: 906–909

Borg S, Kuonde H, Magnusson E, Sjöqvist B 1980 Salsolinol and salsoline in cerebrospinal lumbar fluid of alcoholic patients. Acta Psychiatrica Scandinavica S 286, 62: 171–177

Borhanmanesh F, Haghighi P 1970 Pregnancy in patients with cirrhosis of the liver. Obstetrics and Gynaecology 36: 315–324

Brown S W, Amit S, Smith B 1980 Examination of the role of tetrahydro-isoquinoline alkaloids in the mediation of ethanol consumption in rats. Advances of Experimental Medicine & Biology 126: 103–120

Carlsson C, Häggendal J 1967 Arterial noradrenaline levels after ethanol withdrawal. Lancet 2: 889 (letter)

Chang T M, Ta-Min Chang, Chey William Y 1980 Radio-immunoassay of secretin. A critical review and current status. Digestive Diseases Sciences July: 27 (7): 529–530

Chapin R E, Briese G R, Mueller R A 1980 Possible mechanisms of reduction of plasma luteinizing hormone by ethanol. Journal of Pharmacology and Experimental Therapeutics 1: 6–10

Chin J H, Goldstein D B 1977 Drug tolerance in biomembranes: a spin label study of the effects of ethanol. Science 196: 684–685

Chopra I J, Solomon D H, Copra V, Young R T, Guadalupe N, Chua Teco 1974 Alterations in Circulating Thyroid Hormones and Thyrotropin in Hepatic Cirrhosis: Evidence for Euthyroidism despite Subnormal Serum Tri-iodothyronin. Journal of Clinical Endocrinology 39: 501–511

Cicero T J, Bell R D, Meyer E R, Badger T M 1980 Ethanol and Acetaldehyde directly inhibit testicular steroidogenesis. Journal of Pharmocology and Experimental Therapeutics 213: 228–233

Cicero T J, Meyer E R, Bell R D 1979 Effect of ethanol on the hypothalamic and pituitary luteinizing hormone axis and testicular steroidogenesis. Journal of Pharmocology and Experimental Therapeutics (2): 208–210

Cohen G, Collins M A, 1970 Alkaloids from catecholamines in adrenal tissue: Possible role in alcoholism. Science 167: 1749–1751

Davis V E, Brown H, Huff J A, Cashaw J L 1967 Ethanol-induced alterations of norephinephrine metabolism in man. Journal of Laboratory and Clinical Medicine 69: 787–799

Davis V E, Brown H, Huff J A, Cashaw J L 1967 The alteration of serotonin metabolism to 5-hydroxytryptophol by ethanol ingestion in man. Journal of Laboratory and Clinical Medicine 69: 132–140

Dreiling D A, Richman A, Fradkin N F 1951 The role of alcohol in the aetiology of pancreatitis: a study of the effect of intravenous ethyl alcohol on the external secretion of the pancreas. Gastroenterology 20: 636

Duncan C Diétrich R A, 1980 A critical evaluation of tetrahydroisoquinoline induced alcohol preference in rats. Pharmacology, Biochemistry and Behaviour 13 (2): 265–81

Ellis F W 1966 Effects of ethanol on plasma corticosterone levels. Journal of Pharmocology and Experimental Therapeuts 153: 121–127

Elwin C E 1969 Stimulation of Gastric Acid secretion by Irrigation of the Antrum with some Aliphatic Alcohols. Acta Physiologica Scandinavica 75: 1–11

Fink R S, Adrian T E, Marjot D H, Bloom S R 1983 Increased plasma pancreatic polypeptide in chronic alcohol abuse. Clinical Endocrinology 18: 417–421

Fink R S, Short F, Marjot D H, James V H T 1981 Abnormal Suppression of Plasma Cortisol during the Intravenous Infusion of Dexamethosone to Alcoholic Patients. Clinical Endocrinology 15: 97–102

Frajria R, Angela A 1977 Alcohol induced pseudo-Cushing's syndrome. Lancet 1: 1050–1051

Glikahri R H, Hottunen M O, Hařkönen M, Leino T, Helenius T, Liewendahl K, Karowen S L 1978 Acute effects of Alcohol on anterior pituitary secretion of the trophic hormones. Journal of Clinical Endocrinology 46: 714–720

Gordon G G, Southern A L 1977 Metabolic effects of alcohol on the endocrine system. In: C S Lieber (ed) Metabolic aspects of alcoholism. MTP Press, Lancaster, p 249–302

Gordon G G, Southern A L, Altman K, Rubin E, Lieber C S 1976 The effect of alcohol administration on sex hormone metabolism in normal men. New England Journal of Medicine 295: 793–797

Green J R B, Snitcher E J, Mowat N A O, Ekins R P, Rees L H, Dawson A M 1977 Thyroid Function and thyroid regulation in euthyroid men with chronic liver disease: evidence of multiple abnormalities. Clinical Endocrinology 7: 453–461

Greenberg G R, McCloy R F, Adrian T E, Chadwick V S, Baron J H, Bloom S R 1978 Inhibition of pancreas and gallbladder by pancreatic polypeptide. Lancet 2: 1280–2

Hacki W H, Greenberg G R, Bloom S R 1978 Role of secretin in man. In: Bloom S R (ed) Gut hormones. Churchill Livingstone, Edinburgh, p 182–192

Hall R, Ormston B J, Besser G M, Cryer R J, McKendrick M 1972 The thyrotrophin — releasing hormone test in diseases of the pituitary and hypothalamus. Lancet 1: 759–763

Heaton F W, Pyrach C C, Bersford R W, Martin D F 1962 Hypomagnesaemia in chronic alcoholism. Lancet 2: 802–805

Hirschovitz B J, Pollard H M, Hartwell J W, London J 1956 The Action of Ethyl Alcohol on Gastric Acid Secretion. Gastroenterology 30: 244–256

Hughes J N, Coste T, Perret M F, Sebaoun J, Modigliani E 1980 Hypothalamo-Pituitary Ovarian Function in Thirty-One Women with Chronic Alcoholism. Clinical Endocrinology 12: 543–551

Ibragimov V 1967 Some biochemical blood parameters in cases of chronic alcoholism. Vrach Delo 6: 134–135

Irvine W T, Watkins D B, Williams E J 1960 The mechanisms by which alcohol stimulates acid secretion. Gastroenterology 39: 41–47

Jones M K, Hatcher E M 1980 Congitive defecits in women alcoholics as a function of gynaecological status. Journal of Studies on Alcoholism-January, 4: 140–6

Kalbfleisch J M, Lindeman R D, Ginn H E, Smith W O 1963 Effects of ethanol administration on urinary excretion of magnesium and other electrolytes in alcoholic and normal subjects. Journal of Clinical Investigation 42: 1471–1475

Kallner G 1981 Assessment of thyroid function in chronic alcoholics. Acta Medica Scandinavica 209: 93–6

Krawitt E L 1975 Effects of ethanol ingestion on duodenal calcium transport. Journal of Laboratory and Clinical Medicine 85: 4 665–671

Lindholm J, Fabricius-Bjerre N, Bahnsen P, Boiesen L, et al 1978a Sex steriods and sex-hormone binding globulin in males with chronic alcoholism. European Journal of Clinical investigation 8: 273–276

Lindholm J, Fabricius-Bjerre N, Bahnsen P, Boiesen L, et al 1978b Pituitary-testicular

function in patients with chronic alcoholism. European Journal of Clinical Investigation 8: 269–272
Linkola J, Fyhrquist F, Glikahri R 1979 Renin, aldosterone and cortisol during ethanol intoxication and hangover. Acta Physiologica Scandinavica 106: 75–82
Linkola J, Fyhrquist F, Nieminen M M, Weber J H, Tontti K 1976 Renin-aldosterone axis in ethanol, intoxication. European Journal of Clinical Investigation 6: 191–194
Linkola J, Glikahri R, Fyhrquist F, Wallenius M 1978 Plasma vasopressin in ethanol intoxication. Acta Physiologica Scandinavica 104: 180–187
Llanos O L, Swierczek J S, Teichmann R K, Rayford B L, Thompson J C 1977 Effect of alcohol on the release of secretin and pancreatic secretion. Surgery 81: 661–667
Magraf H W, Moyer C A, Ashford L E, Lavalle L E 1967 Adrenocortical function in alcoholics. Journal of Surgical Research 7: 55–62
McDonald J T, Margin S 1976 Wine vs ethanol in human nutrition 1. Nitrogen and calcine balance. American Journal of Clinical Nutrition 29: 1093–1103
Mendelson J H, Mello N K, Ellingboe 1981 Acute alcohol intake and pituitary gonadal hormones in normal human female. Journal of Pharmacology and Experimental Therapeutics 218: 23–26
Mendelson J H, Ogata M, Mello N K 1971 Adrenal function and alcoholism I Serum cortisol Psychosomatic Medicine 33: 145–157
Merry J, Marks V 1972 The effect of alcohol, barbiturate and diazepamon hypothalamic pituitary-adrenal function in chronic alcoholics. Lancet 2: 990–992
Mezey E, Potter J J, Merchant C R 1979 Effect of ethanol feeding on bone composition in the rat. American Journal of Clinical Nutrition 32 (i): 25–29
Mezey E, Jow E, Slattin R E, Tobon F 1970 Pancreatic function and intestinal absorption in chronic alcoholism. Gastroenterology 59: 657–664
Myers R D, Melchior C L 1977 Alcohol drinking: Abnormal intake caused by tetrahydropapaveroline infusion in the brain. Science 196: 554–555
Nilsson B E, Westlin N E 1973 Changes in bone mass in alcoholics. Clinical Orthopaedics and Related Research 90: 229–232
Nilsson B E 1970 Conditions contributing to fracture of the femoral neck. Acta Chirurgica Scandinavica 136: 383–384
Ogata M, Mendelson J H, Mello N K, Majchrowicz E 1971 Adrenal function and alcoholism II Catecholamines. Psychosomatic Medicine 33: 159–180
Oslen R E, Gursey D, Vester J W 1960 Evidence for a defect in tryptophan metabolism in chronic alcoholism. 263: 1169–1174
Paffenbarger R S, Wing A L, Hyde R T 1974 Chronic disease in former college students XIII Early precursors of peptic ulcer. American Journal of Epidemiology 100: 307–315
Palasciano G, Tiscornia O M, Herge G, Sarles H 1974 Chronic alcoholism and endogenous cholecystolamine-pancreozymine (CCK-PZ). Biomedicine (Express) 21: 94–97
Perman E S 1960 Observation on the effect of ethanol on the urinary excretion of histamine, 5-hydroxyindoleacetic acid, catecholamines and 17 hydroxy-corticosteroids in man. Acta Physiologica Scandinavica 51: 62–67
Rees L, Besser G M, Jeffcoate W J, Goldie D J, Marks V 1977 Alcohol Induced Pseudo Cushings Syndrome. Lancet 1: 726–728
Roggin G M, Iber F L, Linscheer W G 1972 Intraluminal fat digestion in the alcoholic. Gut 13: 107–111
Roginsky M S, Zanzi I, Cohn S H 1976 Skeletal and lean body mass in alcoholics with and without cirrhosis. Calcified Tissue Research 21: (Supplement) 386–391
Rosalki S B 1974 Determination de la gamma-glutamyl transpeptidase chez les alcooliques et chez les bureurs d'habitude. Proceedings of the colloquium, Early diagnosis of alcoholism, Paris. Boehringer, Mannhum
Sandler M, Bonham Carter S, Hunter K R, Stern O M 1973 Tetrahydroisoquinoline alkaloids: in vivo metabolites of L dopa in man. Nature 241: 439–443
Sarles H, Sahel J, Palasciano G, Capitaine Y, Meullenet J 1980 Alcohol Consumption and the Human Pancreas. Les colloques de l'Inserm. Alcohol and the Gastrointestinal tract. Inserm 95: 289–314
Smals A G H, Njo K T, Knoben J M, Ruland C M, Kloppenborg P W E 1977 Alcohol induced Cushing Syndrome. Journal of the Royal College of Physicians 12: 36–41

Smals A G, Kloppenborg P W, Njo K T, Knoben J M, Ruland C M 1976 Alcohol-induced Cushingoid syndrome. British Medical Journal 2: 1298
Smith A N, Nyhos L M, Dalgliesh C E, Dutton R W, Lennox B, Macfarlene P S 1957 Further Observations on the endocrine aspects of argentaffinoma. Scottish Medical Journal 2: 24–38
Smith J J 1951 The effect of alcohol on the adrenal ascorbic acid and cholesterol of the rat. Journal of Clinical Endocrinology 11: 792
Stokes P E 1973 Adrenocortical activation in alcoholics during chronic drinking. Annals of the New York Academy of Sciences 215: 77–83
Straus E, Urbach H J, Yalow R S 1975 Alcohol-stimulated secretion of immuno-reactive secretin. New England Journal of Medicine 293: 1031–1032
Stuart D D, Schultz A L 1969 Thyroid Function Tests Stimulating Grave's Disease in Alcoholic Hepatitis. Annals of Internal Medicine 89: 514–515
Saville P D 1965 Changes in bone mass with age and alcoholism. Journal of Bone and Joint Surgery 47A: 492–499
Van Thiel D H, Lester R 1979 The effect of chronic alcohol abuse on sexual function. Clinics in Endocrinology & Metabolism, November 8: 499–510
Van Thiel D H, Lester R 1976 Alcoholism: its effect on hypothalamic pituitary gonadal function. Gastroenterology 71: 318–327
Van Thiel D H, Lester R, Sherens R J 1974 Hypogonadism in alcoholic liver disease. Evidence for a double defect. Gastroenterology 67: 1188–1199
Van Thiel D H, Gavaler J S, Lester R 1974 Ethanol inhibition of vitamin A metabolism in the testes: possible mechanism for sterility in alcoholics. Science 186: 941–942
Walsh M J, Truitt E B, Davis V E 1970 Acetaldehyde Mediation in the Mechanism of Ethanol Induced Changes in Norephinephrine Metabolism. Molecular Pharmacology 6: 416–424
Williams G A, Bowser E N, Hargis G K, Kukreja S C, Shah J H, Vora N M, Henderson W J 1978 Effect of ethanol on parathyroid hormone and calciton in secretion in man. Proceedings of the Society of Experimental Medicine and Biology 159(2): 187–197
Wright J 1978 Endocrine effects of alcohol. Clinics in Endocrinology and Metabolism 7: 2, 351–367
Wright J W 1974 Pituitary function in chronic alcoholism. MSc thesis, University of Surrey

Richard Fink

Cardiovascular effects of alcohol

This chapter will review clinical and subclincial alcoholic cardiomyopathy, alcohol-induced hypertension, the effect of alco hol consumption on coronary artery disease and thrombosis in alcoholism.

CLINICAL ALCOHOLIC CARDIOMYOPATHY

Early history

The association of chronic alcoholism and heart disease has been recognised for over 100 years. Wood's treatise (Wood, 1855) first mentioned alcohol as a causative factor in heart failure, and Freidereich, 1861) described idiopathic cardiac hypertrophy in association with chronic alcoholism. In 1884, Bollinger presented a study to the Medical Society of Munich, decribing 1000 autopsies performed by the pathology laboratory of the University of Munich, which showed that 46 (4.6 per cent) of the 1000 cases had died from idiopathic cardiac hypertrophy. Bollinger determined that the amount of beer consumed per capita in Munich in 1882 was 432 litres/capita/year, whereas overall beer consumption in Germany was 88 litres/year. He therefore suggested that the observed cardiac changes represented the toxic effect of habitual beer consumption. BY 1906 Graham Steel had also recognised alcohol as a potential cardiac toxin (Steel, 1906), and the term alcoholic heart disease was used for the first time in 1902 by John McKenzie in his work *'The Study of the Pulse'*.

The similarity between alcoholic heart disease and beri-beri heart disease

Following description by Aalsmer & Wenkebach (1929) of beri-beri heart disease (right heart failure, hyperkinetic circulation and oedema responding to nutritional therapy) the similarity between it and alcoholic heart disease (heart failure responding to nutritional therapy) led to the belief that both conditions were variations of the same nutritional disorder (Blankenhorn et al, 1946).

This view was challenged in 1957 by a study (Bridgen, 1957) which showed that only 5 of 50 subjects with clinical alcoholic cardiomyopathy responded to the administration of thiamine. Recently, invasive catheterisation studies and metabolic investigations (see below) have confirmed that alcohol is directly toxic to cardiac muscle in vitamin replete well-nourished individuals.

Clinical features of alcoholic cardiomyopathy

Age, race, sex

All studies of alcoholic cardiomyopathy show a preponderance of male patients within the age range 35–65 years (Bridgen, 1957; Bridgen & Robinson, 1964; Evans, 1964). The race and social class of patients reflect the location at which the study was performed rather than a predeliction of the disease for a particular group. Bridgen & Robinson (1964) described cases belonging to social classes 3 and 4 typical of the Whitehall area of London. Evans (1959) on the other hand, found his cases of alcoholic cardiomyopathy in social classes 1 and 2 Tobin et al (1967) studied subjects drawn from the rural area of America where of his total of 38 patients, 29 were negro men, 5 negro women and 4 were white men.

Drinking history

In his initial study Bridgen (1957) suggests that 'huge' quantities of spirits were consumed over many years and that symptoms appeared more rapidly in patients consuming spirits. In his later and larger study, however, he states that 10 years or more of heavy alcohol consumption was required for the development of alcoholic cardiomyopathy, and emphasized the injurious effect of all types of alcohol (Bridgen & Robinson, 1964). Evans 1964) studied businessmen and professional individuals, and confirmed that cardiomyopathy occurred irrespective of the form in which the alcohlic beverage was consumed.

Symptoms

The illness may be heralded by the insidious or abrupt onset of breathlessness. In many cases these symptoms spontaneously improve and, as the majority of alcoholics are heavy smokers, such complaints may be attributed to chronic airways disease. Palpitations which tend to occur at night are also prevalent at the early stage of the disease. Non-specific symptoms include generalised chest pain, sweating, haemoptysis and abdominal pain (Burch & de Pasquale, 1969; Burch & Giles, 1971).

Routine biochemistry

Clinical alcoholic cardiomyopathy is associated with generalised abnormality of routine serum enzyme tests (Burch & de Pasquale, 1969). Increased aspartate transaminase activity may be observed but is non-specific because similar elevation can result from concomitant liver and muscle disease. The same applies to total lactate dehydrogenase determination.

Electrophoretic determination of the serum activity of the 'cardiac' isoenzymes, lactate dehydrogenase 1 (LD 1) and creatine kinase MB (CK-MB) was carried out in two patients with clinical alcoholic cardiomyopthy and in neither case was abnormal isoenzyme activity detected (Fink, Marjot & Rosalki, 1978). This suggests a functional disturbance of cardiac muscle in such patients rather than cell membrane necrosis leading to liberation of intracellular enzymes.

Morbid anatomy and histopathology

Gross pathology

The heart is enlarged in most cases, hypertrophy involving the left and right ventricles. In view of the known susceptibility of the alcoholic to venous thrombosis, it is also interesting to note that endomycardial mural thrombosis, particularly in the atria, is a common finding (Bridgen & Robinson, 1964; Bulloch et al, 1972).

Microscopic and electronmiscroscopic changes

On histoligical examination, myocardial cells show some necrosis and inflammation considerable fatty infiltration, vacuolation, fibre hypertrophy and fibre degeneration. The lipd material has been analysed using histochemical techniques and is thought to consist mainly of triglyceride (Burch & de Pasquale, 1969). Electronmicroscopy shows mitochondrial damage characterised by loss of cristae and accumulation of inclusion bodies. Other changes include swelling of the sarcoplasmic reticulum and accumulation of glycogen (Hibbs et al, 1975; Alexander, 1967). Loss of oxidative enzymes including cytochrome oxidase, succinic dehydrogenase, lactic dehydrogenase, malic dehydrogenase and D P N — diaphorase activity have been reported (Burch & de Pasquale, 1969).

Haemodynamic changes

Changes found on cardiac catheterisation are significantly different from normal values, but are not specific for alcoholic cardiomyopathy. Right heart catheterisation reveals elevation of ventricular and-diastolic pressure, pulmonary capillary wedge pressures and cardiac index values (Reagan et al, 1969), while left chamber catheterisation shows similarly abnormal pressure profiles.

Treatment

Follow-up studies by Demakis (Demakis et al, 1974) have show that the response to treatment is improved if the disease process is detected early in the course of its development. For practical purposes this entails maintaining a high index of suspicion in relation to cardiac function in heavy drinkers; especially in those complaining of non-specific symptoms such as cough, breathlessness, chest pain and sweating (a useful early feature reflecting autonomic discharge associated with early cardiac decompensation). All heavy drinkers displaying these symptoms should undergo haemodynamic assessment to establish objective evidence of early dysfunction. Unfortunately the serum activities of cardiac specific isoenzymes CK-MB and LD-1 do not show diagnostic changes in patients with alcohol induced cardiac damage, and therefore are valueless as screening procedures for this disorder (see above). Once the diagnosis of alcoholic cardiomyopathy is made, complete withdrawal of alcohol is absolutely necessary as further consumption results in rapid progressive decompensation and death as a result of congestive heart failure, arrhythmia or pulmonary emboli (Burch & Giles, 1971). Concurrent measures include correction of vitamin deficiencies (such as thiamine deficiency) by instituting a regular nutritious diet and abolition of smoking.

Patients with cardiac failure resulting from alcoholic cardiomyopathy are treated in the conventional manner with oxygen, digitalis and diuretics. Burch (Burch & Giles, 1971) has emphasized that the clinical progress of such patients is frequently complicated by metabolic and thrombotic complications.

The metabolic problems chiefly arise as a result of electrolyte imbalance. Beer drinkers in particular may present with hyponatraemia (Hilden & Svendsen, 1975) and in alcoholics generally diarrhoea and vomiting produce hypokalaemia. These abnormal changes may be exacerbated by the use of frusemide and may restrict the use of this efficient method of reducing fluid overload. Thrombotic disease may arise from cardiac arrhythmias, or changes in platelet aggregability (this is considered below).

Prognosis

Demakis (Demakis et al, 1974) followed up 57 patients with alcoholic cardiomyopathy for an average of 40.5 months. 15 improved, 12 remained stable and 30 deteriorated. A significantly greater proportion of patients who abstained from alcohol showed improvement. Deaths occurred in 24 individuals who died in an average time of 36 months. Burch (Burch & Giles, 1971) followed 37 patients with clinical alcoholic cardiomyopathy for a mean per iod of 6.25 years and reported that 16 individuals died during this period.

SUBCLINICAL CARDIOMYOPATHY

Post-mortem examination of alcoholic subjects who had been asymptomatic during life and who had died from non-cardiac causes, showed a high incidence (90 per cent) of cardiac fibrosis which did not appear to be related to vascular narrowing or any cause other than the toxic effect of alcohol (Schenk & Cohen, 1970). Such evidence of subclinical cardiac damage was also found in an asymptomatic alcoholic when mitochondrial and sarcoplasmic degeneration was observed on elctronmicroscopy of cardiac muscle biopsy material (Schmalbruch & Dume, 1969). Many workers have also shown that asymptomatic, detoxified, vitamin replete alcoholics also show haemodynamic evidence of cardiac dysfunction (Asokan, Frank & Witham, 1972; Gould et al, 1969; Reagan et al, 1969; Fink, Marjot & Rosalki; 1978; Gould et al, 1973; Levi et al, 1977; Spodick, Piggott & Chirife, 1972; Matthews et al, 1981).

Biochemical changes in coronary sinus blood

Cardiac muscle metabolism may be studied by measuring biochemical differences between coronary artery and coronary sinus blood samples obtained during catheterisation procedures. Wendt (Wendt et al, 1966) studied in this manner 11 abstinent, vitamin replete asymptomatic alcoholics before and after all subjects had consumed 6 ozs of vodka. Compared to basal values, results after alcohol ingestion showed an overall decline in the lactate/pyruvate ratio. These results suggested inhibition of glycolysis, and under these circumstances a changeover to the oxidation of free fatty acids would be expected. Both Wendt (Wendt et al, 1966) in humans and Reagan (Reagan et al, 1966) in dogs, showed that this did not occur during alcohol ingestion and that the preferred substrate was triglyceride. The myocardial extraction of this lipid is certainly increased during alcohol consumption, but evidently oxidation does not balance the rate at which triglyceride is imported, as abnormal triglyceride infiltration of the myocardial cell is observed on histochemical study. One possible mechanism for impaired oxidation could be mitochondrial damage and loss of oxidative enzymes. This is supported by results (Wendt et al, 1965) showing increased activity of intra-mitochondrial enzymes, malate and lactate dehydrogenase in coronary sinus blood samples obtained from abstinent alcoholics.

With regard to loss of intracellular ions, alcohol in dogs results in significant increases of the concentration in coronary sinus blood samples of potassium and phosphate (Reagan & Koroxenides, 1966).

PATHOGENESIS OF IMPAIRED CARDIAC CONTRACTILITY PRODUCED BY ALCOHOL INGESTION

A number of possible causes of impaired contractility will be discussed. The effect of alcohol-induced increase in plasma osmolality; alcohol induced mitochondrial damage; abnormal sarcolemmal binding of calcium; the toxic effect of acetaldehyde on cardiac tissue.

Alcohol-associated increase in plasma osmolality

The effect of hyperosmolar solutions on cardiac contractility was described by Koch Weser (1963) who observed reduction of cardiac papillary muscle contraction, when the osmolality of fluid bathing an experimental preparation was increased by 100 mmol/Kg. Alcohol is osmotically active and Reagan (Reagan et al, 1964) showed that cardiac contractility declined by 70 per cent of control values following a 30 per cent increase in plasma osmolality associated with a blood alcohol level of 95 mg/de. To separate the osmotic from metabolic effects of alcohol these workers produced similar changes in osmolarity with sucrose infusion and recorded the same changes in haemodynamic values. The mechanism responsible for this effect is unknown, but may reflect intracellular dehydration with loss and abnormal concentration of intracellular electrolytes. While alcohol induced hyper-osmolarity might explain the acute depression of myocardial contractility, it does not explain the presence of impaired contractility observed in abstinent alcoholics (see above).

Mitochondrial damage

Excess alcohol ingestion is associated with degeneration of mitochondrial membranes and loss of intra-mitochondrial enzyme systems (see above). This could explain failure of glycolysis and free fatty acid metabolism, with insufficient production of energy to meet myocardial requirements.

Abnormal sarcolemmal binding of calcium

Muscular contraction and relaxation results from interaction between actin and myosin filaments mediated by calcium released from endoplasmic reticulum. Bing (Bing et al, 1974) therefore studied calcium transport in cardiac muscle cells from dogs fed alcohol for 6 months. Abnormal sarcolemmal binding and release were found and this was possibly related to reduction in mitochondrial oxygen consumption. Whether this abnormality is responsible to any great extent for the observed impaired contractility associated with alcohol is unknown, because the animals studied by Bing did not show significant abnormality on haemodynamic testing.

Toxic effect of acetaldehyde

Schreiber (Schreiber et al, 1971) investigated the effect of alcohol and acetaldehyde on the incorporation of C^{14} — lysine into cardiac protein. Ethanol, at a concentration of 250 mg/dl which normally reduces hepatic albumin synthesis, did not alter the intra-ventricular free lysine pool in either ventricle, or reduce incorporation of C^{14} — lysine into cardiac protein. Acetaldehyde on the other hand, at a plasma concentration of 3.5 mol/l, significantly inhibited the incorporation of C^{14} — lysine into cardiac protein. One problem with this explanation however is that acetaldehyde levels obtained in the experiment exceed that normally found in chronic alcoholics (0.04–0.15 mol/l) (Majchrowicz & Mendelson, 1970).

ALCOHOL-INDUCED HYPERTENSION

A number of studies have alluded to the association between alcohol consumption and arterial hypertension (Dauber et al, 1967; Kannel & Sarlie, 1974), but these findings were considered inconclusive because of small numbers, lack of diversity of subjects and relatively small changes of blood pressure among drinkers. However, with study of large, diverse populations, the evidence appears to be very strong that alcohol ingestion in excess of 6 drinks/day is a risk factor for hypertension (Klatsky et al, 1977; Ramsay, 1977; Beevers, 1977).

Natural history of alcohol induced hypertension

Saunders (Saunders, Beevers & Paton, 1981) studied 132 alcoholics on admission to an alcohol unit, and for varying periods of abstinence. On admission both systolic and diastolic blood pressure was elevated in 51.5 per cent of cases and, during the ensuing period of alcohol withdrawal, greatest elevation of blood pressure was noted in patients experiencing severest withdrawal symptoms. With resolution of withdrawal symptoms and on discharge some 11 days later, hypertension was only found in 12 patients. Of the patients who were abstinent for 1 year and who presented for follow-up, 12 were normotensive. Of the patients who had resumed drinking, increases of blood pressure were noted.

The natural history of alcohol induced hypertension in non-alcoholics has not been reported. Presumably, this will also prove to be reversible on cessation of drinking, unless secondary renal damage had occurred. In his study of alcoholics, Saunders (above) showed this complication occurred in 9 patients and was likely to be the cause of irreversible hypertension in these individuals.

Basis for alcohol-induced hypertension

Biochemical factors

Current understanding derives from a single study which correlates blood pressure measurement with metabolic studies in 35 alcoholics studied on days 1, 4 and 7 after admission for detoxification (Bannan et al, 1981). Mean blood pressure on day one correlated with plasma cortisol concentration, but there was no correlation with plasma renin activity or dopamine β-hydroxylase concentration. However, subsequent falls in blood pressure correlated significantly with reduction in dopamine-β-hydroxylase activity, a plasma marker of synaptic catecholamine release. These findings suggest that blood pressure elevations in alcoholics are dependent on plasma cortisol levels during alcohol ingestion, and that catecholamine release is also a possible causative factor. Studies of changes in the renin-angiotensin axis during alcohol consumption by normal individuals have been published (see Ch. 14), but their clinical significance is not clear as blood pressure measurements were not made at the time blood sampling occurred.

Alcohol is osmotically active and a 30 per cent increase in plasma osmolarity is found for example, is association with blood alcohol levels of 95 mg/dl. The possibility that this property of alcohol is responsible for blood pressure elevation is suggested by previous experimental work (Holland, Sundsten & Sawyer, 1959; Lasser et al, 1960) which showed significant increments in systolic and diastolic pressure in animals receiving intra-arterial infusions of hypertonic saline solutions. This response was diminished by injection of phentolamine (an alpha receptor blocking agent), but was independent of alteration in circulating volume induced by infusion. This was shown by maintaining constant circulating volumes through occlusion of femoral vein venous return. The duration of blood pressure elevation following experimental infusion of hypertonic solutions is very brief (10 seconds) and further work is required to establish whether this mechanism is of significance in alcohol induced hypertension in humans.

ALCOHOL AND CORONARY HEART DISEASE

The popular belief that alcohol ingestion is 'good for the circulation' has received support from recent studies showing that regular drinkers are less susceptible to myocardial infarction than non or occasional drinkers. Thus in English civil servants, death from myocardial infarction was lower in men consuming moderate quantities of alcohol per day (9–34 g) than in non-drinkers (Marmot et al, 1981) and a similar protection from fatal myocardial infarction emerged from large scale European (St Legar, Cochrane & Moore, 1979) and Yugoslav studies (Kozararevic et al, 1980). Protection from non-fatal myocardial infarction is also associated with moderate alcohol consumption, but the relationship between alcohol ingestion and protection from angina or coronary insufficiency is much weaker (Yano, Rhoades & Kagan, 1977). This suggests that drinking protects against the precipitation of acute myocardial infarction, but does not inhibit development of coronary artery disease, a theory supported by an autopsy study which failed to show correlation between pre-mortem alcohol consumption and independent assessment of coronary atherosclerosis at post-mortem examination (Yano, Rhoades & Kagan, 1977).

Despite this recent evidence of beneficial effect of alcohol consumption on the incidence of myocardial infarction and death from myocardial infarction, previous workers have in fact reported that alcohol intake was a risk factor for coronary artery disease (Dyer A et al, 1977), while others showed no relationship between the two (Pell & D'Alonzo, 1968). In general, however, where a positive relationship between coronary thrombosis and alcohol consumption had been revealed, the population studied consisted of heavy drinkers rather than individuals consuming moderate quantities of alcohol. The reasosons for different results between various studies is discussed by Dyer (Dyer et al, 1977) and Marmot (Marmot et al, 1981).

A possible explanation for the prevention of myocardial infarction is the inhibition of platelet aggregability which follows ingestion of ethanol (Hutton & Fink, 1981). Coronary vasodilatation is a further possibility, although the effect of ethanol on coronary blood flow is a contentious issue which is reviewed by Bing (Bing & Tillmans, 1977).

THROMBOEMBOLIC DISEASE IN ALCOHOLICS

Although moderate levels of alcohol ingestion are associated with protection from ischaemic heart disease, ethanol excess is a risk factor for peripheral (Haselager & Vreecken, 1977) and cerebrovascular thrombosis (Lee, 1979). These circulartory disorders are the third most common cause of death among alcoholics (Tashiro & Libiscombe, 1963; Dahlgren & Myrhed, 1977; Nichols, Edwards & Kyle, 1974).

Pathogenesis of thromboembolic disease

Mechanisms which may encourage thrombosis in alcoholics include dehydration, cardiac arrhythmias and cardiac failure. Blood coagulation factors show significant increases in factor XI activity and levels of antithrombin III during the first week of abstinence (Wellerstedt et al, 1977). Other workers (Haselager & Vreecken, 1977) described 'rebound' thrombocytosis in 7 alcoholics approximately 7 days after complete alcohol withdrawal and found clinical deep vein thrombosis and pulmonary embolism in 5. Thromboembolic disease could also reflect platelet hyperaggregability. Of interest is the finding (Hutton et al, 1981) of significant platelet hyperaggregability in alcoholics one week after alcohol withdrawal.

Further work is required to show whether increased circulatory thrombosis in alcoholics occurs during the withdrawal period. Some indication that it does is suggested by a report (Hillbom & Markku, 1978) of cerebrovascular accidents in young people. This showed that of 76 consecutive cases of CVA in patients under 40 years, illness was preceded by alcohol ingestion in 15 per cent of cases.

CONCLUSION

The effect of alcohol on the cardiovascular system is traditionally considered in relation to clinical cardiomyopathy, particularly from vitamin deficiency. This chapter has shown the importance of the direct-toxic effect of alcohol or its metabolites on the myocardium and draws attention to the other important disorders which may result from chronic ethanol excess: subclinical alcoholic cardiomyopathy, alcohol-induced hypertension, coronary artery disease and thromboembolic disease.

REFERENCES

Aalsmer W C, Wenkebach K R 1929 Herz und Kreislaut bei der Beri-Beri. Krankheit, Wien. Archives of Internal Medicine 16: 193–272

Alexander C S 1966 Idiopathic heart disease II. Electron microscopic examination of myocardial biopsy specimens in alcoholic heart disease. American Journal of Medicine 41: 229–234

Asokan S K, Frank M J, Witham A C 1972 Cardiomyopathy without cardiomegaly in alcoholics. American Heart Journal 84: 13–18

Bannan L T, Beevers A, Paton J B, Saunders J B, Walters J R F 1981 Hypertension and alcohol withdrawal. Clinical Science 62 (3): 37P

Beevers D G 1977 Alcohol and hypertension. Lancet 2: 114–115

Bing R J, Tillmans H 1977 The effect of alcohol on the heart. Metabolic aspects of alcoholism. MTP Press, Lancaster; p 117–134

Bing R J, Tillmans H, Fauvel J M, Seeler K, Mao J C 1974 The effect of prolonged alcohol administration on calcium transport in heart muscle of the dog. Circulatory Research 35: 33–38

Blankenhorn M A, Vilter C F, Scheinker I M, Austin R S 1946 Occidental beri-beri heart disease. Journal of the American Medical Association 131: 717–726

Bollinger O 1884 Uber die Haufigkeit und Ursachender idiopathischen Herzhypertrophie in Munchen. Deutsch Med Wochenstr 10: 180

Bridgen W, Robinson J, 1964 Alcoholic Heart disease. British Medical Journal 1: 1283–1289

Bridgen W 1957 Uncommon myocardial diseases. The non-coronary cardiomyopathies. Lancet 2: 1243–1249

Bulloch R T, Pearce M B, Murphy M L, Jenkins B J, Davis J L 1972 Myocardial lesions in idiopathic and alcoholic cardiomyopathy — study by ventricular septal biopsy. American Journal of Cardiology 29: 15–25

Burch G E, Giles T G 1971 Alcoholic cardiomyopathy. Concept of disease and treatment. American Journal of Medicine 150: 141–145

Burch G E, De Pasquale N P 1969 Alcoholic cardiomyopathy. American Journal of Cardiology 23: 723–731

Dahlgren L, Myrhed M 1977 Alcoholic females. II, Causes of death with reference to sex difference. Acta Psychiatrica Scandinavica 56: 81–91

Dauber J R, Kannel W B, Kagan A et al 1967 In: Stamber J (ed) Environmental factors in hypertension, epidemiology of hypertension. Grene & Stratton, New York, p 255–288

Demakis J G, Proskey A, Rahimtoola S H, Jamil M et al 1974 The natural course of alcoholic cardiomyopathy. Annals of Internal Medicine 80: 293–297

Dyer A, Stamler J, Ogelsby P, Berkson D et al 1977 Alcohol consumption, cardiovascular risk factors and mortality in two Chicago epidemologic Studies. Circulation 25 (6): 1067–1074

Evans W 1959 The electrocardiogram of alcoholic cardiomyopathy. British Heart Journal 21: 445–456

Evans W 1964 Alcoholic cardiomyopathy — progress in cardiovascular. Disease 7: 151–171

Fink R S, Marjot D H, Rosalki S B 1979 Detection of alcoholic cardiomyopathy by serum enzyme and isoenzyme determination. Annals of Clinical Biochemistry 16: 165–166

Friedreich N 1861 Handbuch der Speziellen Pathologie und Therapie Die Krankheiten des Herzens. Erlangen. Ferdinand Enke,

Gould L, Reddy R, Goswami K, Venkataraman K, Gombrecht R F 1972 Cardiac effect of two coektails in normal man. Chest 63: 943–947

Gould L, Zahir M, Shariff M, Dilieto M 1969 Cardiac haemodynamics in alcoholic heart disease. Annals of Internal Medicine 71: 543–553

Haselager E M and Vreeken J 1977 Rebound thrombocytosis after alcohol abuse: a possible factor in the pathogenesis of thromboembolic disease. Lancet 1: 774–75
Hibbs R G, Ferrans V J, Black W C. Weilbaecher D G, Walsh J J, Burch G E 1975 Alcoholic cardiomyopathy. An electron microscopic study. American Heart Journal 69: 766–779
Hilden T, Svendsen T L 1975 Electrolyte disturbances in beer drinkers: a specific 'hypo-osmolality syndrome'. Lancet 2: 245–246
Hillbom M, Markku, 1978 Does ethanol intoxication promote brain infarction in young adults? Lancet 2: 1181–1183
Holland R C, Sundsten J W, Sawyer C H 1959 Effects of intracarotid injections of hypertonic solution on arterial pressure in the rabbit. Circulation Research VII: 713–720
Hutton R A, Fink R S, Wilson D T, Marjot D H 1981 Platelet hyperaggregability during alcohol withdrawal. Clinical and Laboratory Haematology 3: 223–229
Kannel W B, Sarlie P 1974 Hypertension in Framingham. In: Paul O (ed) Epidemiology and control of hypertension. Stratten Intercontinental Medical, New York, p 553–592
Klatsky A L, Friedman G P, Siegelaub A B, Gerard M J 1977 Alcohol consumption and blood pressure. New England Journal of Medicine 296: 1194–1200
Koch-Weser J 1963 Influence of osmolarity of perfusate on contractility of mammalian myocardium. American Journal of Physiology 204: 957–962
Kozararevic Dj, McGee D, Vojvodic N, Racic Z, Dawber T, Gordon T, Zukel W 1980 Frequency of alcohol consumption and morbidity and mortality. Lancet: 613–616
Lasser R P, Schoenfield M R, Allen D F, Friedberg C K 1960 Reflex circulatory effects elicited by hypertonic and hypotonic solutions injected into femoral and brachial arteries of dogs. Circulation Research 8: 913–919
Lee K 1979 Alcoholism and cerebrovascular thrombosis in the young. Acta Neurologica Scandanavica 59 (5): 270–4
Levi G F, Quadri A, Ratti S, Basagni M 1977 Pre-clinical abnormality of left ventricular function in chronic alcoholics. British Heart Journal 39: 35–37
Mackenzie J 1902 The study of the pulse. Pentland, Edinburgh, 237
Marmot M O, Rose G, Shipley M J, Thomas B J 1981 Alcohol and Mortality: a U-shaped curve. Lancet 1: 580–583
Majchrowicz E, Mendelson J H 1970 Blood concentration of acetaldehyde and ethanol in chronic alcoholics. Science 168: 1100–1102
Matthews E C, Gardini J M, Henry W L et al 1981 Echocardiographic abnormalities in chronic alcoholics with and without overt congestive heart failure. American Journal of Cardiology 47: 570–578
Nicholls P, Edwards E, Kyle E 1974 Quarterly Journal for studies of Alcoholism 35: 841–855
Pell S, D'Alonzo C A 1968 The prevalence of chronic disease among problem drinkers. Archives Environmental Health 16: 679–680
Ramsay L E 1977 Liver dysfunction in hypertension. Lancet 2: 111–114
Reagan T J, Koroxenides G, Moschos C B, Oldewurtel H A, Lehan P H, Hellems H K 1966 The acute metabolic and haemodynamic responses of the left ventricle to ethanol. Journal of Clinical Investigation 45: 270–280
Reagan T J, Leivinson G E, Oldewurtel H A, Frank M J, Weisse H B, Moschos C B 1969 Ventricular function in non cardiacs with alcoholic fatty liver: role of ethanol in the production of cardiomyopathy. Journal of Clinical Investigation 48: 397–407
Reagan T J, Weisse A B, Oldewurtel H A, Hellems H K 1964 The hyperosmotic effects of ethanol and sucrose on the left ventricle. Journal of Clinical Investigation 43: 1289–1290
St Leger A S, Cochrane A L, Moore F 1979 Factors associated with cardiac mortality in developed countries with particular reference to the consumption of wine. Lancet: 1: 1017–1020
Saunders J B, Beevers D G, Paton A 1981 Alcohol induced hypertension. Lancet 2: 653–656
Schmalbruch H, Dume T 1969 Clinically inapparent changes in the human myocardial cell caused by alcoholism. Archives Kreislautfarsch 58: 202
Schenk E A, Cohen J 1970 The heart in chronic alcoholism. Pathologia et Microbiologia 35: 96–104
Schreiber J S, Bridgen K, Oratz M and Rothschild M A 1972 Ethanol, aldehyde and myocardial protein synthesis. Journal of Clinical Investigation 51: 2820–2826

Spodick D H, Piggott V M, Chirife R 1972 Preclinical cardiac malfunction in chronic alcoholism. New England Journal of Medicine 287: 677–680
Steel G 1906 Textbook on diseases of the heart. Blakiston, Philadelphia, 1906
Tashiro M, Libscombe W R 1963 Mortality experiences of alcoholics. Quarterly Journal for Studies of Alcoholism 24: 203–212
Tobin J R, Driscoll J F, Lim M T, Sutton G C, Szeto P B, Gunnar R M 1967 Primary myocardial disease and alcoholism. The clinical manifestations and course of the disease in a selected population off patients observed for 3 or more years. Circulation 37: 754–764
Wallerstedt S, Cederblad G, Korsan-Bengsten K, Olsson R 1977 Coagulation factors and other plasma proteins during abstinence after heavy alcohol consumption in chronic alcoholics. Scandinavian Journal of Gastroenterology 12: 649–655
Wendt V E, Ajluni R, Bruce T A, Prasad A S, Bing R J 1966 Acute effects of alcohol on the myocardium. American Journal of Cardiology 17: 804–812
Wendt V E, Wu C, Balcon R, Doty G, Bing R 1965 Haemodynamic and metabolic effects of chronic alcoholism in man. American Journal of Cardiology 15: 175–184
Wood G B 1885 A treatise on the practice of medicine. Lippincott, Philadelphia, Vol 2, p 168
Wu K K, Hoak J C 1975 Increased platelet aggregates in patients with transient ischaemic attacks. Stroke 6: 521–524
Yano K, Rhoades G C, Kagan A 1977 Coffee, alcohol and risk of coronary heart disease among Japanese men living in Hawaii. New England Journal of Medicine 2 (97): 405–409

Index

Note: page numbers of chapter titles are in bold type

Pancreatitis, 138, 240–241, 253–254

Val Ash 2NOHA.